616.8482 VIE

SOUTHERN GENERAL HOSPITAL

KU-733-483

SGH001016

LIBRARY
SOUTHERN GENERAL HOSPITAL
This book is due for return on or before the last date shown below.

616.8482 VIE

Manual of Spine Surgery

Uwe Vieweg • Frank Grochulla

Editors

Manual of Spine Surgery

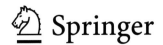 Springer

Editors
Dr. Uwe Vieweg
Clinic for Spinal Surgery
Sana Hospital Rummelsberg
Schwarzenbruck
Germany

Dr. Frank Grochulla
Department for Spinal Surgery
Hospital for Orthopaedics
Trauma Surgery and Spinal Surgery
Euromed Clinic
Fürth
Germany

Illustrator
Atelier Erfurth
Bad Dürrheim
Germany

ISBN 978-3-642-22681-6   ISBN 978-3-642-22682-3   (eBook)
DOI 10.1007/978-3-642-22682-3
Springer Heidelberg New York Dordrecht London

Library of Congress Control Number: 2012936152

© Springer-Verlag Berlin Heidelberg 2012

This work is subject to copyright. All rights are reserved by the Publisher, whether the whole or part of the material is concerned, specifically the rights of translation, reprinting, reuse of illustrations, recitation, broadcasting, reproduction on microfilms or in any other physical way, and transmission or information storage and retrieval, electronic adaptation, computer software, or by similar or dissimilar methodology now known or hereafter developed. Exempted from this legal reservation are brief excerpts in connection with reviews or scholarly analysis or material supplied specifically for the purpose of being entered and executed on a computer system, for exclusive use by the purchaser of the work. Duplication of this publication or parts thereof is permitted only under the provisions of the Copyright Law of the Publisher's location, in its current version, and permission for use must always be obtained from Springer. Permissions for use may be obtained through RightsLink at the Copyright Clearance Center. Violations are liable to prosecution under the respective Copyright Law.
The use of general descriptive names, registered names, trademarks, service marks, etc. in this publication does not imply, even in the absence of a specific statement, that such names are exempt from the relevant protective laws and regulations and therefore free for general use.
While the advice and information in this book are believed to be true and accurate at the date of publication, neither the authors nor the editors nor the publisher can accept any legal responsibility for any errors or omissions that may be made. The publisher makes no warranty, express or implied, with respect to the material contained herein.

Printed on acid-free paper

Springer is part of Springer Science+Business Media (www.springer.com)

Preface

This book has become necessary as a consequence of the rapid expansion of non-instrumented and instrumented spine surgery using different minimally invasive and non-fusion techniques. To do justice to this development, this book aims to present the different techniques to spinal surgeons (orthopaedics and neurosurgeons) in a clear and instructive way using detailed illustrations. The success of any spinal operation depends on good definition of the indications, consideration of the contraindications, technical and organisational factors, correct preoperative preparation and positioning of the patient and good operating technique. The description of different open, less invasive or minimally invasive techniques with more than 600 illustrations will provide the spinal surgeons useful guidelines for their use. We appreciate the valuable contributions from all the authors, and we also thank the staff of our publisher, Springer-Verlag Heidelberg, for their assistance and cooperation.

Uwe Vieweg
Frank Grochulla

Contents

Contributors

Sashin Ahuja Consultant Spinal Surgeon, University Hospital of Wales, Llandough Hospital, Cardiff, UK

Edward Bayley Department of Spinal Surgery, The Centre for Spinal Studies and Surgery, Queens Medical Centre, University Hospital NHS Trust, Nottingham, UK

Christof Birkenmaier, M.D., Ph.D. Department of Orthopedic Surgery, Großhadern Medical Center, University of Munich, Munich, Germany

Bronek Boszczyk, M.D., DM The Centre for Spinal Studies and Surgery, Queens Medical Centre, University Hospital NHS Trust, Nottingham, UK

Bernhard Bruns, M.D. Department of Neurosurgery, Hospital Meiningen, Meiningen, Germany

Paulo Tadeu Maia Cavali, M.D. Department of Spinal Surgery, Unicamp University, Campinas, Sao Paulo, Brazil

Michael A. Finn, M.D. Department of Neurosurgery, School of Medicine, University of Colorado, Aurora, CO, USA

Oliver Gonschorek, M.D. Department of Spine Surgery, Trauma Center, Berufsgenossenschaftliche Unfallklinik Murnau, Murnau, Germany

Frank Grochulla, M.D. Department for Spinal Surgery, Hospital for Orthopaedics, Trauma Surgery and Spinal Surgery, Euromed Clinic, Fürth, Germany

Ulrich Hahn, M.D. Department for Trauma and Orthopedic Surgery, Medical Center Geldern, Geldern, Germany

Felix Hohmann, M.D. Department for Spine Therapy, Hessingpark Clinic, Augsburg, Germany

Annette Kienle, M.D., Ph.D. Mechanical Implant Testing, SpineServ GmbH & Co. KG, Ulm, Germany

Stefan Kroppenstedt, M.D., Ph.D. Department of Spinal Surgery, Center of Orthopedic Surgery, Sana Hospital Sommerfeld, Kremmen, Germany

Palaniappan Lakshmanan Consultant Spinal Surgeon, Sunderland Royal Hospital, Sunderland, UK

Robert Morrison, M.D. Department of Spine Surgery, Sana Hospital Rummelsberg, Schwarzenbruck, Germany

Jürgen Nothwang, M.D. Department of Traumatology and Orthopedics, Rems-Murr-Kliniken gGmbH, Schondorf, Germany

Luca Papavero, M.D., Ph.D. Clinic for Spine Surgery, Schön Clinic Hamburg, Hamburg, Germany

Tobias Pitzen, M.D., Ph.D. Department of Spine Surgery, SRH Klinikum Karlsbad-Langensteinbach, Karlsbad, Germany

Christoph Röder, M.D., Ph.D., M.P.H. Institute for Evaluative Research in Orthopaedic Surgery, University of Bern, Bern, Switzerland

Sebastian Ruetten, M.D., Ph.D. Center for Spine Surgery and Pain Therapy, Center for Orthopaedics and Traumatology, St. Anna-Hospital, Herne, Germany

Khalid Saeed, MBBS, FRCSI (Neurosurgery) Department of Spinal Surgery, New Cross Hospital, The Royal Wolverhampton Hospitals NHS Trust, Wolverhampton, UK

Stefan Schären, M.D. Department of Orthopaedic Surgery and Spine Surgery, University Hospital, Basel, Switzerland

Meic H. Schmidt, M.D., FACS Division of Spine Surgery, Department of Neurosurgery, Clinical Neurosciences Center, University of Utah, Salt Lake City, UT, USA

Kirsten Schmieder, M.D., Ph.D. Department of Neurosurgery, University Hospital Mannheim, University of Heidelberg, Mannheim, Germany

Werner Schmoelz, Ph.D. Department of Trauma Surgery and Sports Medicine – Biomechanics, Medical University Innsbruck, Innsbruck, Austria

Christian Schultz, M.D., M.B.A. APEX SPINE Center, Munich, Germany

Christoph J. Siepe, M.D., Ph.D. Department of Spine Surgery, Schön Klinik München Harlaching, Spine Center, Munich, Germany

Steffen Sola, M.D. Department of Neurosurgery, University of Rostock, Rostock, Germany

Uwe Vieweg, M.D., Ph.D. Clinic for Spinal Surgery, Sana Hospital Rummelsberg, Schwarzenbruck, Germany

Karsten Wiechert, M.D. Department of Spine Therapy, Hessingpark Clinic, Augsburg, Germany

Michael Winking, M.D., Ph.D. Department of Spine Surgery, ZW-O Spine Center, Klinikum Osnabrück, Osnabrück, Germany

Thomas Zweig, M.D. Institute for Evaluative Research in Orthopaedic Surgery, University of Bern, Bern, Switzerland

Definition and Trends of Modern Spinal Surgery

1

Uwe Vieweg

1.1 Introduction and Core Messages

Spine surgery is a field of operative medicine. The spine calls for a variety of different surgical access techniques because of its elongated shape and the varying anatomic situations in its different regions. Pathologies and their localisation, and also technological development, have given rise to numerous surgical procedures, e.g., microscopic and endoscopic discectomy, percutaneous instrumentation, endoscopically guided instrumentation, complex anterior–posterior spinal reconstruction, dynamic procedures (disc and nucleus replacement) and also procedures incorporating biological processes (stem cell therapy, growth factors, etc.). Spine surgery is a unique surgical specialty typically involving both orthopaedic and neurosurgical specialists. Rather than developing still further as a separate, highly specialised, surgical discipline spine surgery should be seen within the overall therapeutic context and should join forces with other areas of therapy to provide interdisciplinary treatment of the spine for the benefit of patients.

1.2 Definition

Spine surgery refers to the area of surgery concerned with the diagnosis and treatment of spinal disorders. This surgical subspecialty is concerned with the management of disorders of the spine, employing both operative and non-operative

U. Vieweg, M.D., Ph.D.
Clinic for Spinal Surgery, Sana Hospital Rummelsberg,
90593 Schwarzenbruck, Germany
e-mail: uwe.vieweg@yahoo.de

forms of treatment to preserve and restore function. Spine surgery is used to treat diseases and injuries affecting different structures in the spinal column and may therefore be indicated for a variety of spine problems. Generally, surgery may be performed for degenerative disorders, trauma, instability, deformities, infections and tumours. With regards to epidemiology and health economics these problems affecting the body's central structural axis, particularly the degenerative disorders, are among the major challenges facing the health systems of modern industrialised countries. Spine surgery is thus crucially important. In most cases it is performed with the purpose of correcting an anatomical lesion or stabilising the spine, if the patient has not shown significant improvement with conservative treatments. Spine surgery is performed by neurosurgeons and by orthopaedic and trauma surgeons. Operations involving the spine may also be carried out by radiologists (vertebroplasty, kyphoplasty) or general surgeons. Recent advances have led to a number of technical developments which are now employed to aid spine surgery, including:

- Spinal navigation
- Fluoroscopy
- Spinal implants
- Bone substitutes, stem cells and growth factors
- Endoscopy
- Microscopy
- Neurophysiological monitoring
- Improved instruments and retractors
- High frequency surgery.

In the USA, back pain is the most common cause of activity limitation in people younger than 45 years. Back pain is the fifth-ranking cause of admission to hospital and the third most common reason for surgery [1, 2, 7]. The United States has the highest rate of spine surgery in the world, but spine surgery shows wider geographic variations than most other procedures [1, 2].

U. Vieweg, F. Grochulla (eds.), *Manual of Spine Surgery*,
DOI 10.1007/978-3-642-22682-3_1, © Springer-Verlag Berlin Heidelberg 2012

Table 1.1 Some major national and international spine organisations

Name of society	Abbreviation	Founded	Administrative office	Number of members	Specialties	WWW	Journals publications
North American Spine Society	NASS	1984	Burr Ridge/ Washington, USA	>5,000	Orthopaedic surgery, neurosurgery neurology, radiology, research	Spine.org	*The Spine Journal, The Spine Line*
AANS/CNS-Joint Neurosurgical Committee on Spine	AANS/CNS	2003	Washington, USA	>1,430	Neurosurgery	Spinesection. org	
American Board of Spine Surgery	ABSJ	1997	New York, USA	–	Neurosurgerys, orthopaedic surgery	American Board of SpineSurgery. org	*Journal of American Board of Spine Surgery*
EuroSpine- Spine Society of Europe	EuroSpine	1998	Zürich, Ulster, Switzerland	530	Neurosurgery, orthopaedic surgery	Eurospine.org	*European Spine Journal*
Deutsche Wirbelsäulengesellschaft	DWG	2005	Ulm, Germany	770	Orthopaedics, traumatology, spinal surgery, neurosurgery physical medicine, rehabilitation, research, anesthesiology, pain management and various	DWG.org	*European Spine Journal*
AO Spine	AOSpine	2003	Duebendorf Switzerland	>4,500	Orthopaedics, neurosurgery research	AOSpine.org	*InSpine Evidence-Based Spine Surgery*
Cervical Spine Research Society	CSRS	1973	Rosmont, IL, USA	>200	Biomechanical engineering, neurology, neurosurgery, radiology, orthopaedic surgery	CSRS.org	*The Cervical Spine.* Lippincott Raven
International Society for the Study of the Lumbar spine	ISSLS	1998	Gothenburg, Sweden	>380	Orthopaedics, neurosurgery, radiology, neurology,	ISSLS.org	*The Lumbar Spine* Lippincott Williams & Wilkins
Scoliosis Research Society	SRS	1966	Milwaukee, USA	>1,000	Orthopaedics, neurosurgery, others	srs.org	
Association of European Research Groups for Spinal Osteosynhesis	ARGO	1996	Strasbourg, France	–	Orthopaedics, neurosurgery radiology, neurology, anatomy	Argospine.org	*ARGO Spine News and Journal EJOST*
The Spine Arthroplasty Society	SAS	1999	Aurora, IL, USA	1,400	Orthopaedics, neurosurgery, research, others	Spine Arthroplasty.org	*SAS Journal*

1.2.1 Spine Organisations and Societies

In recent years, a number of scientific associations and societies have been founded by different surgeons to encourage applied research in the area of spine surgery (see Table 1.1). Germany's first such organisation was founded in 1955 under the name Deutsche Gesellschaft für Wirbelsäulenforschung (German Society for Spine Research). In 2006, in Munich, this society amalgamated with its sister organisation, the Deutsche Gesellschaft für Wirbelsäulenchirurgie (German Society for Spine Surgery), to form the Deutsche Wirbelsäulengesellschaft (DWG, German Spine Society).The North American Spine Society (NASS) (founded 1984) is one of the largest scientific organisations concerned with the diagnosis and treatment of spine diseases. NASS is a multidisciplinary medical organisation dedicated to fostering evidence-based ethical spine care by promoting education, research and advocacy. NASS has more than 5,000 members from many different disciplines including orthopaedic surgery, neurosurgery, physiatry, neurology, radiology, anaesthesiology, research, physical therapy and other spine care professions. The EuroSpine (former: European Spine Society (ESS), European Spinal Deformity Society (ESDS)) was founded 1998 in Innsbruck, Austria. The aims of EuroSpine, the Spine Society of Europe (ES), are to stimulate the exchange of knowledge and ideas in the field of research, prevention and treatment of spine diseases and related problems and to coordinate efforts undertaken in European countries for further development in this field. The ES with the support of the EuroSpine Foundation introduces a European education plan for spine specialists to foster excellence in spinal care (see EuroSpine Courses, www.Eurospine.org).

The AO Foundation (Arbeitsgemeinschaft für Osteosynthesefragen=Association for the Study of Internal Fixation, commonly called AO) was established in 1958 by a group of Swiss surgeons to address diseases and injuries to the musculoskeletal system and has now grown to become a highly influential worldwide organisation. Distribution and sales of all AO products is done through Synthes via a subsidiary! From March 2006, Synthes acquired existing Synthes-branded products from the AO Foundation. Within the AO Foundation, a group of spine surgeons led by John Webb, Max Aebi and Paul Pavlov supported by the AO's industrial partners pushed for greater autonomy for the spine surgeons within the AO. As a consequence of this development, AO Spine International was established in June 2003. Today AO Spine has a membership of around 4,500 surgeons, researchers and allied spine professionals. The American Board of Spine Surgery (ABSS) and the American College of Spine Surgery were established in 1997 and 1999, respectively. The ABSS sets standards for professional training and certification in spine surgery, promoting quality assurance, while the American College of Spine Surgery encourages, sponsors and accredits suitable training programmes. Its primary goal is to assist the public and the medical profession by setting educational and postgraduate training requirements for spine surgeons and by promoting continuing quality assurance programs. As the list in Table 1.1 demonstrates, a great many organisations have come into being, sometimes in competition with one another. They include purely scientific non-profit organisations, scientific societies allowing links with industry and bodies representing particular professional interests (boards and academies). For some of these organisations, where the profiles are similar, fusion may be an interesting option for the future to enable resources to be employed more effectively.

1.3 Trends of Spinal Surgery

In recent years, two trends have developed in spine surgery. These are *minimally invasive and/or less invasive spine surgery* (*MISS and LISS*) and *non-fusion technology*. In the future developments in regenerative medicine, using a variety of biological processes such as stem cell applications for improved bone fusion, growth factors and replacement disc tissue, may become spine surgery's next trend (Table 1.2).

1.3.1 Minimally Invasive and Less Invasive Spine Surgery

Minimally invasive techniques have given rise to a whole new range of technology aimed at reducing surgical trauma. Minimally invasive procedures such as percutaneous treatments in outpatient settings are becoming more and more popular. The techniques of minimally invasive and less invasive spinal surgery have earned a permanent place in the operative treatment of the spine. In essence, minimally invasive spine surgery involves operating through small incisions, usually with the aid of endoscopic or microscopic visualisation. These procedures provide surgical options that address pathological conditions in the spinal column without producing the types of morbidity commonly seen in open surgical procedures. MISS and LISS are gentle, quick, efficient and economical. The advantages are low blood loss, small skin incisions, reduced post-operative pain, minimal damage to skin and muscles, faster and better rehabilitation and a more rapid return to normal activities. The ventral spine can be treated with the aid of special retractor systems and modern implants, surgically addressed operating with endoscopic assistance or entirely endoscopically. The dorsal spine can be accessed from the dorsal side, either percutaneously or with the aid of special retractor systems.

1.3.2 Non-fusion Techniques

Non-fusion techniques aim to provide stabilisation while maintaining the mobility and function of the spine and eliminating the pain caused by the damaged spinal disc. Individuals who have already undergone spinal fusion may develop problems in the vertebrae and discs next to the fusion site (so-called 'adjacent level' degeneration) even when the fusion itself has been entirely successful. These problems tend to develop several years after initial surgery. When segments of the spine are fused together, the segments next to the fusion are subjected to increased forces. This is one reason why spinal disc or nucleus replacement and dynamic stabilisation are being developed. Total disc replacement in the lumbar spine, using an artificial disc, is the most advanced non-fusion technique currently in use, but other procedures such as nucleus replacement, posterior dynamic stabilisation and interspinal distraction are also used. The aim of total disc replacement is to relieve low back and leg pain due to disc degeneration and restore the motion of the spine. The artificial disc is a device made of two base plates connected with or without a pivot. This structure allows a different wide range of movements. The new motion preservation technologies of spine arthroplasty could offer significant advantages, including the maintenance of range of motion and mechanical characteristics, restoration of natural disc height and spinal alignment, significant pain reduction and prevention of adjacent segment degeneration [3]. Dynamic stabilisation describes the treatment method of achieving stabilisation by maintaining the disc with a controlled motion segment [4]. Dynamic stabilisation can be achieved using graft ligament systems, pedicle screw–based systems, facet replacement systems and interspinous process spacers.

Table 1.2 Simplified list of approaches and available operating techniques (decompression, fusion, non-fusion) for different spinal levels

Level	Anterior approaches				Posterior approaches			
		Decompression	Fusion	Non-fusion		Decompression	Fusion	Non-fusion
C0–C2	Transoral	Resection of the odontoid	Plate	No	Midline	Laminectomy and	Rod-screw	No
	Extraoral	Resection of the vertebral body	Plate	No	Posterolateral	hemilaminectomy	Screw plate	No
			Transarticular screw				Transarticular screw Wiring	
C3–C7	Anterolateral	Discectomy	Plating	Artificial disc	Midline	Laminectomy and	Rod-Screw	Laminoplasty
		Uncoforaminotomy	Cage/spacer implantation		Posterolateral	hemilaminectomy	Screw Plate	
		Resection of the vertebral body	Vertebral body replacement			Foraminotomy		
T1–T12	Sternotomy	Discectomy	Plate	No	Midline	Laminectomy and	Rod-Hook	No
	Thoracotomy	Resection of the vertebral body	Cage/spacer implantation			Costtransversectomy	Rod Screw	
	– Classic		Vertebral body replacement			Hemilaminectomy		
	– Mini-open							
	– Endoscopic							
L1–S1	Anterior	Discectomy	Plating	Artificial disc	Midline	Laminectomy	Rod-screw system	Interspinous spacer
		Resection of the vertebral body	Cage	Nucleus replacement	Posterolateral	Hemilaminectomy	Screws	Pedicle screw–based systems
			Vertebral body replacement			Foraminotomy	Screw plate system	Facet replacement systems
	Anterolateral	Resection of the vertebral body	Plating	Nucleus replacement				
		Discectomy	Cage					
			Vertebral body replacement					

1.3.3 Outlook

The future of spine surgery will be determined by further developments in spinal navigation and by the introduction of various minimally invasive, partially percutaneous, techniques and new implants. Fusion techniques and fusion materials will change considerably. The implants will increasingly be made of various partially absorbable biomaterials. Microelectromechanical systems and the use of growth factors or genetic techniques will be part of daily practice. In the more distant future, the solutions will probably lie more in disc repair by cell biology than in replacement with mechanical hardware. The future will show whether disc regeneration by injected chondrocytes, or application of molecules such as anticatabolics, non-chondrogenic mitogens, chondrogenic morphogens and intracellular regulators, is a real option for early tissue repair surgery, as is currently being considered for more disabling and advanced degenerative disc disease [5, 6, 8]. New techniques are being developed to fight the degenerative process itself. Among these is gene therapy, which could provide long-term delivery of molecules to retard or even reverse degenerative processes. All these developments will mean that the various pathological processes in the spine can be treated on a much more individual basis. There will be individualised spinal surgery, in some cases rigid, in others dynamic and function preserving or a combination of the two. In order to prepare the surgeons of the future, medical training will have to include a subspecialisation in spinal surgery. A higher level of training in general and specialised spinal surgery must be guaranteed [6]. The ever-growing socioeconomic pressure resulting from the increasing frequency of spinal diseases and their consequences is driving forward the development of differential diagnostic procedures and efficient targeted treatment. This pressure will become more acute in the coming years as the average age of the population increases and the financial resources of health systems decrease. The future of spine surgery must also lie in interdisciplinary efforts to prevent spinal disease. *Over the coming decades, the subspecialisation of this area will progress almost by law, starting with professional subspecialisation and working towards developing spine surgery as a separate speciality. However, the future of spine surgery must also lie in interdisciplinary efforts to prevent spinal disease. Rather than developing still further as a separate, highly specialised, surgical discipline, spine surgery should be seen within the overall therapeutic context and should join forces with other areas of therapy to provide interdisciplinary treatment of the spine for the benefit of patients.*

References

1. Praemer A, Furnes S, Rice DP (1992) Musculoskeletal conditions in the United States. AAUS, Rosemont, pp 1–99
2. Taylor VM, Deyo R, Cherkin DC, Kreuter W (1994) Low-back pain hospitalization: recent United States trends and regional variations. Spine 19:1207–1213
3. Shibata KM, Kim DH (2006) Historical review of spinal arthroplasty and dynamic stabilizations. In: Kim DH, Cammisa FP, Fessler RG (eds) Dynamic reconstruction of the spine. Thieme, New York/Stuttgart, pp 1–16
4. Freudiger S, Dubois G, Lorrain M (1992) Dynamic neutralisation of the lumbar spine confirmed on a new lumbar spine stimulator in vitro. Arch Orthop Trauma Surg 119:127–132
5. Kaech D (2008) Future perspectives in spine surgery. ArgoSpine News J 19:77
6. Vieweg U (2005) Stabilization in spine surgery-past, present, and future. BackUp 1:1–2
7. Debure A (1992) Modern trends in spinal surgery. J Bone Joint Surg Br 74:6–8
8. Deyo RA, Mirza SK (2006) Trends and variations in the use of spine surgery. Clin Orthop Relat Res 443:139–146

Principles of Surgical Stabilisation of the Spine

Tobias Pitzen

2.1 Introduction and Core Message

Within this chapter, we will illuminate the problems connected with the definition of spinal instability which is basic to understand the mechanics of spinal stabilisation. The principles of external and internal spinal stabilisation will be explained shortly. Moreover, we will describe principles of spinal stabilisation mainly based on the localisation of the pathology and the stabilising effect of implants. Finally, we will explain, how a patient may be mobilised following spinal stabilisation.

2.2 Spinal Stability and Instability

The human spine is a complex structure, consisting of 'rigid' bodies (vertebrae), connected by flexible components (ligaments and discs). The main functions of the human spine are:

1. To maintain an upright posture under a huge variety of loading mechanisms and situations
2. To protect the neural elements (nerve roots, spinal cord)

According to White and Panjabi, spinal stability is defined as 'the ability of the spine under physiological loads to limit patterns of displacement so as not to damage or irritate the spinal cord band nerve roots and to prevent incapacitating deformity, pain or deficits due to structural changes' [15]. Conversely, spinal instability may be defined as absence of spinal stability. Consequently, spinal instability may result in the loss of normal posture (Fig. 2.1) and second in pain, next

in damage to the neural structures. To prevent or treat these, spinal instability calls for spinal stabilisation. If performed correctly, spinal stabilisation will transfer the unstable spine into a stable spine. Within this chapter, the main principles (to the author's opinion) for spinal stabilisation will be illuminated.

2.3 How to Diagnose 'Spinal Instability'?

Although the above definition on spinal instability is probably the best ever given, it is difficult to translate into measurable distances and angles [8, 14]. Especially in degenerative diseases, it may be more than even difficult to judge segmental instability. In, however, tumour or trauma spine conditions, it is at least more obvious if a spinal segment is unstable:

- Large defects within the vertebral body (Figs. 2.1 and 2.2)
- Wedge-shaped vertebral bodies, affection of 2 or 3 'columns' as described by Denis [1]
- Horizontal translation of more than 3.5 mm
- Angulation more than 11° (Fig. 2.1)
- Disruption of the disc and the ligaments as diagnosed by MRI scans

They may indicate spinal instability, especially if combined with local pain and neurological deficits.

2.4 Spinal Stabilisation with Respect to the Localisation of Pathology

As rule of thumb, any kind of anterior pathology (Figs. 2.1 and 2.2) is probably treated in the best way by anterior approach, decompression and fixation, any kind of posterior pathology (Fig. 14.1) by posterior approach, decompression, fixation. Combined instability due to combined pathology

T. Pitzen, M.D., Ph.D.
Department of Spine Surgery, SRH Klinikum Karlsbad,
Strasse des Friedens 102, 76307 Karlsbad, Germany
e-mail: tobias.pitzen@kkl.srh.de

U. Vieweg, F. Grochulla (eds.), *Manual of Spine Surgery*,
DOI 10.1007/978-3-642-22682-3_2, © Springer-Verlag Berlin Heidelberg 2012

9

Fig. 2.1 Kyphotic deformity of the spine due to a large defect within the L2 vertebral body and consequently, disruption of the posterior ligaments. (**a**) Sagittal MRI scan and (**b**) sagittal CT reconstruction

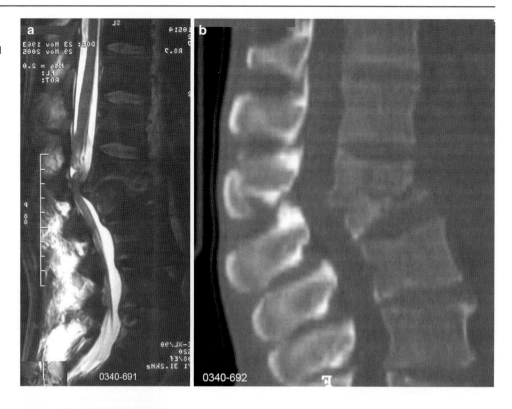

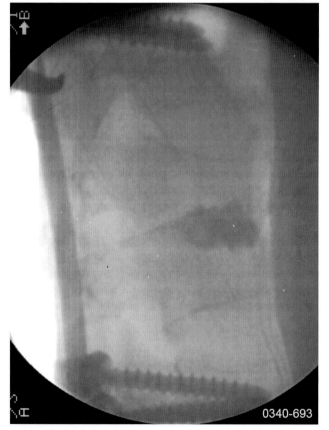

Fig. 2.2 Following posterior pedicle screw-rod fixation, the spine is realigned and – at least temporarily – able to resists bending moments against flexion–extension, lateral bending and axial rotation. However, due to the anterior defect indicated by contrast dye, axial loading (lifting the patient up) should not be performed

usually calls for combined AP-fixation (Fig. 2.3). However, a lot of exceptions are to be noted.

2.5 First Steps in Spinal Stabilisation Procedures (External Stabilisation, Realignment, Decompression)

For external stabilisation, the patient's spine must be immobilised (first by external means, i.e., immobilisation mattress, orthesis) as soon as severe instability is suspected or diagnosed. However, please keep in mind, that any kind of external fixation – even a Halo – allows some degree of motility within the cervical spine [2]. Everybody involved in the patient's treatment must be familiar with the fact, that his/her spine is considered to be unstable. Care must be taken, if the patient is transported, for example to the operating room or intubated for surgery.

Realignment may be performed as a closed or open procedure [7]. Closed procedures usually include traction on the cervical spine, applied by external force, brought to the head by a fixed clamp [13]. In addition, manoeuvres including some degree of re-inclination or inclination, or rotation may be added according to the patient's individual trauma mechanism. There is, however, always the risk of dislocation of bone or disc fragments that may compress the spinal cord. Thus, closed reduction is not recommended by the author, even if not accompanied by neuro-monitoring. To the authors' opinion, it is safer to perform an open reduction after decompression of the neural structures.

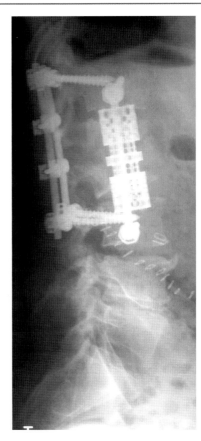

Fig. 2.3 After cage insertion and lateral screw-rod fixation, the spine now resists loading in axial compression. This is an example for combined, anterior posterior stabilisation due to a combined anterior–posterior instability

2.6 Internal Stabilisation of the Spine

Following decompression and realignment of the spine, several implants may be used to stabilise the spine. It is, however, difficult to select the appropriate type of instrumentation. The following aspects may help to select the appropriate type of implant(s) for internal stabilisation of the spine.

2.6.1 Preferred Implants for Posterior Spine Stabilisation

The preferred implants for posterior spine stabilisation are facet screws (within the cervical spine) or pedicle screws (all over the spine), connected by rods (and there is a possibility to use cross connectors to fix both rods with each other). There are different pros and cons for both types of screws: pedicle screws have a higher pullout force and give a better three-dimensional fixation than facet screws, meaning that a pedicle screw-rod fixation usually resists higher loading forces than a facet screw-rod fixation [6]. However, the mechanical strength of facet screw-rod fixation is usually sufficient for cervical spine stabilisation. The complication rate of pedicle screws is

much higher than for facet screws [5, 12]. As an alternative to screw-rod constructs, different types of hooks or wires may be used to fix a segment, but the mechanical superiority of modern screw-rod constructs is undebatable. Whatever has been used for posterior stabilisation procedure, the final construct must stabilise the spine against flexion–extension, lateral bending and axial rotation and distraction. Posterior instrumentation systems, however, are usually not performed to stabilise against axial loading or compression.

2.6.2 Preferred Implants for Anterior Spine Stabilisation

If anterior decompression was necessary, then anterior stabilisation must follow. In case of disc excision, the disc may be replaced by a piece of tricortical bone graft, by a cage or – in case of degenerative instability – by a disc prosthesis. In case of vertebral body resection, this may be replaced again by a piece of tricortical bone graft or a cage, usually filled with bone graft or bone substitute. Such cage or bone graft mainly stabilises against compression and does stabilise against flexion and to some smaller degree to lat bending and rotation – but never against loading the spine in extension if the anterior longitudinal ligament has been cut. Adding an anterior plate (or an anterior screw-rod fixation within the thoracolumbar spine) to this construct, however, adds stability in extension. The combination of cage, anterior plate and monosegmental posterior fixation by facet screw-rod systems usually immobilises a spinal segment even if all ligaments are destroyed [9]. Keep, however, in mind the so-called junctional regions (especially cervicothoracic or thoracolumbar) of the spine usually require longer constructs (Figs. 2.4 and 2.5).

2.6.3 Posterior Versus Anterior Stabilisation

As a rule of thumb, posterior stabilisation of the spine is usually indicated if the posterior aspects of the spine are destroyed (Fig. 2.1). It is obvious from Fig. 2.2 that the posterior stabilisation is – at least temporarily – sufficient to fix the spine after realignment. However, anterior stabilisation using a cage or bone graft and a plate is usually – and also in this case – required, if the anterior aspect of the spine is affected, which is also obvious from Fig. 2.2. The large defect as indicated by contrast dye must be bridged by an implant to carry the axial compression load applied to the spine Fig. 2.3 [4]. Again, there is no doubt that posterior instrumentation systems like facet screw-rod or – even more pronounced – pedicle screw-rod fixation provides much more three-dimensional stability (stability in flexion–extension, lateral bending and axial rotation) than anterior stabilisation [11]. Thus, if there is an extremely unstable situation,

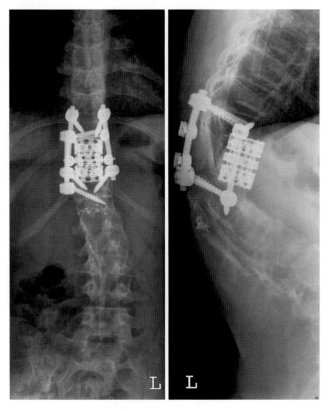

Fig. 2.4 Lateral and AP X-ray of the thoracolumbar spine region of a 12-year-old girl having undergone a spondylectomy of the 11th thoracic vertebra. As a result of a short segment stabilisation within the TL-junctional region using a cage, lateral screw-rod fixation and posterior screw-rod fixation, both sagittal and coronal profil of the spine could not permanently be stabilised

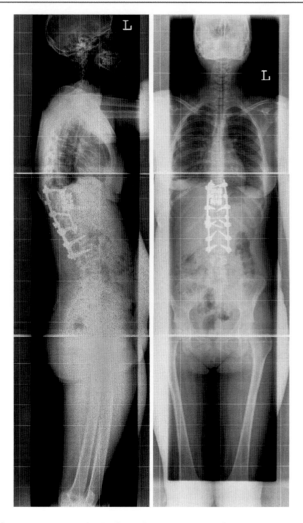

Fig. 2.5 Lateral and AP view of the whole spine following anterior–posterior revision of the above case. As can be seen, the cage is now able to carry the axial load of the whole body, the screw-rod fixations could stabilise the spine in all three dimensions

then a posterior instrumentation usually provides better fixation. That is why posterior stabilisation is usually the first step in fixing an extremely unstable spine.

However, anterior interbody stabilisation (using any type of a cage or even a bone graft) provides much more stability against axial loading or compression. Anterior plating provides three-dimensional stability and is especially useful if additional stability vs. extension loading (reclination of the head) is required. Thus, if stabilisation against compression is needed, then a cage or bone graft should be inserted and a plate is helpful to provide stability against extension.

2.7   How Implants Work

Posterior stabilisation systems (such as pedicle screw-rod systems or facet screw-rod systems) are performed:

- To stabilise the segment(s) in all directions (flexion–extension, rotation, lateral bending),
- But not to stabilise against compression loading.

Anterior interbody systems (cages, disc prosthesis) are performed:

- To transfer axial compression load between two vertebral bodies
- To restore height within one or more segments
- To prevent kyphotic angulation
- To stabilise the segment(s) in flexion, rotation and lateral bending (not in extension in case of the ant. long. ligament resected)

Anterior plates and anterior screw-rod systems are performed:

- To add additional stabilisation to a cage construct, especially in extension after resection of the resected ant. long. ligament, thus
- To prevent a cage from dislodgment

2.7.1 Should a Rigid (Constrained), Semi-rigid or Dynamic Implant Be Used?

Within a rigid implant construct, there is no motility between the components of the construct, that is between screws and plate of an anterior cervical plate system. Conversely, there is some motility between the components of a semi-constrained or even dynamic system. As a consequence, some surgeons may prefer rigid implants in patients suffering from extremely unstable spine segments. There is, however, some evidence, for example in a cervical spine trauma model, that dynamic plates are at least equal to rigid ones with respect to three dimensional stabilisations [3]. Moreover, speed of fusion is significantly higher, and rate of implant complication is significantly lower in the presence of a dynamic plate. Conversely, loss of correction is more pronounced if dynamic plates are used [10].

2.8 Temporary Versus Permanent Stabilisation

So far, principles of temporary stabilisation of the spine have been described; however, keep in mind that these implants will fail (break, dislocate) if there is no bony healing between the adjacent vertebral bodies. Only bony bridging between the fixed vertebrae will result in permanent stability (Fig. 2.6). Thus, autologous bone graft should be harvested from the iliac crest or elsewhere and transplanted at the posterior and anterior site – whatever has been exposed, both anterior and posterior if possible. If no autograft is available, then use some kind of bone substitute. Note, that the graft is in contact with the patient's bone and avoid non-steroidal anti-inflammatory drugs, steroids, smoking for the time of bone healing.

2.9 Mechanism of Trauma

To analyse the mechanism of trauma may also help to select the appropriate type of instrumentation. The appropriate instrumentation will stabilise the spine by acting against the forces and moments that have caused the injury. This means, however, that we must illuminate this mechanism of trauma. The following example may help: A 38-year-old male was involved into a traffic accident. He complained about severe neck pain. A small wound was seen at his forehead. CAT scans (sagittal reconstruction, Fig. 2.7) did not show any dislocation or fracture. A lesion with the anterior longitudinal ligament and the disc, however, was seen in the MRI (Fig. 2.8). As a summary from this short – but sufficient – information, it may be concluded that hyperextension (wound at the forehead) was the main injury vector to resulting in destruction of the disc and the anterior longitudinal ligament. Thus, the disc must be excised and replaced by a bone graft

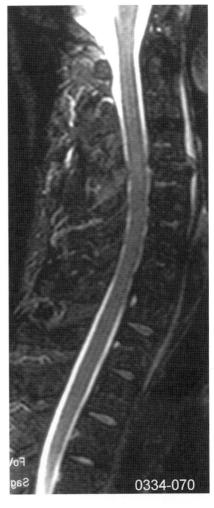

Fig. 2.6 Bone bridging C4–C6 following replacement of the C5 vertebral body using a tricortical iliac crest graft. A permanent stabilisation was achieved by bony bridging

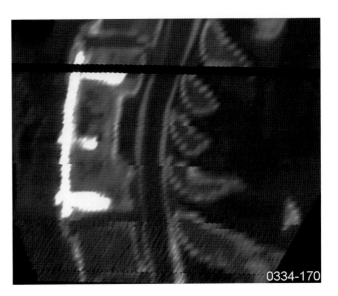

Fig. 2.7 CAT-scan of the cervical spine of the patient described above. No bony destruction

Fig. 2.8 CT (**a**) and MRI (**b**) of the cervical spine of the patient mentioned within the text. Destruction of the anterior longitudinal ligament and the disc C3–C4

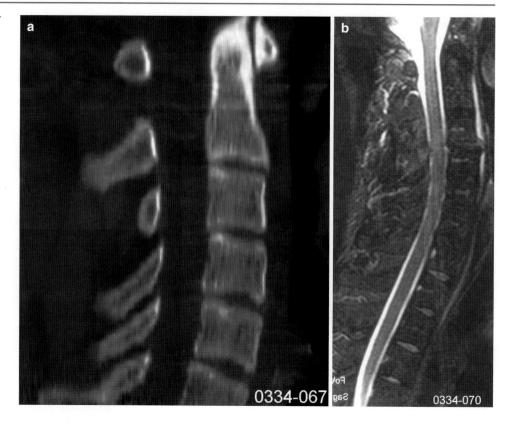

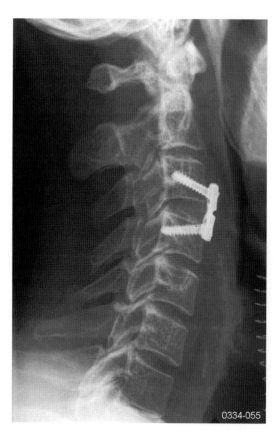

Fig. 2.9 Lateral X-ray of the cervical spine of the above mentioned patient

or cage. As a further consequence, the ideal fixation must be able to work against extension, which is an anterior plate. Due to the fact, that the disc must be replaced, the complete type of instrumentation is a cage or bone graft, and an additional anterior plate (Fig. 2.9).

2.10 Loading the Construct After Surgery

As long as no bony fusion is apparent via computed assisted tomography, we must be careful when mobilising the patient. Mechanics of the implants/construct may give valuable information concerning 'What is allowed and what is forbidden'. Two examples may help:

1. A patient, in whom a vertebral body reconstruction has been performed using a cage, may be loaded in compression. If all the posterior ligaments are intact, then flexion, lateral bending and rotation may be without major danger. There is, however, limited stability in extension! Adding a plate enlarges stability in extension.
2. A patient, in whom spondylitis destructed a disc and major parts of the adjacent vertebral bodies, underwent posterior instrumentation using a pedicle screw-rod system (Fig. 2.2). Although such instrumentation will result in three dimensional stability and stability against distraction, there is no stability in compression. Thus, this patient should not walk around or sit, however may be rotated.

Thus, be familiar with the biomechanics of the implants.

References

1. Denis F (1995) The three column spine and its significance in the classification of acute thoracolumbar injuries. Spine 20:1122–1127

2. Dickmann CA, Crawford NA (1998) Biomechanics of the craniovertebral junction. In: Dickmann CA, Spetzler RF, Sonntag VKH (eds) Surgery of the craniovertebral junction. Thieme, New York, pp 59–80

3. Dvorak MF, Pitzen T, Zhu Q (2005) Anterior cervical plate fixation: a biomechanical study to evaluate the effects of plate design, endplate preparation, and bone mineral density. Spine 30:294–301

4. Goel VK, Clausen JD (1998) Prediction of load sharing among spinal components of a C5–C6 motion segment using the finite element approach. Spine 23:684–691

5. Kast E, Mohr K, Richter HP et al (2006) Complications of transpedicular screw fixation in the cervical spine. Eur Spine J 15:327–334

6. Kothe R, Rüther W, Schneider E et al (2004) Biomechanical analysis of transpedicular screw fixation in the subaxial spine. Spine 29:1869–1875

7. Ordonez BJ, Benzel EC, Naderi S et al (2000) Cervical facet dislocation: techniques for ventral reduction and stabilization. J Neurosurg 92:18–23

8. Panjabi MM, White AA, Johnson RM (1975) Cervical spine mechanics as a function of transection of components. J Biomech 8:23–32

9. Pitzen T, Lane C, Goertzen D et al (2003) Anterior cervical plate fixation: biomechanical effectiveness as a function of posterior element injury. J Neurosurg 99:84–90

10. Pitzen TR, Chrobok J, Stulik J et al (2009) Implant complications, fusion, loss of lordosis, and outcome after anterior cervical plating with dynamic or rigid plates: two-year results of a multi-centric, randomized, controlled study. Spine 34:641–646

11. Schmidt R, Wilke HJ, Claes L et al (2003) Pedicle screws enhance primary stability in multilevel cervical corpectomies: biomechanical in vitro comparison of different implants including constrained and nonconstrained posterior instrumentations. Spine 28:1 821–1828

12. Sekhon LH (2005) Posterior cervical lateral mass screw fixation: analysis of 1026 consecutive screws in 143 patients. J Spinal Disord Tech 18:297–303

13. Sutton DC, Silveri CP, Cotler JM (2000) Initial evaluation and management of the spinal injury patient. In: Surgery of spinal trauma. Lippincott Williams & Wilkins, Philadelphia, pp 113–127

14. White AA, Johnson RM, Panjabi MM (1975) Biomechanical analysis of clinical stability in the cervical spine. Clin Orthop 109:85

15. White AA III, Panjabi MM (1990) Clinical biomechanics of the spine, 2nd edn. JB Lippincott, Philiadelphia

Implant Materials in Spinal Surgery

3

Werner Schmoelz

3.1 Introduction and Core Message

Generally, biomaterials used in orthopaedic surgery can be classified in three groups: metals, ceramics and polymers. Ideally, material properties of orthopaedic implants should have a low elastic modulus close to cortical bone, high wear resistance, high strength, high corrosion resistance, high fracture toughness and high ductility. Unfortunately, no material is standing out in all desirable properties and some of the characteristics such as low elastic modulus and high strength are even opposing. Therefore, the material chosen for any kind of implant is depending on its specific requirements which are most important and necessary for the particular function of the implant. This may lead to different components of one implant being manufactured of different materials to best suit its intended application. In the last century, spinal implants were mainly manufactured of metal alloys such as stainless steel, pure titanium and titanium-aluminium-vanadium. In recent years, developments in the field of non-metallic biomaterials lead to the application of new materials such as PEEK and composite materials.

3.2 Definition

Orthopaedic implant materials can be grouped to the more general description of biomaterials. A consensus of experts in biomaterial science defined the term biomaterial as a non-viable material used in a medical device, intended to interact with biological systems [12].

Generally, biomaterials used in orthopaedic surgery can be classified in three groups: metals, ceramics and polymers. Ideally, material properties of orthopaedic implants should have a low elastic modulus close to cortical bone, high wear resistance, high strength, high corrosion resistance, high fracture toughness and high ductility. Unfortunately, no material is standing out in all desirable properties and some of the characteristics such as low elastic modulus and high strength are even opposing. Therefore, the material chosen for any kind of implant is depending on its specific requirements which are most important and necessary for the particular function of the implant. This may lead to different components of one implant being manufactured of different materials to best suit its intended application. In the last century, spinal implants were mainly manufactured of metal alloys such as stainless steel, pure titanium and titanium-aluminium-vanadium. In recent years, developments in the field of non metallic biomaterials lead to the application of new materials such as PEEK and composite materials.

3.3 Physical Characteristics

3.3.1 Strength

The ability of a material to withstand an applied stress is called strength. Yield strength refers to the point in the stress strain curve after which plastic deformation occurs. Strength of a material may vary with the stress (compressive, tensile or shear) applied. For most orthopaedic implants' fatigue strength is the most relevant criterion, as it refers to the

W. Schmoelz, Ph.D.
Department of Trauma Surgery and Sports Medicine – Biomechanics,
Medical University Innsbruck,
Anichstrasse 35, 6020 Innsbruck, Austria
e-mail: werner.schmoelz@uki.at

U. Vieweg, F. Grochulla (eds.), *Manual of Spine Surgery*,
DOI 10.1007/978-3-642-22682-3_3, © Springer-Verlag Berlin Heidelberg 2012

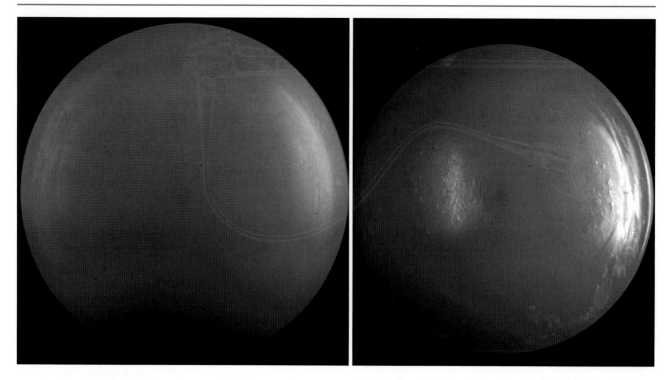

Fig. 3.1 PE core of a total disc replacement after test in a wear simulator. *Left*: unloaded control specimen. *Right*: loaded test specimen showing circular wear at the *right hand side*

materials ability to withstand alternating stresses under cyclic loading. This is especially important during the daily routine of the patient. Strength of a metallic material is depending on its microstructure and can be altered in the fabrication process (casting, forging, annealing, etc.)

3.3.2 Flexibility: Elastic Modulus

The elastic modulus describes the magnitude at which a material deforms when subjected to stress. It is determined from the linear slope of a stress-versus-strain curve. In order to minimize stress shielding, the elastic modulus of implants should be in the range of cortical bone.

3.3.3 Corrosion Resistance

Degradation of materials into its constituent atoms caused by electrochemical reactions with its surroundings is called corrosion. The human body fluids present a very hostile environment to metals making corrosion resistance an important aspect in the biocompability of a material. The occurrence of small holes in the surface due to break-up of the corrosion-resistant oxide film is called pitting corrosion. Crevice corrosion can occur in rod/screw or plate/screw connections of

spinal instrumentation through development of a local chemistry causing corrosion [11], while galvanic corrosion results from two different metals with different electrode potentials and the body fluid forming a voltage cell.

3.3.4 Wear Resistance

Relative motion between two surfaces in contact causes erosion of the material called wear. In contrast to corrosion, wear is produced by a mechanical action in form of contact and motion causing the removal of small particles from a surface (see Fig. 3.1). Wear debris can induce inflammatory reactions causing local bone loss and threatening implant fixation (see Fig. 3.2). Generally, the amount of wear increases with the applied load and decreases with the hardness of the worn surface.

3.3.5 Biocompatibility

Generally, biocompatibility is defined as the ability of a material to perform with an appropriate host response in a specific application [12]. For orthopaedic implants, this can be interpreted as the property of being biologically compatible by not producing a toxic, injurious or immunological response in the human body. However, it should be considered, that biocompatibility refers to a specific material and not to a device, which is often composed of more than one material.

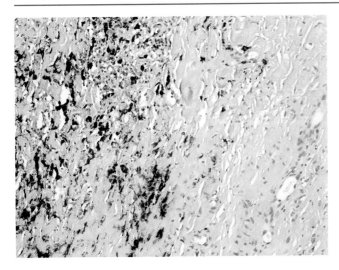

Fig. 3.2 Tissue responses to metal wear particles next to an implant

3.4 Commonly Applied Implant Materials

The bulk of orthopaedic implants used for skeletal reconstructions (e.g., plates, screws, rods and joint replacements) are manufactured of metallic biomaterials. This is due to their ability to withstand high and also dynamic loads. In order to improve implant fixation and/or cell ingrowth, the anchoring surfaces can be roughened, precoated or refined with porous coatings.

An excerpt of material properties of commonly used implant materials and its comparison to cortical bone is listed in Table 3.1. Further information on chemical composition and additional material properties can be found in the references.

3.5 Metals

The majority of implants used in spinal instrumentation (screws, rods, hooks, vertebral body replacements, etc.) are manufactured of metallic materials. They provide high tensile, compressive, shear and fatigue strength, biocompatibility, corrosion and wear resistance required in the application of load bearing implants in orthopaedic surgery. Flexibility and strength of a metallic alloy also depends on the fabrication processes (casting, cold and hot forging). After fabrication, the material properties can be enhanced by heat treatment (annealing). Wear resistance of metals can be further improved by processes such as nitriding and ion implantation.

3.5.1 Stainless Steel

The most commonly used stainless steel is 316L (ASTM F138, F139). It is composed of iron, carbon, chromium, nickel and molybdenum. While the carbon content is kept low, the alloying additions improve the corrosion resistance. While stainless steel has been and is used in fracture plates, pedicle instrumentation and screws, a trend towards Titanium (Ti)-based implants due to the superior biocompatibility was seen in recent years. However, stainless steel implants still gain a worldwide popularity due its cost-effectiveness compared to Ti-based alloys.

3.5.2 Cobald Chromium Alloys

The most commonly used cobald-chromium alloys are cobald-nickel-chromium-molybdenum (CoNiCrMo, ASTM F562) and cobalt-chromium-molybdenum (CoCrMo, ASTM

Table 3.1 Mechanical material properties of implant materials

Material	ASTM designation	Elastic modulus in GPa	Yield strength in MPa	Ultimate strength in MPa
Metals				
Stainless steel [3]	F55, F56, F138, F139	190	331–1,213	586–1,350
CoCr alloys [3]	F75, F562	210–232	448–1,500	951–1,795
Ti alloys				
CPTi [2]	F67	110	485	760
Ti-6Al-4V [3]	F136	116	896–1,034	965–1,103
Ti-35Nb-7Zr-5Ta [4]	–	55	596	
Polymers				
PMMA [9]	F451–99	1.8–3.3	35–70	38–80
PEEK [5, 6]	F2026–02	3.6–13	12–60	70–208
UHMWPE [8]	F648	0.5–1.3	20–30	30–40
Ceramics				
Alumina [7]	F603–83	380	310–3,790	310–3,790
Zirconia [5]	F1873–98	201	420–7,500	420–7,500
Cortical bone [1, 10]	–	12–20	114	133–205

F75). While chromium improves the corrosion resistance, molybdenum increases the strength and makes it strong, hard, biocompatible and corrosion resistant. Due to these characteristics, it is used in joint replacements and fracture stabilisations requiring a long service life. However, the high percentage of nickel in CoNiCrMo raises concerns of possible toxicity by wear particles.

3.5.3 Titanium Alloys

First attempts to use titanium as orthopaedic implant material dates back to the late 1930s. Commercially pure titanium (CPTi, ASTM F67) and the titanium alloy (Ti-6Al-4V, ASTM F136) are among the most common applied titanium-based materials. The increased biocompability and corrosion resistance of titanium-alloys compared to stainless steel and CoCr alloys is attributed to a stable oxide film protecting it from corrosion. The elastic modulus of titanium alloys is closer to bone and approximately half of stainless steel and CoCr alloys, while their strength generally exceeds that of stainless steel. Due to the lower resistance to wear compared to CoCr alloys, Ti-alloys are hardly applied as bearing material.

An advantage of Ti-based alloys is their feature to produce fewer artefacts in computer tomography (CT) and magnetic resonance imaging (MRI) scans. Currently, attempts in material research are being made to reduce the elastic modulus of Ti-based alloys to further approximate that of cortical bone.

3.6 Ceramics

Ceramics are characterized by a high wear resistance, low friction and good biocompability, but also reduced fracture toughness. Therefore, they are mainly used for bearing surfaces in joint replacements. The most commonly used ceramics in total hip arthroplasty are Zirconia (ZrO_2) and Alumina (Al_2O_3). Other forms of ceramics used in orthopaedics are hydroxyapatite and glass ceramics in the form of implant coatings.

3.7 Polymers

Generally, considering all types of medical applications, polymers form the largest group of biomaterials. For polymers used in orthopaedic implants, the most important characteristics for choosing a specific polymer are yield stress, wear rate and creep resistance.

3.7.1 Polyethylene (PE)

Low friction coefficient, low wear rate and resistance to creep of PE in the form ultra-high molecular weight polyethylene (UHMWPE) are the reasons for PE being the most common bearing material in total joint arthroplasty (TJA). It was initially introduced in total hip replacements by Sir J. Charnley, later adopted for total knee replacements and recently for total disc replacements.

3.7.2 Poly-methyl Methacrylate (PMMA)

Plexiglas is the trade name of another, to the general population's more known form of PMMA. For orthopaedic application, PMMA was first applied in the fixation of the hip stems and acetabular components in hip arthroplasty. Nowadays, injectable PMMA cements are available with varying viscosity, depending on their application. They are characterized by a high resistance to creep, sufficient yield strength and their capability to from a structural interface with surrounding bone. In spinal surgery, they are applied in vertebroplasty and kyphoplasty procedures and in selected cases, for implant fixation of pedicle screws in patients suffering from osteoporosis.

3.7.3 Poly-ether-ether-ketone (PEEK)

Initially developed for demanding engineering application and widely used in aerospace and automotive industries, PEEK was commercially available as biomaterial at the end of last century. Mechanical properties of PEEK composites can be adapted to its desired application by addition of carbon fibres and even exceed those of titanium alloys. In spinal instrumentation, PEEK and PEEK composites are commonly applied in fusion cages and in some designs for pedicle screws and internal fixator rods. Its radiolucency allows the assessment of bony fusion without typical artefacts seen caused by metallic implants.

References

1. Ashman RB, Cowin SC, Van Buskirk WC et al (1984) A continuous wave technique for the measurement of the elastic properties of cortical bone. J Biomech 17:349–361
2. Breme J, Biehl V (1998) Metallic biomaterials. In: Black J, Hastings G (eds) Handbook of biomaterial properties. Chapman & Hall, London, pp 135–213
3. Brunski JB (2004) Classes of material used in medicine. In: Rater BD, Hoffmann AS, Schoen FJ, Lemons JE (eds) Biomaterials science: an introduction to materials in medicine. Elsevier/Academic, London, pp 137–153

4. Geetha M, Singh AK, Asokamani R et al (2009) Ti based biomaterials, the ultimate choice for orthopaedic implants – a review. Prog Mater Sci 54:397–425

5. Hallab NJ, Wimmer M, Jacobs JJ (2008) Material properties and wear analysis. In: Yue JJ, Bertangnoli R, McAfee PC, An HS (eds) Motion preservation surgery of the spine. Saunders/Elsevier, Philadelphia, pp 52–62

6. Kurtz SM, Devine JN (2007) PEEK biomaterials in trauma, orthopedic, and spinal implants. Biomaterials 28(32):4845–4869

7. Li J, Hastings G (1998) Oxide bioceramics: inert ceramic materials in medicine and dentistry. In: Black J, Hastings G (eds) Handbook of material properties. Chapman & Hall, London, pp 340–354

8. Park J, Lakes RS (2007) Biomaterials – An introduction, 3rd edn. Springer Science + Business Media, New York

9. Polymers: a property database. http://www.polymersdatabase.com/. Accessed 2010

10. Reilly DT, Burstein AH (1974) Review article. The mechanical properties of cortical bone. J Bone Joint Surg Am 56:1001–1022

11. Vieweg U, van Roost D, Wolf HK et al (1999) Corrosion on an internal spinal fixator system. Spine 24:946–951

12. Williams DF (1986) Definitions in biomaterials. In: Proceedings of a consensus conference of the European society for biomaterials, Chester, 3–5 March 1986. Elsevier, New York

Mechanical and Biomechanical Testing of Spinal Implants

4

Werner Schmoelz and Annette Kienle

4.1 Introduction and Core Message

Mechanical and biomechanical testing provides crucial information about the safety, effectiveness and function of spinal implants. Mainly static and dynamic tests are carried out. While mechanical tests may be carried out according to testing standards or in some cases to individual testing procedures, biomechanical tests should be conducted according to published recommendations or in case of dynamic testing, as individual test procedures. In order to allow for direct comparison between testing laboratories, it should be strived for standardised testing. However, as standardised loading often simplifies the in vivo occurring conditions, more physiological testing can be carried out additionally and may become the next improved testing standard. Mechanical testing focuses mainly on the safety issue, while effectiveness and function of an implant can be tested in a biomechanical setup. Each type of implant generally requires specific mechanical and biomechanical tests depending on its design, material, indication and function. In general, mechanical testing can be subdivided in static and dynamic fatigue testing as well as special types of testing such as wear or corrosion testing. Biomechanical testing concentrates on quasi-static and short-term dynamic testing mostly in interaction with biological tissue.

W. Schmoelz, Ph.D. (✉)
Department of Trauma Surgery,
and Sports Medicine – Biomechanics,
Medical University Innsbruck,
Anichstrasse 35, 6020 Innsbruck, Austria
e-mail: werner.schmoelz@uki.at

A. Kienle, M.D., Ph.D.
Mechanical Implant Testing, SpineServ GmbH & Co. KG,
89077 Ulm, Germany
e-mail: annette.kienle@spineserv.de

4.2 Mechanical Testing

4.2.1 Static Testing

Almost all new implants require static mechanical testing. A spinal artificial disc, for example will probably not receive clearance without static compression, subsidence, creep, luxation and expulsion testing. While compression and subsidence testing are well prescribed in ASTM standards [3, 4], creep, luxation and expulsion need to be investigated according to individual testing protocols. The ASTM F 2077 and ASTM F 2346 standards propose static axial compression until failure to test a spinal intervertebral implant's strength [4] (see Fig. 4.1). This standardised loading protocol allows for comparison between testing laboratories. However, the test results are difficult to interpret since uniaxial loading does not represent the normal, multiaxial loading of the spine. Objective safety requirements are non-existent, and therefore results have to be compared with those from competitive implants. Unfortunately, such data is scarce in the scientific literature, and the databases used by regulatory authorities are mostly non-public. Therefore, new implants are often directly compared with an already approved predicate device, which is similar in shape, materials and indications. If there is no predicate device available, the results may also be interpreted based on the scientific literature. This, however, requires a scientific background of the testing laboratory.

ASTM or ISO standards do not cover all testing procedures needed to characterise the implant's safety. Expulsion tests with artificial discs for example are among these tests. In these cases, individual testing procedures have to be developed, resulting in different designs from testing laboratory to testing laboratory. This complicates comparisons between results. On the other hand, non-standardised procedures can be adapted to the individual needs of the implant and to the physiological loading of the spine, which facilitates interpretation of the results.

U. Vieweg, F. Grochulla (eds.), *Manual of Spine Surgery*,
DOI 10.1007/978-3-642-22682-3_4, © Springer-Verlag Berlin Heidelberg 2012

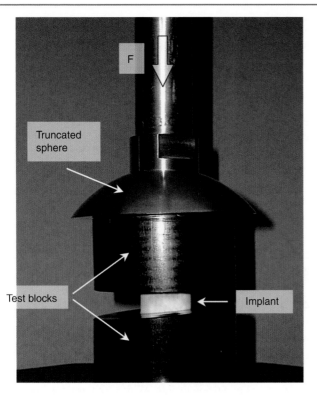

Fig. 4.1 Test setup for axial compression testing according to ASTM F 2077 [2]. A uniaxial load is applied to the implant through a truncated sphere and two test blocks, which represent the adjacent vertebral bodies

4.2.2 Dynamic Fatigue Testing

Dynamic testing is relevant to characterise the implant's risk of failure due to repetitive cyclic loading. A new posterior stabilisation device, for example is commonly tested in a vertebrectomy model according to ASTM F 1717 [1] (see Fig. 4.2). Two "vertebral bodies" made of ultra-high molecular weight polyethylene positioned with a large gap in between represent a bisegmental spinal segment after complete resection of the middle vertebral body. The implant spans this gap and transfers all load between both "vertebral bodies", which is an extreme "worst-case". Therefore, the run-out loads, i.e., the maximum loads tolerated without implant failure, are small compared to the in vivo loads. Thus, similar to static testing, comparative data are essential. The vertebrectomy model is well established for anterior and posterior stabilisation systems of the spine; however, semi rigid fixation devices, such as an internal fixator, which allows some movement, cannot be tested in this model since these implants rely on anterior support. A new ISO standard addresses this requirement [9]. Anterior support is simulated using springs (see Fig. 4.2). This also helps in interpreting the results since the loading conditions become more physiological. Such improvements of testing standards are under development

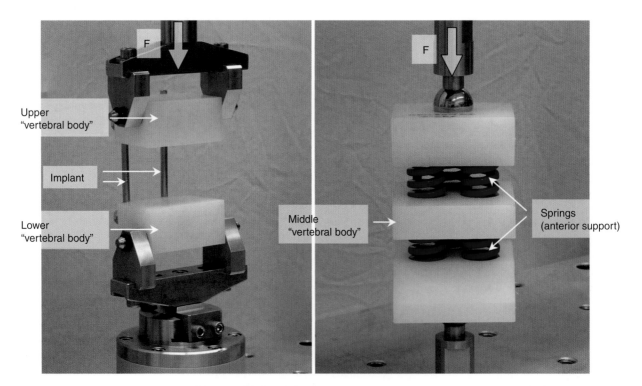

Fig. 4.2 *Left*: "Vertebrectomy model" according to ASTM F 1717 [1]. The implant spans a gap (vertebrectomy) between two "vertebral bodies". *Right*: Testing according to ISO/FDIS 12189 [9]. The middle vertebral body is not removed. Springs assure for anterior support (on this photograph, the implant itself cannot be seen since it is mounted to the posterior side of the construct)

also for other types of motion preserving implants such as facet joint or nucleus replacements.

Besides the test setup, the number of loading cycles also needs to be adapted to the in vivo situation. The number of loading cycles usually ranges between 2.5 and 10 millions. 2.5 million cycles are used for implants, which are implanted into the human body only for a few weeks or months, while 10 million loading cycles are generally used for "permanent" implants such as artificial discs. It is stated that 5 million loading cycles represent about 2–2.5 years in a patient's life [1, 2]. Ten million cycles of "extreme" loading, as applied for wear testing, are said to represent 80 years [5]. Unfortunately, scientific data are scarce on this topic.

4.3 Biomechanical Testing

4.3.1 Quasi-Static Flexibility Testing

Biomechanical in vitro testing assessing the immediate post-implantational effectiveness and function of spinal instrumentation in a treated segment should be carried out using pure bending moments according to the recommendations of spinal implant testing [12, 17]. Several research groups implemented the concept of pure moment loading in different setups. The concept induces rotational motion in one of the main motion planes (lateral bending, flexion/extension and axial rotation) while the remaining five degrees of freedom are allowed to move freely (see Fig. 4.3). During loading, the bending moment and the intersegmental motion are recorded continuously using a six-component load cell and a three-dimensional motion analysis system. The standard outcome parameters to evaluate biomechanical effects of the applied instrumentation are the range of motion (RoM) and the neutral zone (NZ). The load transfer or the change of load transfer of an instrumented segment compared to the intact motion segment can be assessed by measurements of the intradiscal pressure [15, 16] or instrumented internal fixator rods [6, 14]. For more physiological loading of the spine, an axial preload induced by the upper body mass and/or muscle forces acting on the spine may be included in the test setup [13]. Upon its introduction, this was named "follower load". However, the application of a follower load also has some drawbacks, as shear forces due to the subjective placement of the follower load can be induced. Additionally, experiments carried out with and without a follower load generally reported the same effects of spinal instrumentation on RoM and NZ for both test setups, except for different absolute magnitudes [11]. Therefore, in order to allow comparison of test results obtained in different laboratories for different spinal instrumentations, loading protocols other than pure moment should be carried out in addition and not

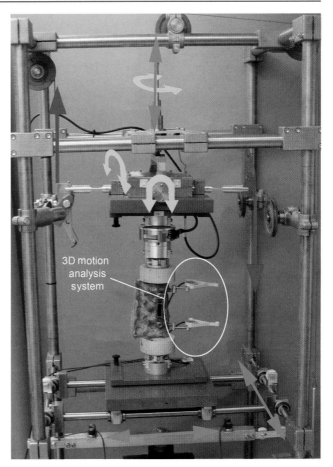

Fig. 4.3 Custom built test bench to apply pure moments. *Green arrows* show translational degrees of freedom, *yellow arrows* show rotational degrees of freedom and *red arrows* show force couple to induce pure moments

instead. A common method to compensate for inter-specimen variation and to highlight the effect of instrumentation on the RoM of a treated segment is normalisation, in which the RoM of a treated segment is reported as percentage of the native untreated motion segment.

4.3.2 Dynamic Loosening of Implants

To investigate long-term effectiveness and function of spinal instrumentation, various custom-built test setups in servohydraulic material testing machines have been used (see Fig. 4.4). These setups are intended to investigate implant anchorage and to provoke loosening at the implant–bone interface by repetitive loading, which can be of particular interest in the treatment of patients suffering from reduced bone quality. Generally, biomechanical tests intending to provoke implant failure or loosening apply a cyclic force–controlled loading protocol simulating from a few days up to

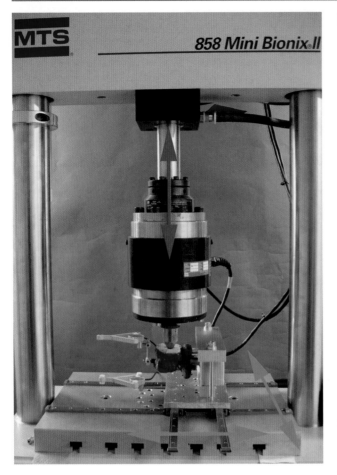

Fig. 4.4 Experimental test setup to provoke loosening of pedicle screws. *Green arrows* show translational degree of freedom and *red arrows* show load application

several months of in vivo loading. In order to accelerate the in vivo occurring loosening/failure of the implant-bone interface, different loading protocols can be applied. A constant force, while the location of load application is varied [10] or a stepwise increasing load protocol, with a fixed point of load application [7] are often used. To provoke loosening and show a correlation of the number of load cycles to failure and the bone mineral density, a continuously increasing force-controlled loading protocol [8] is best suited to show differences in implant anchorage of various fixation and screw designs.

References

1. ASTM F1717-11A (2011) Standard test methods for spinal implant constructs in a vertebrectomy model. Current edition approved July 1, 2011. Published July 2011, pp 1–20
2. ASTM F2077-11 (2011) Test methods for intervertebral body fusion devices. Current edition approved July 15, 2011. Published August 2011, pp 1–9
3. ASTM F2267-04 (Reapproved 2011) (2011) Standard test methods for measuring load induced subsidence of intervertebral body fusion device under static axial compression. Current edition approved Dec. 1, 2011. Published January 2012, pp 1–7
4. ASTM F2346-05 (Reapproved 2011) (2011) Standard test methods for static and dynamic characterization of spinal artificial discs. Current edition approved Dec. 1, 2011. Published January 2012, pp 1–10
5. ASTM F2423-11 (2000) Standard guide for functional, kinematic and wear assessment of total disc prostheses. Current edition approved July 1, 2011. Published August 2011, pp 1–9
6. Cripton PA, Jain GM, Wittenberg RH et al (2000) Load-sharing characteristics of stabilized lumbar spine segments. Spine 25:170–179
7. Disch AC, Knop C, Schaser KD et al (2008) Angular stable anterior plating following thoracolumbar corpectomy reveals superior segmental stability compared to conventional polyaxial plate fixation. Spine (Phila Pa 1976) 33:1429–1437
8. Ferguson SJ, Winkler F, Nolte LP (2002) Anterior fixation in the osteoporotic spine: cut-out and pullout characteristics of implants. Eur Spine J 11(6):527–534
9. ISO 12189:2008(E) (2008) Implants for surgery – Mechanical testing of implantable spinal devices – Fatigue test method for spinal implant assemblies using an anterior support. Published 29 Feb 2008, pp 1–19
10. Kettler A, Schmoelz W, Shezifi Y et al (2006) Biomechanical performance of the new BeadEx implant in the treatment of osteoporotic vertebral body compression fractures: restoration and maintenance of height and stability. Clin Biomech (Bristol, Avon) 21(7):676–682
11. Niosi CA, Zhu QA, Wilson DC et al (2006) Biomechanical characterization of the three-dimensional kinematic behaviour of the Dynesys dynamic stabilization system: an in vitro study. Eur Spine J 15(6):913–922
12. Panjabi MM (1988) Biomechanical evaluation of spinal fixation devices: I. A conceptual framework. Spine 13:1129–1134
13. Patwardhan AG, Havey RM, Carandang G et al (2003) Effect of compressive follower preload on the flexion-extension response of the human lumbar spine. J Orthop Res 21:540–546
14. Rohlmann A, Bergmann G, Graichen F et al (1997) Comparison of loads on internal spinal fixation devices measured in vitro and in vivo. Med Eng Phys 19:539–546
15. Schmoelz W, Huber JF, Nydegger T et al (2006) Influence of a dynamic stabilisation system on load bearing of a bridged disc: an in vitro study of intradiscal pressure. Eur Spine J 15:1276–85
16. Wilke HJ, Neef P, Caimi M et al (1999) New in vivo measurements of pressures in the intervertebral disc in daily life. Spine 24:755–762
17. Wilke HJ, Wenger K, Claes L (1998) Testing criteria for spinal implants: recommendations for the standardization of in vitro stability testing of spinal implants. Eur Spine J 7:148–154

Spinal Retractors

Luca Papavero

5.1 Introduction and Core Messages

Open surgical retractors provide continuous, unobstructed access to surgical sites. They unavoidably push the retracted tissue increasing intra-tissue pressure and reducing perfusion.

Ischemic damage tends to increase as time and pressure increase. The resultant ischemia can damage the compressed tissues if perfusion is not restored within reasonable time periods ranging, depending on the tissue types and their locations, from tens of seconds (brain) to several minutes or more (muscle). Unless the surgeon provides for repetitive removal or reduction of pressures that are applied by retraction, there is no available option for preventing this problem. Tubular retractors inserted via a transmuscular route cause less increase of the intramuscular pressure, less postoperative muscular damage seen on the MRI and less postoperative analgesic consumption. They seem to provide a valuable alternative in certain spinal surgeries. Radiolucent retractor blades allow for an unobstructed view of the surgical target area. Furthermore, bony anatomy is visualized more detailed because it becomes the most dense structure in the X-Ray beam.

5.2 Definition

Most self-retaining retractors have an elongated rack bar and two retracting arms: a fixed retracting arm and a movable retracting arm. Both arms typically extend in a direction normal to the rack bar. The movable arm can be displaced along the rack bar using a crank, which also acts as a torque lever, to activate a pinion mechanism. Two blades are provided, usually below the retractor arms. The basic design and mechanism for separating the two or more spreader or retractor arms have remained relatively unchanged since the first introduction of retractors. The relationship between increased intramuscular pressure (IMP), reduced intramuscular blood flow (BF), and low back pain (LBP) has been shown in a rat model where a balloon increased IMP of the lumbar paraspinal muscles and decreased intramuscular BF [1]. Compared to sham groups, at 1 day after balloon insertion, IMP for the balloon group was significantly higher while intramuscular BF was lower. Expression of pain mediating substance P in the L1 DRG was also significantly greater for the balloon group. Furthermore, compared to normal lumbar paraspinal muscles, at 1 h after insertion, muscles of the balloon group showed edematous fibers. At 1, 7, and 28 days after insertion, muscle fibers displayed edema, inflammatory cell infiltration, and clear atrophy. Prolonged use of self-retaining retractors causes reduction in muscle function and is suspected to increase scar tissue generation and postoperative spinal muscle dysfunction [2]. Muscle injury is closely related to muscle retraction and

L. Papavero, M.D., Ph.D.
Clinic for Spine Surgery, Schön Clinic Hamburg,
Dehnhaide 120, 22081 Hamburg, Germany
e-mail: lpapavero@schoen-kliniken.de

relaxation during lumbar disk surgery [3]. After lumbar laminectomy, total duration of muscle retraction greater than 60 min is associated with significant worse VAS scores for back pain and ODI and SF-36 scores for disability at 6 months after surgery. However, no relationship between outcome parameters and retractor type, operating surgeon, and wound length has been demonstrated [4]. The reported data refer to standard retractors. The insertion of open retractors via a subperiosteal approach has been compared in cadaver and clinical studies with the transmuscular insertion of tubular retractors. The latter showed a significantly lower increase of IMP in lumbar paraspinal muscles. Furthermore, significantly less muscle edema was seen on MRI in the minimally invasive group six months after surgery [5]. The analgesic consumption after lumbar microdiscectomy was less when the disk herniation had been removed via a transmuscular approach by tubular retractor than via the subperiosteal route by an open retractor [6].

5.3   Classification of Retractors

Due to the myriad of retractors and their modifications used in spinal surgery, any classification must be necessarily incomplete. Therefore, the criteria presented in the following are tentative.

(a) *Holding mechanism*
   1. Hand-held
   2. Self-retaining
   3. Table-fixed
(b) *X-Ray imaging*
   1. Opaque (stainless steel)
   2. Semilucent (titanium, aluminum)
   3. Lucent (PEEK, carbon)
(c) *Muscle/bone contact*
   1. Subperiosteal
   2. Transmuscular
(d) *Anatomical region*
   1. Cervical
   2. Thoracic
   3. Lumbosacral
(e) *Approach to the spine*
   1. Anterior
   2. Lateral
   3. Posterior

Of course, a retractor may be defined by several parameters crossing the various criteria of classification. Furthermore, the individual surgical experience may favor the use of a spreader designed, for example, for the anterior cervical approach in dorsal lumbar transmuscular pedicle screw insertion. On the other hand, a tubular retractor originally designed for lumbar disk herniation surgery may be fruitfully used for minimally invasive anterior odontoid screwing [7].

5.4   Clinical Examples

A very limited selection of retractors is presented with keywords highlighting the most interesting features of their application. The examples represent an author´s choice which reflects necessarily only a fragment of the experience of the spine community.

The author is well aware of the fact that many readers will miss their workhorses and apologizes in advance. However, an exhaustive presentation of retractors would be beyond the scope of this chapter.

5.5   Cervical Spine

Transoral approach: self-retaining; ring-type with independent blades (Fig. 5.1).

Anterior subaxial approach: self-retaining with equal, opposite retraction force; radiolucent blades top or side loading (Fig. 5.2a). Alternative: ring-type table-fixed retractor (Fig. 5.2b).

Posterior subaxial approach: self-retaining (Adson, Gelpi) for conventional open approach. Frequent release of the retractor (e.g., sharp Gelpi) performing cervical laminoplasty has been demonstrated to reduce significantly postoperative axial neck pain ($P < 0.025$) and hypotrophy of the neck muscles ($P < 0.001$) compared to continuous opening of retractor (e.g., blunt Adson) (Fig. 5.3a) [8]. Table-fixed tubular retractor for transmuscular approach (dorsolateral foraminotomy, lateral mass screw insertion, Fig. 5.3b).

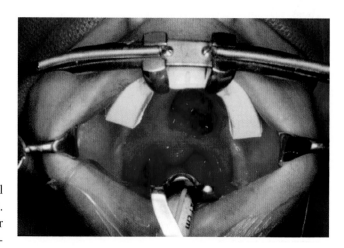

Fig. 5.1 Oral intubation with a flexometallic tube positioned at the *bottom* of the mouth. The mouth is kept open with a gag that rests against the upper dental arch (rubber protection!) and depresses the tongue (avoid squeezing between the tongue blade and the teeth!). Examples: Crockard (Codmann, USA), Spetzler-Sonntag (Aesculap, Germany) (Courtesy of img.medscape.com)

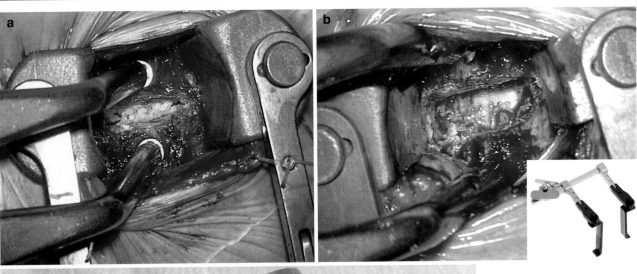

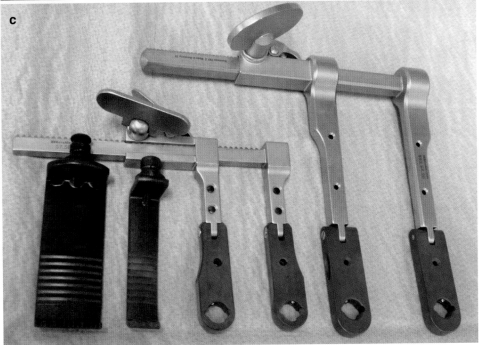

Fig. 5.2 (**a**) Classical cervical spreader with radiolucent blades (Medicon, Germany). In order to miniaturize the approach the function of the up-down blades can be substituted by the distraction screws. (**b**) The width of the lateral blades has been reduced from 24 to 12 mm. The black parts are made of PEEK (The Invisible, Medicon, Germany). (**c**) Comparison of conventional vs. miniaturized cervical retractors. The black parts are radiolucent

5.6 Thoracic Spine

Lateral approach: table-fixed ring-type retractor; blades of aluminum; pins for blade fixation into the vertebral bodies (Fig. 5.4).

Posterior approach: see lumbosacral spine.

5.7 Lumbosacral Spine

Anterior approach: a table-fixed ring-type is frequently used (see thoracic spine) (Fig. 5.5). An alternative is the self-retaining retractor anchored to the vertebral bodies.

Posterior approach: One of the most popular approaches in spinal surgery. Until 10 years ago, decompression and stabilization have been mostly performed via a subperiosteal bilateral open route. The surgical target area is approached with the aid of familiar bony landmarks. The advantage of this technique is the excellent anatomical view. Disadvantages are the denervation and the postoperative hypotrophy of the paravertebral muscles with functional impairment (Fig. 5.6a).

In percutaneous placement of pedicle screws, the "retractor blades" are inserted into the screw head (Fig. 5.6b).

The classical Caspar-type retractor for lumbar microsurgery combining speculum and counter-retractor (Fig. 5.6c) allows the subperiosteal (inter-laminar, translaminar) as well as the

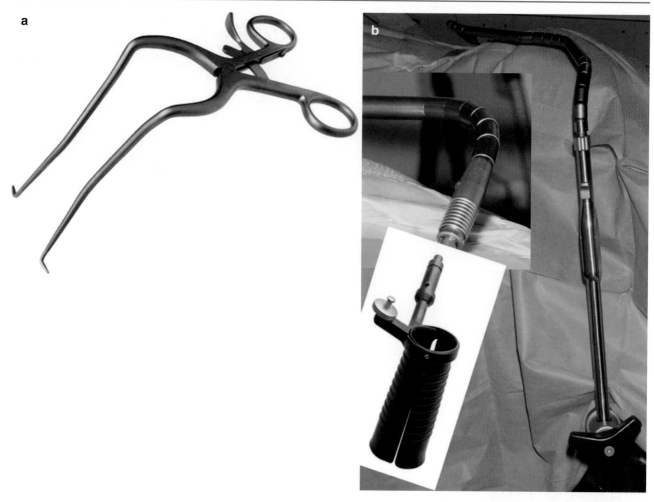

Fig. 5.3 (a) Deep Gelpi retractor (With permission of Aesculap AG, Tuttlingen, Germany) (b) The table-fixed adjustable holding arm, "the snake," holds an expandable tubular retractor in situ. Usually, the cylin- dric retractor is inserted by blunt opening of the paravertebral cervical or lumbar muscles (XS-Mikrodisk, Medicon, Germany) (© by Medicon)

transmuscular approach (paraspinal). The miniaturized edition minimizes further the approach (Fig. 5.6d).

5.8   Conclusions

- The review of the literature indicates that a lot of efforts are being made to address the tissue ischemia related to retraction.
- Experimental surgical retractors with integrated force and oxygenation sensors monitor or report real-time data

to the surgeon. They quantify better the retraction dam- age so "safe" thresholds of magnitude and duration can be defined [9].

- A further promising investigation is the "perfusion stimulating retractor." On this principle, when the capillary blood flow is interrupted for an acceptably short time, perfusion is partially or fully restored shortly after retraction is removed. The cyclic applica- tion and reduction of pressure enable sufficient perfu- sion to be maintained over the course of the surgical procedure.

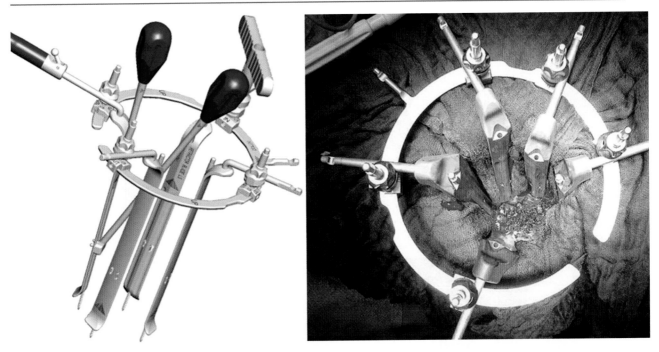

Fig. 5.4 The EndoRing (Medtronic, USA) may be used as a self-retaining, pin-based system or may be attached to existing table based systems. The blade pusher allows the surgeon to safely manipulate the retractor blade(s) while surrounding anatomy is protected behind the blade (a-Illustration, B9 intraoperative situation) (Used with permission from Medtronic International Trading Sarl ©02/12/2010 Medtronic International Trading Sarl)

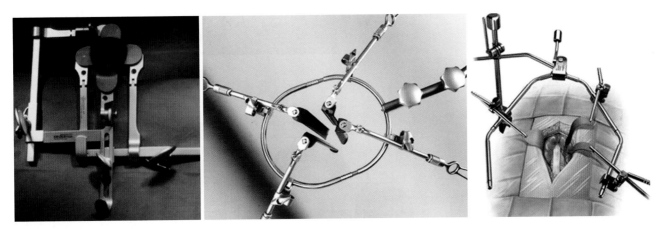

Fig. 5.5 Options for the mini-open approach to the lumbar spine: (*left*) self-retaining (MIASPAS, Aesculap); (*center*) closed ring (actic-o retractor, Aesculap); (*right*) open frame (With permission from Aesculap AG, Tuttlingen, Germany)

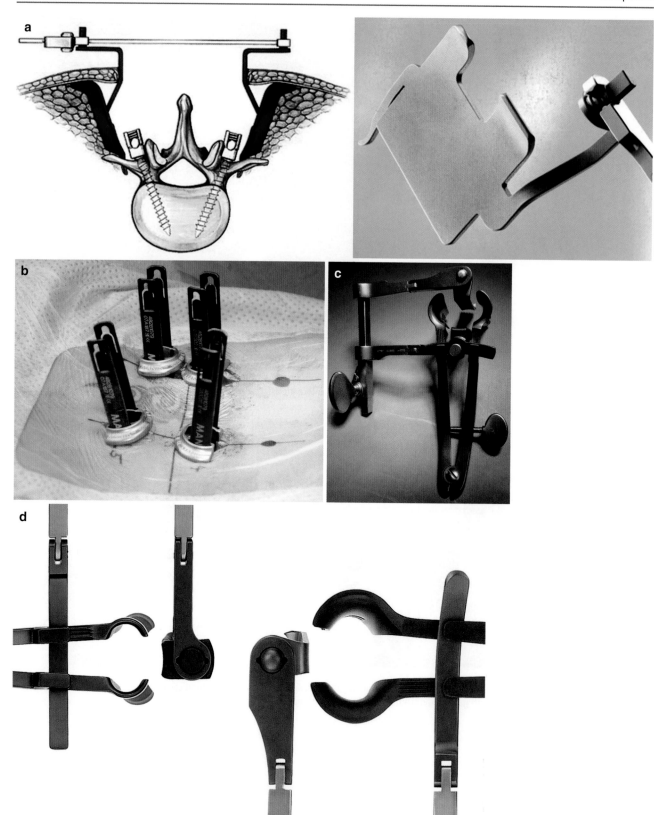

Fig. 5.6 (**a**) The uncommon design of the retractor aims to reduce the skin incision and at the same time, to maximize the lateral retraction of muscle tissue in order to allow unobstructed introduction of pedicle screws (SLR, Aesculap) (With permission from Aesculap AG, Tuttlingen, Germany). (**b**) Following the percutaneous, transmuscular, fluoroscopy aided insertion of the pedicle screw, slim titanium blades are docked into the screw head in order to retract the muscle and to allow the insertion of the rod (Mantis, Stryker). (**c**) The Caspar type retractor has been developed in the seventies and is still one of the most popular retractors in spinal microsurgery. (**d**) The miniaturized Caspar-type retractor (*left*) reduces the length of the skin incision, the amount of muscle dissection and facilitates lateral fluoroscopy because of the blades made of PEEK (Piccolino, Medicon) (© by Medicon)

References

1. Kobayashi Y, Kikuchi S, Konno S et al (2007) Increased intramuscular pressure in lumbar paraspinal muscle and low back pain. Poster 101 at EuroSpine, 25–28 Oct 2007, Brussells
2. Taylor H, McGregor A, Medhi-Zadeh S et al (2002) The impact of self-retaining retractors on the paraspinal muscles during posterior spinal surgery. Spine 27:2758–2762
3. Kotil K, Tunckale T, Tatar Z et al (2007) Serum creatine phosphokinase activity and histological changes in the multifidus muscle: a prospective randomized controlled comparative study of discectomy with and without retraction. J Neurosurg Spine 6:121–125
4. Datta G, Gnanalingham K, Peterson D et al (2004) Back pain and disability after lumbar laminectomy: is there a relationship to muscle retraction? Neurosurgery 54:1413–1420
5. Stevens K, Spenciner D, Griffiths K et al (2006) Comparison of minimally invasive and conventional open posterolateral lumbar fusion using magnetic resonance imaging and retraction pressure studies. J Spinal Disord Tech 19:77–86
6. Brock M, Kunkel Ph, Papavero L (2008) Lumbar Microdiscectomy: Subper iosteal vs. transmuscular approach and influence on the early postoperative analgesic consumption. Eur Spine J 17:518–522
7. Hott JS, Henn JS, Sonntag VK (2003) A new table-fixed retractor for anterior odontoid screw fixation: technical note. J Neurosurg 98(Suppl 3):294–296
8. Yokohama T (2003) Release of the muscle retractors can reduce axial symptoms after cervical laminoplasty. Poster presented at the 31st annual meeting cervical spine research society, CSRS, 11–13 Dec 2003, Scottsdale
9. Fischer G, Saha S, Horwat J et al (2005) Intra-operative ischemia sensing surgical instruments. Poster at Complex medical engineering, 15–18 May 2005, Takamatsu

Stefan Kroppenstedt

6.1 Introduction and Core Messages

Standard fluoroscopy is familiar to most spine surgeons because it provides real-time intraoperative visualization of spinal anatomy. The major limitations of fluoroscopy are occupational radiation exposure and the fact that the images can only be obtained in one plane at a time. Image-guided spinal navigation has evolved as a spinal surgical tool overcoming the limitations of standard fluoroscopy. It has been proven to be a versatile and effective tool for facilitating complex surgical procedures. However, image guidance has its limitations and does not replace the surgeon's own experience and judgment. There are several modalities of spinal image guidance (such as CT-based, fluoroscopy-based, three-dimensional C-arm fluoroscopy), and each has its own advantages and limitations. Pitfalls and errors are related to issues of the accuracy, technique, and overall ease of use of the technology during surgery. A thorough understanding of these problems is required to ensure an effective use of image-guided navigation for spinal surgery.

S. Kroppenstedt, M.D., Ph.D.
Department of Spinal Surgery,
Center of Orthopedic Surgery, Sana Hospital Sommerfeld,
Waldhausstraße 44, 16766 Kremmen, Germany
e-mail: s.kroppenstedt@sana-hu.de

6.2 Fluoroscopy

Fluoroscopy is an X-ray procedure that produces real-time moving images of internal structures through the use of a fluoroscope. Standard fluoroscopy is familiar to most spine surgeons because it provides immediate intraoperative visualization of spinal anatomy. A modern surgical image intensifier (also called C-arm because of its shape) consists of a generator (radiation source), image receiver (intensifier with camera), and a monitor unit (containing a image memory and processing unit) (Fig. 6.1). Today, two monitors are mandatory for surgical machines. The C-arm is fixed on a mobile stand in such a way that it can be moved and turned to all sides (transverse and longitudinal to the patient, orbital movement around the patient, rotation and adjustment of height).

6.2.1 Radiation Protection

Besides the fact that the images can only be obtained in one plane at a time, a further major limitation of fluoroscopy is occupational radiation exposure. Thus, radiation protection is a very important issue. When using X-rays on a patient, a differentiation is made between effective radiation and scattered radiation. Part of the effective radiation is scattered by the patient's body and leaves the body as lower-energy scatter radiation in all directions. In order to protect the user and the parts of the patient's body not being

U. Vieweg, F. Grochulla (eds.), *Manual of Spine Surgery*,
DOI 10.1007/978-3-642-22682-3_6, © Springer-Verlag Berlin Heidelberg 2012

Fig. 6.1 Surgical image intensifier (C-arm) consisting of a generator (*a*), image receiver (*b*), and a monitor unit (*c*) (With permission of Siemens)

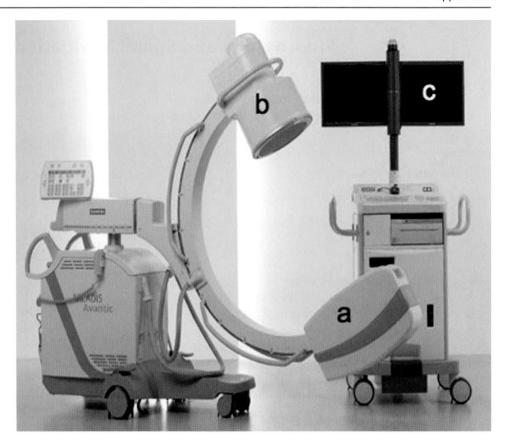

examined from this scattered radiation, the following rules should be observed:

(a) Prevention of scattered radiation
- Keep the radiation times as short as possible.
- Do not start radiation until the emitter and image receiver system are correctly positioned. A laser light visor makes it easier to position the machine without radiation.
- Use pulse techniques for procedures with movement.
- As far as possible, always work with the lowest dose (half-dose program).
- Use the slot or iris diaphragm for gating because the amount of scattered radiation is directly related to the patient volume through which radiation has passed.

(b) Protection from scattered radiation
- Distance is the best radiation protection because radiation decreases by the square of the distance.
- Use radiation protection clothing.
- Cover those parts of the patient's body which are not being examined.

In addition, positioning the image receiver system as close as possible to the patient's body (Focal spot/skin distance is thereby enlarged.) does not only improve the physical image quality but also considerably reduces radiation exposure for the patient [4].

6.3   Tips and Tricks

- Check before every operation that the machine is fully functional.
- After the patient has been positioned (before washing and covering), ensure that a trouble-free use of the C-arm during the operation will be possible.
- Everyone in the room must wear protective clothing.
- Prevent of and protect from scattered radiation.
- Store images with important interim results so that they are available later on for documentation.
- Whenever an image has to be compared with another one, transfer one image to the auxiliary monitor.
- After the operation, save/document the necessary images.

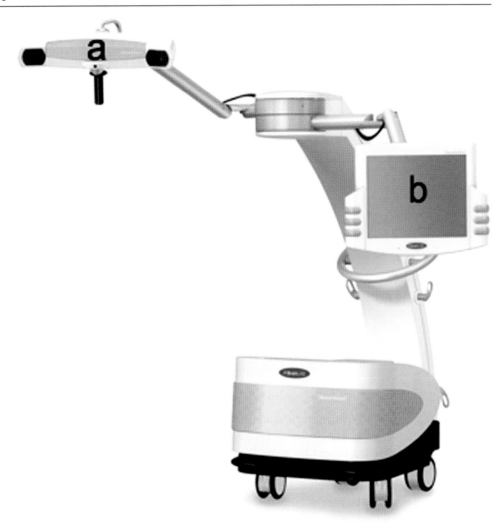

Fig. 6.2 Spinal navigational system with camera (*a*) and workstation monitor (*b*) (With permission of Brainlab)

6.4   Spinal Navigation

Using spinal navigation technology a three-dimensional model of the patient's spine appears on a computer screen with virtual representations of real surgical instruments that the surgeons have in their hand. A variety of spinal navigational systems are available on the market using different imaging modalities for navigation. The common components of most of these systems include an image-processing computer workstation interfaced with two-camera optical localizer (Fig. 6.2), a dynamic reference base (DRB), which is fixed at the patient, and navigated instruments. The camera transmits and tracks infrared light, which is continuously reflected back to the camera by passive reflectors attached to the DRB and the navigated instruments (Fig. 6.3). Alternatively, the infrared light is emitted by a series of LEDs mounted on the DRB and navigated instruments. The tracked infrared light is relayed to the computer workstation. After registration process, the computer workstation provides simultaneous, multiplanar visualization of the spinal anatomy and allows virtually any dedicated or manual calibrated surgical instrument to be tracked in relation to the displayed anatomy in real time (Fig. 6.4) [1]. At present, the various different imaging modalities in use for spinal navigation include: CT, fluoroscopy, the combination of both (CT-Fluoro matching) and 3D-fluoroscopy [2, 3].

6.4.1   Preoperative CT-Based Image Guidance

CT-based navigation systems use a preoperatively acquired CT data set, which has to be transferred to the computer workstation. The computer reconstructs the data into different views. Thus, preoperative surgical planning is possible. Intraoperatively, after surgical exposure, the image-guided

Fig. 6.3 Reference frame (*a*) attached to a spinous process C2 and navigated drill bit (*b*)

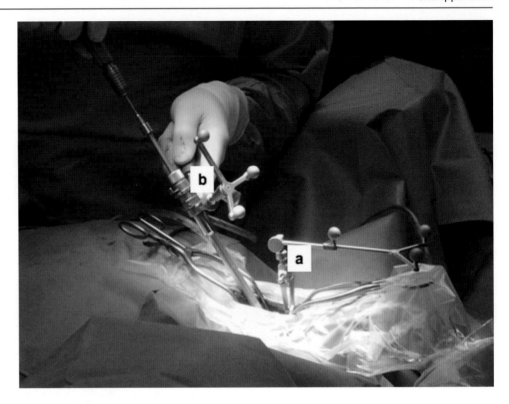

procedure begins with the patient registration. The DRB is attached firmly to the spine. The electrooptical camera tracks the spatial position of the patient by way of signals from DRB. The surface of the vertebral level of interest is touched/scanned with a registration probe (matching Fig. 6.5). This information allows the computer to create a contour map of the vertebra, which is then automatically mapped to CT data. Finally, the accuracy of the system needs to be verified. The probe tip is placed on several anatomic landmarks within the operative field, and the computer workstation monitor displays the virtual probe. The positions of the real and virtual probes had to correspond.

6.4.2 Advantages

- Preoperative surgical planning is possible.
- No occupational radiation exposure.
- Radiolucent table is not a must.

6.4.3 Disadvantages

- Requires a special CT protocol preoperatively.
- Registration process can be difficult and time-consuming.

- Because the CT images are acquired preoperatively with the patient in a different position than at the time of surgery, the preoperative data set may not reflect the intraoperative anatomy on others then the registered level.

6.4.4 Fluoroscopy-Based Image Guidance

Fluoroscopy-based image guidance uses intraoperative fluoroscopic images gained with a C-arm on which a calibration target is attached or temporarily hold into the beam. The images (at least one projection) are automatically transferred to the computer workstation for processing. The computer shows the saved fluoroscopic images that allows for the superimposition of the tracked surgical instruments. In contrast to CT-based navigation, no manual registration (matching) is necessary. Software programs exist that can match a preoperative CT scan with intraoperatively acquired fluoroscopic data (CT-fluoro matching).

6.4.5 Advantages

- Provides real-time intraoperative visualization of the spinal anatomy.
- Suited for minimal access applications.

Fig. 6.4 Workstation screen demonstrating a trajectory for the insertion of a C1–2 transarticular screw (*upper screen*) and a C5 facet screw (*lower screen*)

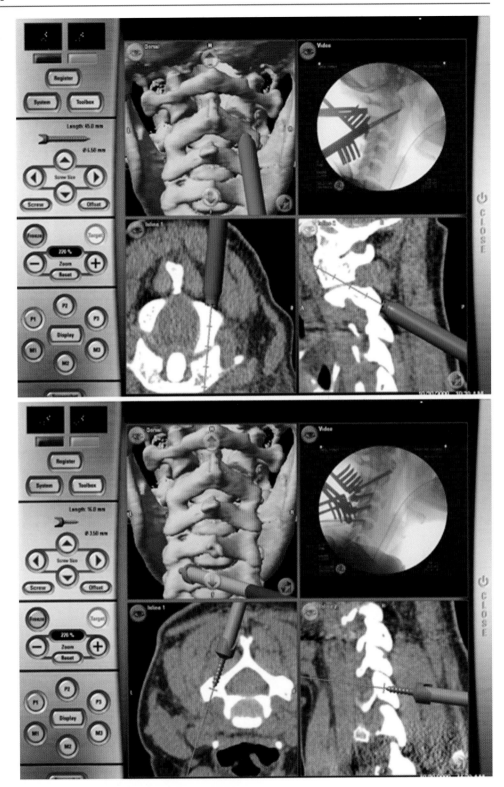

Fig. 6.5 Navigational workstation screen demonstrating a
region matching for C2 vertebra

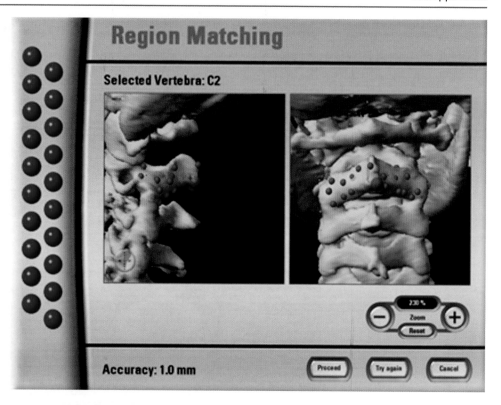

Fig. 6.6 Three-dimensional
C-arm fluoroscopy. The
isocentric C-arm rotates
automated 190° around the
patient (With permission of
Medtronic)

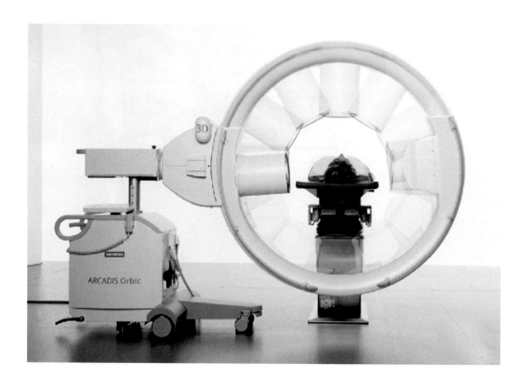

6.4.6 Disadvantages

- Does not offer the axial images that are helpful during CT-based navigation.
- Impaired image quality in certain areas of the spine like the lower cervical or upper thoracic spine and under certain conditions like in patients who are obese, osteopenic, or have spinal deformity.

6.4.7 Preoperative CT-based image guidance, registered with fluoroscopy (CT-Fluoro matching)

The minimally invasive CT-Fluoro matching method uses two intraoperatively acquired fluoroscopy images to register a pre-operatively acquired CT dataset. For this registration the level of interest in the fluoroscopy image and in the CT are fused by the system after a manual prepositioning workflow.

6.4.8 Advantages

- Minimally invasive registration.
- Full CT image quality, 3D reconstructions and axial views.

6.4.9 Disadvantages

- Extra time for pre-positioning steps.
- Final verification of the registration accuracy demanding for minimally invasive cases.

6.4.10 Three-Dimensional C-Arm Fluoroscopy based image guidance

Three-dimensional C-arm fluoroscopy uses an rotating C-arm fluoroscope fitted with a calibration target. An isocentric C-arm is capable of obtaining multiple successive images during an automated partial-rotation around the patient while maintaining the relevant spinal anatomy in the center of the field (Fig. 6.6). Specialized software allows the fluoroscopic images to be reconstructed into axial, sagittal, and coronal views, and the unit can effectively function as a CT scanner.

6.4.11 Advantages

- Reduction of X-ray exposure to surgical team
- Well suited for minimal access applications.

- The 3D C-arm provides three-dimensional reconstructed views of the patient as currently positioned on the operating room table.
- The surgeon-dependent registration step is eliminated.
- As many as three adjacent lumbar levels can be imaged and navigated during each cycle.
- It offers the ability to obtain a postoperative scan while still in the operating room.

6.4.12 Disadvantages

- High radiation exposure to the patient.
- High initial costs.

6.5 Indications

- Spinal fixation procedures are especially useful:
  - Upper cervical and cervicothoracic junction.
  - Deformities.
  - Less invasive/percutaneous approaches.
- En bloc tumor resection.
- Biopsy.

6.6 Contraindications

- Insufficient image quality.
- Verification of the systems accuracy fails.
- Lack of experience in spinal navigation.
- Surgeon is not able to perform the surgical procedure without navigation.

6.7 Technical Prerequisites

- Complete spinal navigation system.
- Carbon table and carbon head clamp/fixation (exception: CT-based navigation).

6.8 Tips and Tricks

- Put the monitor of the C-arm in an ergonomic position directly next to monitor of the workstation. The surgeon must be allowed to look at the monitors easily during the operation.
- Using (3D) C-arm: Before the operation, check if images can be gained without artifacts and position camera to allow for unimpaired line of sight for registration during scan.
- Using CT-based navigation: Check if preoperatively acquired CT data can be used for navigation (e.g., no

artifacts due to CT table); additional use of a standard C-arm can be very helpful.

- DRB has to be fixed tightly to avoid relative movements causing inaccuracies. If the DRB gets loose after registration, registration must be repeated.
- It is strongly recommended to repeat regularly the verification of the systems accuracy, especially before inserting a new screw.
- Position the camera to allow for unimpaired communication between the components (DRB and navigated instruments) while the surgeon can keep his ergonomic position.
- For MIS surgeries: consider placing all relevant wires first, then to continue with screw hole preparation since inserting the k-wires will have less negative influence on the registration accuracy on adjacent levels.

References

1. Holly LT, Foley KT (2007) Image guidance in spine surgery. Orthop Clin N Am 38:451–461
2. Gebhard F, Weidner A, Liener UC, et al. (2004) Navigation at the spine. Injury 35 Suppl 1:35–45
3. Holly LT, Foley KT (2003) Intraoperative spinal navigation. Spine 28:54–61
4. Kreienfeld H, Klimpel H, Bottcher V (2006) Use of X-rays in the operating suite. In: Aschemann D, Krettek C, editors. Positioning techniques in surgical applications. Vol. 4.2. Berlin: Springer; pp. 37–9

Surgical Microscopy in Spinal Surgery

7

Frank Grochulla

7.1 Introduction and Core Messages

Minimally invasive spinal surgery aims to achieve good clinical outcomes, comparable to those of conventional open surgery, while minimizing the risk of iatrogenic trauma resulting from the surgical procedure. Surgical microscopes are one of the most exciting advances in the surgical field. The use of the microscope as a surgical tool was pioneered by Carl Zeiss, a leading German company in the optical and opto-electronic industry. The surgical microscope was first used for ENT surgery in the middle of the 1950s. In the mid-1970s, it was used in spine surgery. Pioneers such as Caspar, Yasargil and Williams were the first spine surgeons to perform microsurgical procedures for the treatment of lumbar disc diseases [1–4]. Since then, the surgical microscope has become an important tool in the field of spinal surgery.

7.2 Definition

The operating microscope used in minimally invasive and microsurgery is a stereoscopic binocular microscope with different magnification levels, giving an upright three-dimensional image. The microscope is used to obtain good visualization of fine structures in the operating field. In the standing type of microscope, a motorised zoom lens system operated by hand or foot controls provides an adjustable working distance. In head-mounted models, interchangeable eyepieces provide the magnification needed. The surgical microscope brings the deep anatomical structures into sharp and brilliant magnified detail, enabling surgeons to perform minimally invasive procedures. It also helps them to preserve important deeper structures and thus to reduce tissue trauma and blood loss (see advantages and disadvantages of loupes and surgical microscopes, Table 7.1). In summary, the microscope is a very helpful tool, enabling the surgeon to perform microsurgical procedures in spinal surgery. Different types of surgical microscope are available. Stand-/floor-type and table-type models are the most common. Wall- and ceiling-mounted surgical microscopes are also available. The two most widely used surgical microscope systems in spine surgery are manufactured by Zeiss and Leica (see Fig. 7.1).

7.3 Advantages

- Simultaneous magnification and illumination of the surgical field
- Three-dimensional magnification
- Coaxial illumination
- Comfortable standing or sitting position for surgeon and assistant (Fig. 7.2), independent of line of sight
- Shared viewing for assistant (teaching)
- Short learning curve
- Smaller skin incisions and less traumatic approaches
- Reduced tissue trauma and blood loss
- Video recording (see Fig. 7.3) for medico-legal and scientific reasons and for teaching

7.4 Disadvantages

Using a surgical microscope has no real disadvantages. However, some aspects should be kept in mind:
- Some "disadvantages" (e.g., hand-eye coordination) are associated with the learning curve of the surgeon and can be avoided by continuous microsurgical education.

F. Grochulla, M.D.
Department for Spinal Surgery, Hospital for Orthopaedics,
Trauma Surgery and Spinal Surgery, Euromed Clinic,
Europa-Allee 1, 90763 Fürth, Germany
e-mail: frank.grochulla@euromed.de

U. Vieweg, F. Grochulla (eds.), *Manual of Spine Surgery*,
DOI 10.1007/978-3-642-22682-3_7, © Springer-Verlag Berlin Heidelberg 2012

Table 7.1 Advantages and disadvantages of loupes and surgical microscopes

	Loupes	Microscopes
Magnification	Limited range and fixed	Greater range and changeable during surgery
Motion	Long surgery causes neck fatigue and movement of loupes	No movement of microscope
Focus	Refocusing is necessary to restart surgery	Microscope in constant focus regardless of surgeon's attention
Illumination	Not parallel to line of vision	Parallel to line of vision and stronger
Deep three-dimensional vision	Limited with smaller skin incisions (<65 mm)	Maintained with even a 25-mm incision
Teaching	Assistants excluded	Assistants included
Surgeon's neck	Fixed in flexion and requiring repositioning. Fatigue during long surgery	Spared, inclinable binocular head can be adjusted

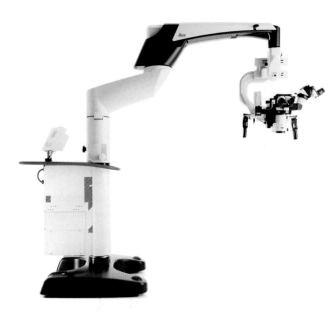

Fig. 7.1 Surgical microscope M525 MS3 (Leica)

- Specially designed retractor systems and instruments are necessary for microsurgery with small skin incisions.
- The visual field is limited. Microsurgery therefore requires meticulous preoperative planning and detailed knowledge of anatomical topography.

7.5 Components of a Surgical Microscope System

7.5.1 Optical System

The optical system of a modern microscope for spine surgery should have the following features:
- At least two tiltable binocular heads for the surgeon and assistant.
- Eyepiece tubes with adjustable interpupillary distance (see Figs. 7.4, 7.5 and 7.6).
- Objective lenses are available with focal lengths from 150 to 400 mm. For spine surgery, 300–400-mm lenses are usual.

7.5.2 Illumination System

The best source of illumination for spinal microsurgery is a xenon light source. This gives a higher light intensity than halogen light sources.

7.5.3 Control System

Surgical microscopes are available with foot or hand controls to adjust magnification, zoom, focus and positioning. Most higher-end equipment comes with motorized foot-controlled focusing as standard, allowing hands-free focusing. Some units also have motorized controls, allowing the surgeon to centre the field of view and tilt the angle of the head assembly via servo motors.

7.5.4 Coupling and Stands

The most advanced principle is the electromagnetic coupling of the microscope to its stand (see Fig. 7.1). This kind of coupling provides comfortable and easy (free floating) controlled movement of the microscope along all axes.

7.5.5 Video Systems and Recording

These are necessary for medico-legal and scientific reasons. High-resolution three-chip digital cameras are used in combination with professional video recording systems.

7.6 Microscope Adjustability

The following features of the surgical microscope can be adjusted:
- Tilt of eyepiece
- Interocular distance
- Eyepiece length
- Focus

Fig. 7.2 Spinal microsurgery in face-to-face position allows the surgeon and assistant to switch position without either sacrificing comfort

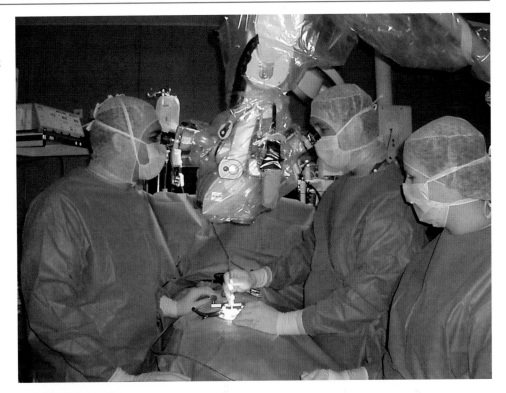

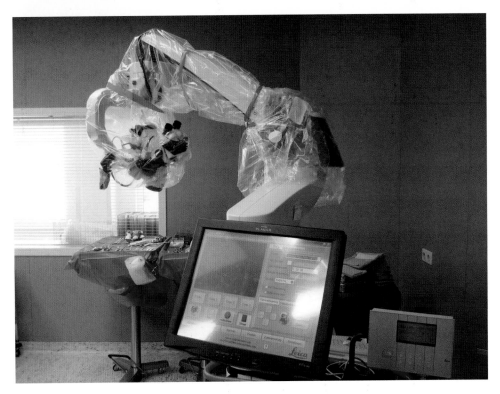

Fig. 7.3 Video- and computer-based recording system

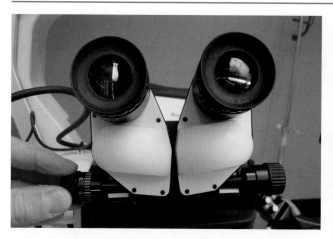

Fig. 7.4 Binocular tubes with adjustable interpupillary distance

- Field and location of autofocus if available
- Zoom/magnification
- Light focus
- Light intensity
- Distance between lens and surgical field
- Degrees of freedom for movement

7.7 Microsurgical Applications

Spinal microsurgery encompasses a wide variety of applications [5] (as listed below):

(a) *Cervical Spine*
  - Anterior cervical decompression and fusion
  - Uncoforaminotomy
  - Total disc replacement
  - Vertebral artery decompression
  - Foraminotomy posterior
  - Laminoplasty

(b) *Thoracic Spine*
  - Anterior transthoracic approaches (discectomy, fractures)
  - Costotransversectomy
  - Discectomy

(c) *Lumbar Spine*
  - Disc herniations
  - Spinal stenosis
  - Foraminal stenosis
  - Synovial cysts
  - Posterior lumbar interbody and transforaminal lumbar interbody fusion preparation
  - Minimally invasive anterior approaches

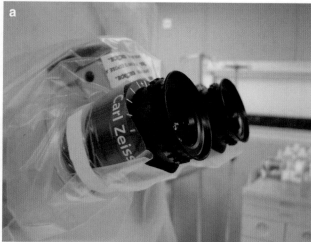

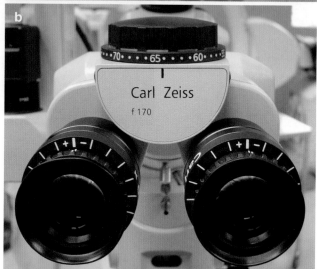

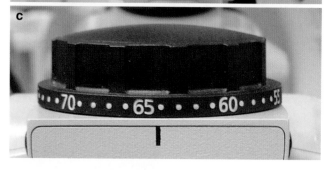

Fig. 7.5 (**a–c**) Sterile adjustment of interocular distance. Adjustments are possible to give the most comfortable position

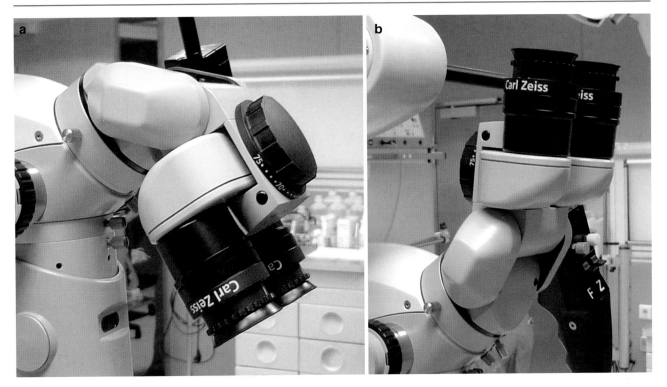

Fig. 7.6 (**a, b**) Adjustment of tilt of binocular head depending on the height of the operating field, the height of the surgeon and the tilt of the microscope

References

1. Caspar W (1977) A new surgical procedure for lumbar disc herniation causing less tissue damage through a microsurgical approach. Adv Neurosurg 4:74–77
2. Mayer HM (2006) Spinal microsurgery. In: Mayer HM (ed) Minimally invasive spine surgery. Springer
3. McCulloch JA, Young PA (1998) The microscope as a surgical aid. In: McCulloch JA, Young PA (eds) Essentials of spinal microsurgery. Lippincott – Raven, Philadelphia
4. Williams RW (1978) Microlumbar discectomy: a conservative surgical approach to the virgin herniated lumbar disc. Spine 3:175–182
5. Yasargil MG (1977) Microsurgical operation of herniated lumbar disc. Adv Neurosurg 7:81

Endoscopy in Spinal Surgery

Uwe Vieweg

8.1 Introduction and Core Messages

An endoscope (from the Greek – éndon – meaning inside and – skopein – meaning to observe) is a device with which it is possible to look at or carry out manipulations within a living organism. Endoscopes may be flexible or rigid. In spine surgery, endoscopes are used both in purely percutaneous applications and with assistance via various minimalized posterior and anterior access routes. For example, they are used with a posterior lumbar access route for endoscopic disc surgery and with anterior thoracic access. The use of endoscopes allows for surgical manoeuvres to be performed through small incisions. The benefits of endoscopic surgery are threefold. Since the incisions are smaller, the recovery from surgery is much quicker. There is also less pain, and there is less damage to the surrounding tissues.

8.2 Definition

Endoscopy is a minimally invasive medical procedure that is used to access the interior surfaces of an organ or preforming spaces by inserting a tube (endoscope) into the body. In the late 1970s and early 1980s, endoscopic techniques were advanced so that they could be used in both diagnosis and treatment of disease. The endoscopic techniques used in other surgical disciplines have now been applied in the treatment of spinal disorders. Improved fibre-optic light sources and the advent of the 3-chip camera have resulted in improvements in visualization of the structures surrounding the spine. By using special endoscopes, instruments and implants, spinal surgeons have been enabled to treat some spinal column disorders with less injury to surrounding tissues. The endoscopic techniques minimize post-operative pain. Thoracoscopes and laparoscopes have been used to perform anterior release of scoliotic or kyphotic deformities and to perform transthoracic microsurgical discectomies. The role of spinal thoracoscopy has expanded to include corpectomy, vertebral reconstruction with internal fixation, hardware application and resection of neurogenic, spinal and paraspinal tumours [1–5]. Advances in interbody fusion cage technology have generated a great deal of interest in laparoscopic techniques [2]. The summary of the most compelling advantages of endoscopic procedures over open surgery are:

- Smaller incisions.
- Less tissue trauma.
- Minimal blood loss.
- Earlier return to activities and work.
- Easier operative approach in obese patients.
- Local or regional anaesthesia can be used in combination with conscious sedation.
- Less post-operative pain medication is required.
- Outpatient surgery is possible.

An endoscope usually consists of:

- *A rigid or flexible optical system* (see Figs. 8.1, 8.2, 8.3c, and 8.4a, b).

  A rigid endoscope transmits images of the object or area being examined through a system of lenses in the endoscope stem to the eyepiece. In flexible endoscopes, the light is usually carried by glass fibres. Such a system may consist of up to 42,000 individual fibres, each of which has a diameter of 7–10 μm.

- *An illumination system*

  The light source is normally outside the body, and the light is typically directed via an optical system. A cold

U. Vieweg, M.D., Ph.D.
Clinic for Spinal Surgery, Sana Hospital Rummelsberg,
90593 Schwarzenbruck, Germany
e-mail: uwe.vieweg@yahoo.de

U. Vieweg, F. Grochulla (eds.), *Manual of Spine Surgery*,
DOI 10.1007/978-3-642-22682-3_8, © Springer-Verlag Berlin Heidelberg 2012

Fig. 8.1 Schematic representation of a flexible endoscope

Fig. 8.2 Schematic representation of a rigid endoscope

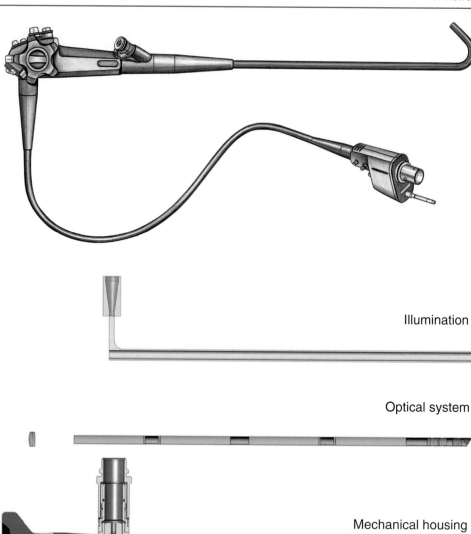

Illumination

Optical system

Mechanical housing

light source is normally used to avoid thermal damage to the organs being examined. Digital image transmission techniques (video endoscopy) may be employed.

- *A lens system*
  This system transmits the image to the viewer from the fibrescope. It allows the surgeon to look both straight ahead and at an angle.
- *A working channel*
  This allows medical instruments or manipulators to be introduced.
- Endoscopes may also be equipped with *suction and irrigation*.

Spinal endoscopy is a procedure in which a small endoscope is passed up through the tailbone into the epidural space

(transhiatal or through the sacral hiatus). This allows direct video imaging of the inside of the spinal canal. Spinal endoscopy is also known as epiduroscopy because the endoscope is looking into the epidural space (see Fig. 8.4a, b). During a spinal endoscopy, an attempt may be made to remove some of the scar tissue or adhesions from around trapped nerves.

Endoscopic spine surgery utilizes dilatation technology to achieve surgical access through the soft tissue (including skin, subcutaneous fat and muscle/fascia) instead of cutting in order to minimize tissue trauma. Beyond the reduced access trauma, the main differences between the endoscopic and the microsurgical microscopic techniques are in the image dimensionality (two-dimensional with endoscopy

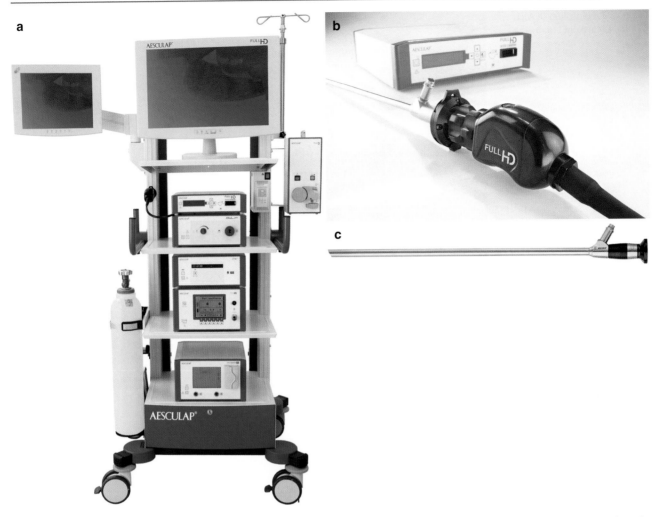

Fig. 8.3 (**a–c**) Video transmission sequence involving 3-chip camera, rigid endoscope with 30° eyepiece, xenon light source, two monitors for surgeon and assistants, video recorder and printer and suction and irrigation unit (With permission of Aesculap AG, Tuttlingen, Germany)

versus three-dimensional in microsurgery). Other differences are employing an angulated and close-up perspective and a straight but remote optical perspective respectively. A number of instrument sets for endoscopic spine surgery are available on the market. They vary considerably in their technical specifications and in the indications they are designed to treat. It is each individual surgeon's responsibility to ascertain that she or he is using an instrument set that is well suited for the planned procedure. While an endoscopic approach to the spine reduces the (visible) trauma of the surgical approach, this minimal invasiveness comes at a price – reduced and two-dimensional visibility in, and limited expandability of, the surgical field. To a large extent, the entry route into the spinal canal or the foramen is dictated by the approach and trajectory chosen and by the local anatomy. Anatomical limitations are set mostly by osseous structures, such as the facet joints, the pedicles and the laminae, but also by the exiting nerve root for foraminal approaches and the vertebral arteries for cervical approaches. In combination with the characteristics of the optical system (angle of view, magnification, etc.), the size of the working channel and the tools available, the anatomy places clear limitations on which areas can be viewed and which lesions can be treated safely. There are burrs, trephines and rongeurs available that allow for the endoscopic resection of bone in order to expand the operative field and enlarge access. However, whenever repositioning of instruments through additional access portals, blind reaming with trephines and excessive bony resection are necessary; the advantages of the minimally invasive procedure over a traditional microsurgical approach are reduced and in some cases may even become a disadvantage. Biplanar fluoroscopy is essential for accurate planning of the approach and for intraoperative control and recording of instrument position.

Fig. 8.4 Epiduroskop (KARL STORZ Endoskope) (**a**, **b**)

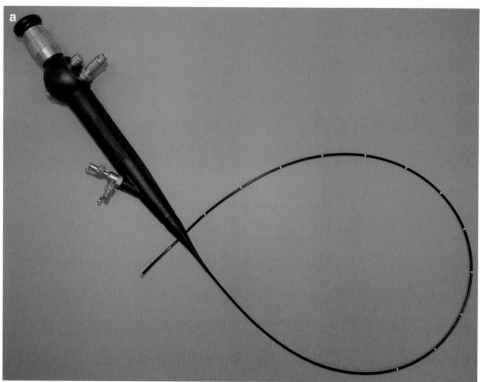

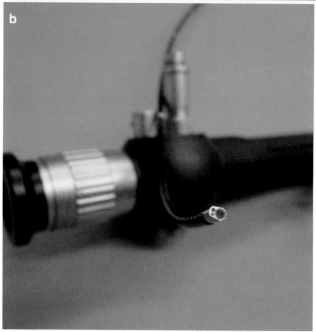

8.3 Types

Endoscopes differ both in their optical systems and in the particular applications for which they are appropriate.

- *Rigid endoscope*

  In a rigid endoscope, the optical system is made up of a series of prisms and lenses arranged in sequence (see Fig. 8.2).

- *Fibre endoscope*

  A fibre endoscope is a flexible endoscope. In this case, the optical system consists of glass fibre bundles. It allows a greater area to be observed and gives a brighter image (see Fig. 8.1).

- *Electronic endoscope*

  The electronic endoscope is a further development of the fibre endoscope. A CCD chip acting as a miniaturized television camera is mounted at its tip and allows an image to be transmitted to a monitor.

- *Chromoendoscope and zoom endoscope*
  A chromoendoscope allows cells to be stained. In gastroenterology, for example, areas of mucous membranes can be sprayed with a harmless pigment such as indigo carmine. This is actually not relevant for spine surgery.

Endoscopic spinal surgery requires coordination of:

- *Endoscopic surgical access*
  Using different thoracoscopic or laparoscopic portals or serial tubular dilators.
- *Operative guidance*
  Intraoperative fluoroscopy is essential to confirm the working level.
- *Endoscopic visualization*
  Digital imaging, endoscopic considerations and illumination.
- *Endoscopic surgical instruments*
  Dissection tools, retractors, irrigation, suction, haemostasis, cautery and endoscopic drills.
- *Spine implants for endoscopic use*

8.4   Endoscopy in Spine Surgery

8.4.1   Anterior Cervical Spine

Endoscopically assisted transoral surgery represents an alternative to standard microsurgical techniques for transoral approaches to the anterior cervicomedullary junction [6].

The anterior approach is very similar to the traditional microsurgical approach, with the neurovascular sheath being positioned lateral to the working channel and the visceral structures medial to the working channel. The tip of the working sleeve is positioned against the anterior longitudinal ligament and the edge of the anterior part of the adjacent vertebral bodies. The disc space can then be passed without performing a discectomy, which is not possible with traditional microsurgery. Herniectomy and, if necessary, removal of osteophytes are carried out with suitable instruments including burrs, trephines, microresectors, various types of forceps, drills, hooks and bipolar microelectrodes. Using this approach, the foraminal areas and the spinal canal can be reached with excellent control of the operating field, but the interpedicular space is not accessible. In the cervical spine – more than in the other segments of the spine – an anterior endoscopic approach facilitates the effective anatomical decompression of the spinal canal and/or the nerve roots (plus in select cases, even the vertebral artery) without requiring replacement of the disc by fusion or arthroplasty.

There is usually no need for a drain or for post-operative immobilization.

8.4.2   Posterior Cervical Spine

The approach and the surgical technique are similar to traditional surgery but are performed using a working tube of varying diameter and the typical endoscopic instruments mentioned for the anterior approach. Fessler et al. [7] have reported on minimally invasive cervical microendoscopic foraminotomy in 25 patients.

8.4.3   Anterior Thoracic Spine

With the aid of thoracoscopy and mediastinoscopy, and using specially adapted trocars and instruments, spine operations can be carried out either entirely endoscopically or with endoscopic assistance. Using thoracoscopy, for example, it is possible to carry out decompression in cases of thoracic disc prolapse or instrumented procedures with additional ventrolateral plating. In 1994, Rosenthal et al. [3] reported the first excision of a herniated thoracic disc by thoracoscopic surgery. Video-assisted thoracoscopic surgery can be used for a variety of spinal indications [11, 12]. The nerve roots and the spinal cord can be decompressed, bone grafts can be placed for interbody fusion, and vertebral body reconstruction and internal fixation can be applied to stabilize the thoracic spine [8] (Figs. 8.5 and 8.6).

8.4.4   Posterior Lumbar Spine

Interlaminar Approach

This approach is very similar to the traditional microsurgical approach. Access to the spinal canal is via a limited flavotomy, and the risks of damaging the dura or neural structures are similar to those applying to the microsurgical approach. Depending on the angle of entry into the interlaminar window in the sagittal plane and the level treated, it may be easy or difficult to actually reach the posterior aspect of the disc. The interpedicular region is very difficult to reach if at all, as is the contralateral side of the ventral epidural space. If the interlaminar window is very small, this approach may not be feasible without resection of the laminar edge and/or the medial aspect of the facet joint, especially with some of the more modern endoscopes that have a larger working channel but also a larger outer diameter.

One clear advantage is the easy convertibility to an open approach.

Posterolateral Approach

This is the best-known foraminal approach to the lumbar spine and can be used for foraminal and extraforaminal disc herniations as well as for intradiscal procedures. It uses an angle of about 60° to the sagittal plane and approaches the

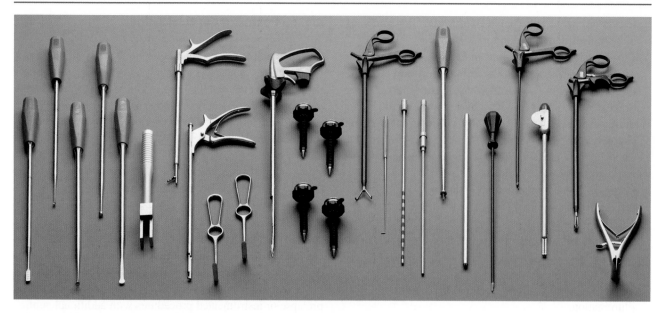

Fig. 8.5 Special long-stemmed instruments for the thoracoscopic preparation of prevertebral structures, discs and bone (Mispas TL, Aesculap) (With permission of Aesculap AG, Tuttlingen, Germany)

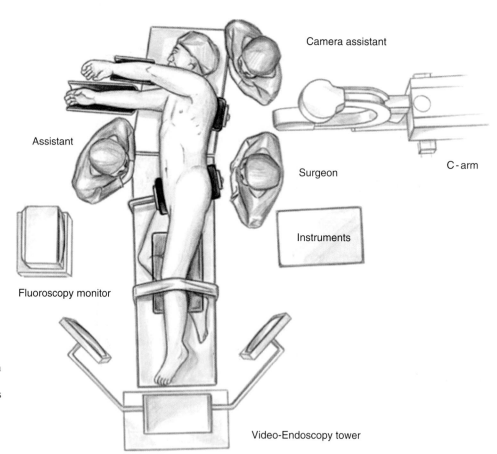

Fig. 8.6 Operating room set-up for endoscopic spine surgery with arrangement commonly used for thoracoscopy. The video monitors are in the surgeon's direct line of sight (With permission of Aesculap AG, Tuttlingen, Germany)

Fig. 8.7 Selective percutaneous endoscopic cervical decompression (PECD) by Dr. Hellinger (With permission of KARL STORZ Endoskope, Germany)

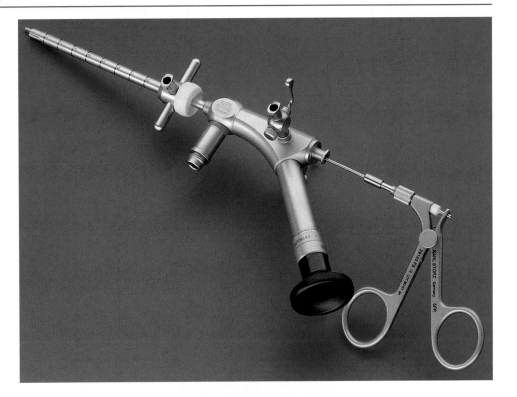

Fig. 8.7 Selective percutaneous endoscopic cervical decompression (PECD) by Dr. Hellinger (With permission of KARL STORZ Endoskope, Germany)

foramen at the level of the disc. It can be performed with the patient either prone or in a lateral decubitus position. The main intraoperative risks are damage to the exiting nerve root (especially where there is advanced loss of disc height) and to blood vessels. To gain adequate access, it is often necessary to ream the lateral aspect of the superior articular process, especially in patients with short pedicles and even without the presence of osteophytes at the facet joint. The ventral epidural space can only be reached in its lateral aspect.

Far or Extreme Lateral Approach

This approach is a more recent development and has largely been pioneered by Ruetten [4]. Using this approach, it is possible to reach the ventral epidural space (with the exception of the interpedicular area) and the foraminal and extraforaminal areas. The foramen is approached at an angle of slightly less than 90° to the sagittal plane. The skin is penetrated at about the level of the facet joints in the coronal plane. The patient should be placed in a prone position. This ensures that there is less interference with the facet joint that occurs with the posterolateral approach, but short pedicles and a large bulging disc can still make it difficult to reach the ventral epidural space. The operative risks are much the same as those applying to the posterolateral approach. There is a higher risk of injury to the dura and the added risk of injury to retroperitoneal organs at the upper lumbar levels. The retroperitoneal anatomy at the level of interest therefore needs to be examined using CT or MRI prior to performing this approach at higher lumbar levels.

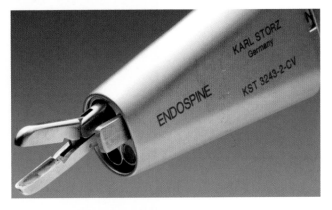

Fig. 8.8 ENDOSPINE operating tube (With permission of KARL STORZ Endoskope, Germany)

8.4.5 Anterior Lumbar Spine

Laparoscopy makes it possible to carry out various surgical procedures on the ventral spine. In 1991, Obenchain [9] performed a laparoscopic L5–S1 discectomy followed, in 1992, by Zdeblick's [2] L5–S1 fusion with laparoscopic placement of an interbody cage. Anterior arthrodesis has been performed by laparoscopic insertion of cages at the L4/L5 and L5/S1 levels [8]. Laparoscopic retroperitoneal techniques have been used for anterior plating to fixate the anterior column rigidly to restore stability [10].

The spinal endoscopy can divided in percutaneous-(see Figs. 8.7, 8.8, 8.9, and 8.10, selective percutaneous

Fig. 8.9 Thoracoscopic spine surgery – set acc. to Rosenthal (With permission of KARL STORZ Endoskope, Germany)

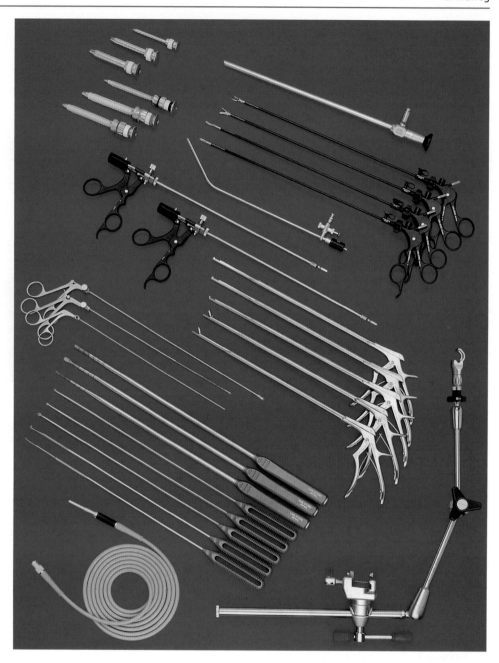

endoscopic cervical decompression, ENDOSPINE operating tube, thoracoscopic spine surgery – set acc. to Rosenthal, percutaneous lumbar transforaminal endoscopy, KARL STORZ Endoskope) or endoscopic-assisted (EASYGO!, KARL STORZ Endoskope) techniques.

8.5 Tips and Tricks

- Endoscopes are precision instruments and must be handled with care. Any damage to the shaft or excessively hard knocks can cause the lenses to become loose or slip inside the instrument. A typical sign of this is clouding of the eyepiece which can lead to a complete breakdown if the endoscope is subjected to further damage.
- The end of the shaft containing the prism must be protected from high temperatures. All manufacturers give their own recommendations, but an upper limit between +65°C and +70°C is common. Some manufacturers achieve upper limits between +150°C and +200°C.
- If the glass fibres in a flexible endoscope are damaged or subjected to extreme bending, the individual glass fibres may break. This causes small black dots to appear in the endoscopic image.
- To learn these techniques, it is essential that surgeons receive adequate training. This includes practice with cadaver and in vivo models, preceptorships and proctorship

Fig. 8.10 Percutaneous lumbar transforaminal endoscopy (With permission of KARL STORZ Endoskope, Germany)

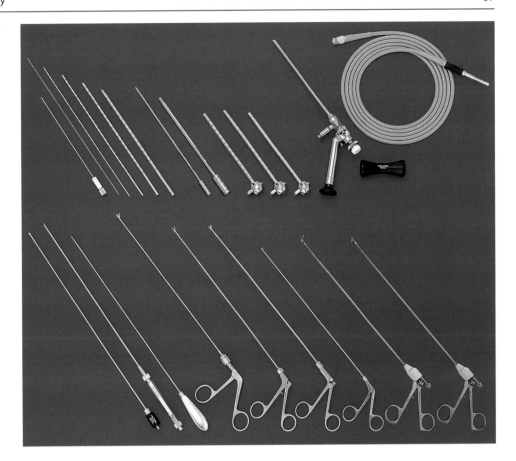

training and, ultimately, teaching in residency and spinal fellowship programs.

References

1. Beisse R, Potulski M, Beger J et al (2002) Entwicklung und klinischer Einsatz einer thorakoskopisch implantierbaren Rahmenplatte zur Behandlung thorakolumbaler Frakturen und Instabilitäten. Orthopade 31:413–422
2. Bohlmann H, Zdeblick T (1988) Anterior excision of herniated thoracic discs. J Bone Joint Surg Am 70:1038–1047
3. Rosenthal D, Rosenthal R, De Simone A (1994) Removal of protruded thoracic disc using microsurgical endoscopy. Spine 19:1087–1091
4. Ruetten S, Komp M, Merk H et al (2008) Full-endoscopic interlaminar and transforaminal lumbar discectomy versus conventional microsurgical technique: a prospective, randomized, controlled study. Spine 33:931–939
5. Ruetten S, Meyer O, Godolias G (2003) Endoscopic surgery of the lumbar epidural space (epiduroscopy): results of therapeutic intervention in 93 patients. Minim Invasive Neurosurg 46:1–4
6. Frempong-Boadu A, Faunce W, Fessler R (2002) Endoscopically assisted transoral-transpharyngeal approach to the craniovertebral junction. Neurosurgery 51:60–66
7. Fessler RG, Khoo LT (2002) Minimally invasive cervical microendoscopic foraminotomy: an initial clinical experience. Neurosurgery 51:37–45
8. Kim DH, Jaikumar S, Kam AC (2002) Minimally invasive spine instrumentation. Neurosurgery 5:15–25
9. Obenchaim TG (1991) Laparoscopic discectomy: case report. J Laparoendosc Surg 1:145–149
10. Mack MJ, Regan JJ, Bobechko WP (1993) Application of thoracoscopy for diseases of the spine. Ann Thorac Surg 56:736–738
11. Raju S, Balabhadra V, Kim DH et al (2005) Thoracoscopic decompression and fixation (MACS-TL). In: Kim DH, Fessler RG, Regan JJ (eds) Endoscopic spine surgery and instrumentation. Thieme, New York
12. Waisman M, Saute M (1997) Thoracoscopic spine release before posterior instrumentation in scoliosis. Clin Orthop 336:130–136

Equipment for Full-Endoscopic Spinal Surgery

9

Sebastian Ruetten

9.1 Introduction and Core Messages

Minimally invasive techniques can reduce tissue damage. Endoscopic operations have advantages which have raised these procedures to the standard in various areas. In arthroscopy, working with rod-lens optics under continuous fluid irrigation has proven valuable. In addition to reduced traumatization, improved visual and light conditions are achieved. Full-endoscopic operations on the lumbar spine can usually be performed uniportal via trans-/extraforaminal or interlaminar approaches. Analogous to the arthroscopy, there is continuous intraoperative irrigation. Since usually only one access is used, the instruments must be inserted through an intra-endoscopic working canal. These days, the equipment available offers operation-technical possibilities comparable to those known from microscope-assisted surgery.

9.2 Definition of Spinal Endoscopy

Full-endoscopic technique is the term for a relatively newly developed method for endoscopic uniportal operations of the lumbar spinal canal and adjacent structures under constant visual control and continuous intraoperative irrigation via a minimally traumatizing access using rod-lens optics with an intraendoscopic working canal. On the lumbar spine, there are existing two different surgical approaches: the trans-/extraforaminal approach through or outside the intervertebral foramen and the interlaminar approach through the interlaminar window.

S. Ruetten, M.D., Ph.D.
Center for Spine Surgery and Pain Therapy,
Center for Orthopaedics and Traumatology,
St. Anna-Hospital, Hospitalstr. 19, 44649 Herne, Germany
e-mail: spine-pain@annahospital.de

9.3 Basic Equipment of Spinal Endoscopy

In addition to standard surgical accessories and small parts, the following basic equipment of the instruments we use (Richard Wolf GmbH, Knittlingen, Germany) is necessary for full-endoscopic operations of the lumbar spine:

- *Rod-lens optics*

  The oval rod-led optics have an outer diameter of maximal 6.9 mm and contain an eccentric working canal with a diameter of 4.1 mm. Moreover, the light source system and an irrigation canal are in the optics unit. The visual angle is 25°. The optics for trans-/extraforaminal and interlaminar accesses differ in their usable length (Fig. 9.1).

- *Access instruments*

  Access is made bluntly in the dilator technique.

  For the trans-/extraforaminal approach, the following instruments are necessary:

  – Spinal needle: for puncture of the target area in or outside the spinal canal

  – Target wire: for subsequent control of the dilators after removal of the spinal needle

  – Dilator: creates the access for the final operation sheath

  – Operation sheath: for insertion of the optics after removal of the dilators

  For the interlaminar approach, the following instruments are necessary:

  – Dilator: creates the access for the final operation sheath

  – Operation sheath: to insert the optics after removal of the dilators

The operation sheaths have a beveled opening which creates a field of vision and work area in an area without clear anatomically preformed hollows. The irrigation fluid is drained off between the oval optics and round operation sheath. The operation sheaths for trans-/extraforaminal and interlaminar accesses differ in their usable length (Fig. 9.2).

U. Vieweg, F. Grochulla (eds.), *Manual of Spine Surgery*,
DOI 10.1007/978-3-642-22682-3_9, © Springer-Verlag Berlin Heidelberg 2012

Fig. 9.1 Rod-lens optics
with intraendoscopic working
canal (With permission from
Wolf Endoscope, Knittlingen,
Germany)

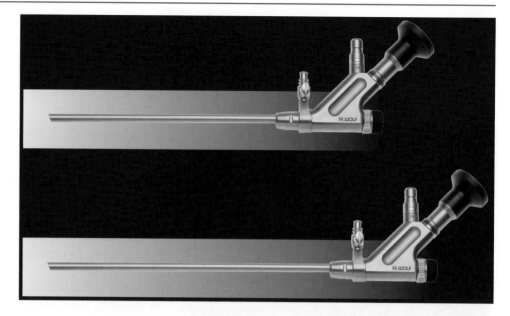

Fig. 9.2 Dilator and operation
sheath (With permission from
Wolf Endoscope, Knittlingen,
Germany)

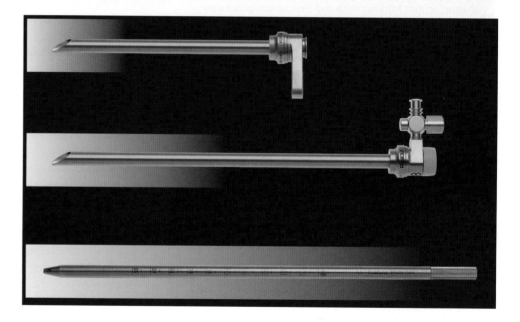

- *Manual instruments*
  The instruments are inserted through the intraendoscopic working canal of the optics. There is a wide variety of punches, shears, rongeurs and other supplies with diameters from 2.5 to 4 mm. The manual instruments for the trans-/extraforaminal and interlaminar approach differ in their usable length (Fig. 9.3).
- *Motor-driven burrs and shavers*
  The burrs and shavers are also inserted via the working canal so that visualization is guaranteed at all times. For bone resection, there are various diamond and normal burrs in ball or oval shapes with various soft-tissue protectors.

The diameter ranges from 2.5 to 4 mm. The shavers for nucleus resection have a diameter of 4 mm (Fig. 9.3).
- *Bipolar coagulation and preparation*
  For intraoperative coagulation and soft-tissue preparation, there are semiactive-flexible, bipolar ball electrodes. They are used with radiofrequency current which can reduce tissue damage in the immediate vicinity of neural structures.
- *Basic unit for endoscopic operations*
  In addition to the operation instruments and the optics, general instruments for endoscopic operations under fluid flow are needed, such as monitor, camera unit, light

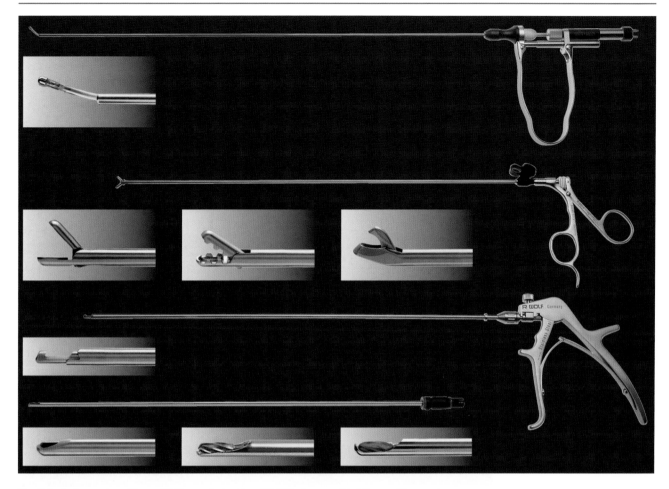

Fig. 9.3 Instruments and burrs (With permission from Wolf Endoscope, Knittlingen, Germany)

source, documentation system, fluid pump, shaver system or radiofrequency generator. Some of the instruments available for arthroscopy or endoscopy can be used (Fig. 9.4).

• *Technical setup in the operating theater*
An X-ray permeable, electrically adjustable operating table and a C-arm are needed. Positioning of the basic units and instruments is made individually and corresponding to the procedure in arthroscopy or endoscopy.

9.4   Tips and Tricks

• Observance of the general indications for the surgical procedure (decompression due to radicular or neurogenic symptoms)
• Observance of the specific indication criteria for the utilization of each approach (trans-/extraforaminal or interlaminar)

Transforaminal [1–3, 5]
– In consideration of abdominal structures performance of a lateral approach to reach the spinal canal sufficiently under constant visualization
– Performance of the approach strictly to the caudal part of the disc level to avoid damaging of the exiting nerve root
– Performance of the extraforaminal approach in cases of intra-/extraforaminal disc herniations or foraminal stenosis
– In cases of insufficient mobility in the spinal canal resection of the ventral bony aspect of the ascending facet

Interlaminar [2–5]
– Performance of the skin incision as medial as possible to facilitate introducing of the endoscope in the spinal canal
– Preparation and identification of the lateral margin of the neural structures before mobilization to avoid damaging of the dura

Fig. 9.4 Endoscopy tower with basic equipment (With permission from Wolf Endoscope, Knittlingen, Germany)

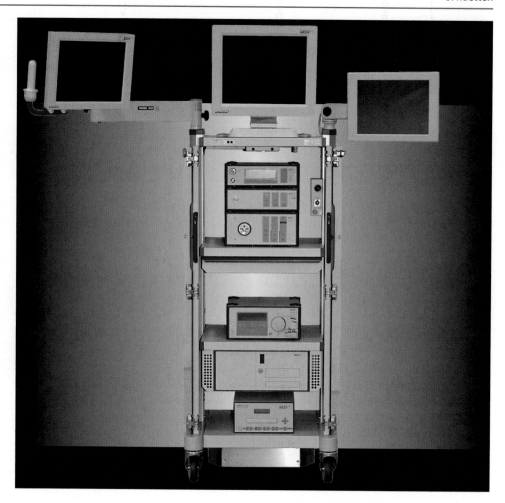

- Avoidance of immoderate retraction for a long time of the neural structures
- In cases of insufficient mobility in the spinal canal or during the approach resection of bony aspect

References

1. Ruetten S, Komp M, Godolias G (2005) An extreme lateral access for the surgery of lumbar disc herniations inside the spinal canal using the full-endoscopic uniportal transforaminal approach. Technique and prospective results of 463 patients. Spine 30:2570–2578
2. Ruetten S, Komp M, Merk H, Godolias G (2007) Use of newly developed instruments and endoscopes: full-endoscopic resection of lumbar disc herniations via the interlaminar and lateral transforaminal approach. J Neurosurg Spine 6:521–530
3. Ruetten S, Komp M, Merk H, Godolias G (2008) Full-endoscopic interlaminar and transforaminal lumbar discectomy versus conventional microsurgical technique: a prospective, randomized, controlled study. Spine 33:931–939
4. Ruetten S, Komp M, Merk H, Godolias G (2009) Surgical treatment for lumbar lateral recess stenosis with the full-endoscopic interlaminar approach versus conventional microsurgical technique: a prospective, randomized, controlled study. J Neurosurg Spine 10:476–485
5. Ruetten S, Komp M, Merk H, Godolias G (2009) Recurrent lumbar disc herniation following conventional discectomy: a prospective, randomized study comparing full-endoscopic interlaminar and transforaminal versus microsurgical revision. J Spinal Disord Tech 22:122–129

Electrosurgery

Uwe Vieweg

10.1 Introduction and Core Messages

In electrosurgery a high-frequency electric current is applied to biological tissue as a means to cut, coagulate, desiccate or fulgurate the tissue. When a current is passed through the tissue, the cell liquid expands and evaporates and the cell explodes, which causes the cutting or coagulation effect. This technique underlies many modern surgical procedures. It is therefore important for spine surgeons to be familiar with its basic physical principles and safety measures.

10.2 Definition

Electrosurgery uses high-frequency energy for cutting, cutting with simultaneous coagulation and coagulation procedures on human tissue (synonyms: HF surgery, diathermia, electrocauterisation, electrosurgery). Today, high-frequency surgery or electrosurgery is an established feature in the different surgical disciplines. Most high-frequency surgical devices now work with frequencies of about 300–600 kHz (see Fig. 10.1). The advantages of high-frequency surgery are that bleeding is minimal, the high working temperature prevents contamination with microorganisms and the surgical procedure requires only a small skin incision.

10.3 Procedures and Devices

- Haemostasis and tissue cutting with high-frequency currents alone (e.g., MBC 200 Söring GmbH)
- Haemostasis and tissue cutting with high-frequency currents and additional helium gas as a carrier for the electric current (e.g., CPC 1,000–1,500–3,000 cold plasma coagulation, Söring GmbH)
- Haemostasis and devitalisation of tissue with high-frequency currents and additional ionised argon gas (e.g., VIO-APC 2 argon plasma coagulation, ERBE Elektromedizin GmbH)
- High-frequency-induced thermotherapy (tissue ablation) with high-frequency currents and hollow insulated-shaft

U. Vieweg, M.D., Ph.D.
Clinic for Spinal Surgery, Sana Hospital Rummelsberg,
90593 Schwarzenbruck, Germany
e-mail: uwe.vieweg@yahoo.de

U. Vieweg, F. Grochulla (eds.), *Manual of Spine Surgery*,
DOI 10.1007/978-3-642-22682-3_10, © Springer-Verlag Berlin Heidelberg 2012

Fig. 10.1 Frequency range for most high-frequency electrosurgical devices

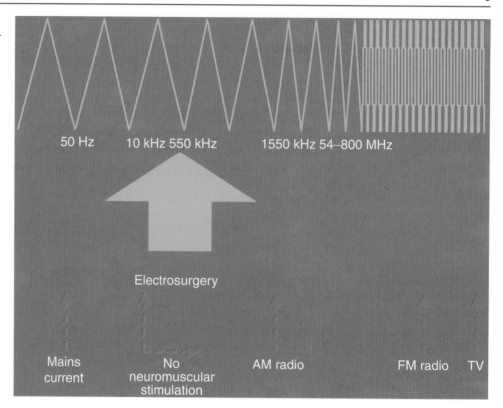

needle electrodes perfused with saline solution (e.g., Elektrotom HITT 106, Integra LifeSciences)
• High-frequency-induced thermotherapy of facet joints, for example, with high-frequency currents supplied through insulated needles specially positioned within the tissue (e.g., MultiGen RF generator, Stryker)

10.4 Manufacturers of High-Frequency Electrosurgical Generators

Aaron Medical Industries, adeor Medical Technologies GmbH, Aesculap AG, Elliquence, ellman International, ERBE Elektromedizin GmbH, Gyrus ENT, Integra LifeSciences, MEGADYNE Medical Products, Naeem Jee Corporation, PEAK Surgical, Schuco, Söring GmbH, Stryker Valleylab.

10.5 Basic Physical Principles [1–5, 8]

When a current is passed through the tissue, the cell liquid expands and the cell explodes and evaporates, which causes the cutting or coagulation effect. Three effects are important when the body is subjected to an electric current: the Faraday effect, the electrolytic effect and the thermal effect. Nerve and muscle cells can be stimulated electrically. In human tissue, the stimulation effect is greatest with an alternating current of approx. 100 Hz. This effect decreases with increasing frequency, thus losing its damaging, or even life-threatening, action.

With high-frequency alternating currents, electrolysis and nerve stimulation occur only to a very small extent. According to Joule's law, the heat ΔQ produced per tissue volume ΔV is directly proportional to the resistivity ρ of the tissue and the square of the current density j. $\Delta Q = \rho \cdot j^2 \cdot \Delta V \cdot \Delta t$. Current densities of $j = 1 - 6 \, \text{A/cm}^2$ are usual. Body tissue has a higher electrical resistance than the metal cutting electrode. The flow of current therefore heats up the surrounding tissue but not the electrode. The effect is particularly strong close to the operating electrode because the whole current flows through a very small cross-sectional area of tissue. At the neutral electrode, the returning current is spread out over a large area and thus causes only slight heating of the tissue. The degree of tissue heating caused by an electric current depends on the following factors: the current density, the resistivity of the tissue and the length of time for which current is applied.

The following variables influence the effect exerted on tissue: power setting, size of electrode, time, manipulation of electrode, type of tissue, waveform and eschar. The smaller the electrode, the greater is the current density. Consequently, the same tissue effect can be achieved with a smaller electrode, even though the power setting is reduced. At any

Fig. 10.2 Illustration of the effects of the two electrosurgical processes – coagulation and incision – on tissue (coagulation: energy dried out by heat-coagulated cell; incision: high energy density, fluid evaporates, cell expands, cell explodes) [6]

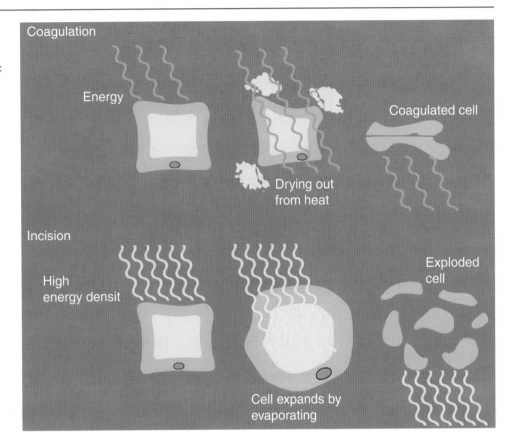

given setting, the longer the generator is activated, the more heat is produced. The greater the heat, the further it will travel to adjacent tissue (thermal spread). Tissues vary widely in resistance. Eschar is relatively high in resistance to current Keeping electrodes clean and free of eschar will enhance performance by maintaining lower resistance within the surgical circuit.

10.6   Effect of High-Frequency Current

The surgical effects of high-frequency currents can be divided into two main groups: cutting and coagulation [1, 3, 5–8]. Cutting severs the tissue, while coagulation dries the tissue out.

- Coagulation is the clotting of protein with reduction of volume and loss of water (see Fig. 10.2). Coagulation can be divided into deep and surface coagulation or into desiccation and fulguration (see Fig. 10.3). Desiccation refers to coagulation induced using an inserted needle electrode (contact coagulation). Fulguration or spray coagulation refers to surface carbonisation or surface coagulation caused by spark discharge from an electrode held close to the tissue (non-contact coagulation). The intra- and extracellular fluid is evaporated by sparks emitted from the tip of the electrode which is held a few millimetres from the

tissue and moved over it. The main difference between fulguration and desiccation is that fulguration does not involve contact between the tissue and the electrode. This effect is primarily used when sealing tissue over a large surface. The depth of coagulation depends on the strength of the current used. If a large current is used, carbonisation occurs and eschar forms which inhibits the spread of the heat to a greater depth. When the electrode is subsequently removed, the burnt tissue is removed as well because it sticks to the electrode tip. However, if a small current and a long duration of action are selected, the tissue around the electrode, down to a depth slightly greater than the diameter of the electrode, is vaporised. Coagulation can also be divided into the following categories depending on the qualities of the current used:

Soft coagulation (<190 V): In this case, no spark or arc of light occurs, and no unwanted cutting is caused. Carbonisation is prevented.

Forced coagulation (*up to* 2.35 kV *peak*): Arcs of light are produced in order to reach a greater coagulation depth. In the process, carbonisation cannot be avoided. Ball electrodes with a small surface area are usually used for this purpose.

Spray coagulation (*up to* 8 kV *peak*): In spray coagulation, long and powerful arcs of light are produced which heat the tissue both exogenously and endogenously. In

Fig. 10.3 Illustration of the effects of the two electrosurgical processes – coagulation and incision – and their subgroups (pure cut, blend cut, desiccation, fulguration) [6]

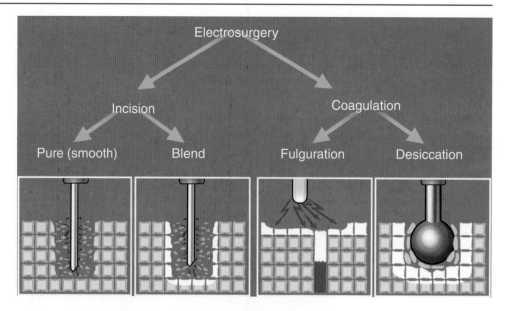

this process, no spark or arc of light occurs, and no unwanted cutting is caused.

- Incision involves cutting of tissue with high-frequency current and electrodes with a small surface area. Explosive evaporation of cellular fluids at the site of the cut severs the tissue and coagulates it at the cut edges (see Fig. 10.2). Incisions are divided into pure cuts and blend cuts (see Fig. 10.3). A pure or smooth incision (cut) exerts as little lateral haemostatic effect as possible.

10.7 Electrode Configurations

Modern, high-frequency electrosurgical devices transfer electrical energy to human tissue via a treatment electrode (in a bipolar or monopolar configuration) that remains cool (see Table 10.1). In the bipolar configuration, the voltage is applied to the tissue using special forceps of which one tine is connected to one pole of the generator, and the other tine is connected to the other pole of the generator. When a piece of tissue is held with the forceps, a high-frequency electric current flows between the tines, heating the intervening tissue. In monopolar electrosurgery, the active electrode is in the surgical site. The patient return electrode is attached somewhere else on the patient. The current must flow through the patient to the patient return electrode. In the monopolar configuration, the patient is in contact with the return electrode, a relatively large or a flexible metalized plastic pad which is connected to the generator. The surgeon uses a pointed electrode to make contact with the tissue. The electric current flows from the electrical tip through the body to the return electrode and then back to the electrosurgical generator.

10.8 Safety Measures

- Insulation
  The patient must lie fully insulated on the operating table (dry drapes, plastic mats, etc.). He/she must also be insulated from all metal items and any tubes capable of conducting electricity. Dry cellulose pads are necessary in skin folds, breast folds and between extremities. For high-power surgical uses under anaesthesia, the monopolar modality relies on good electrical contact between return electrode and the body. If contact with the return electrode is insufficient, severe burns (third degree) can occur in areas of poor contact with the return electrode or where contact is made with grounded metal objects serving as an unintended return path.

- Position and type of neutral electrode
  The neutral electrode should be placed as close to the operating area as possible, and should have good contact with the patient tissue. So-called split return electrodes should always be used. These monitor the contact quality of the return electrode to the patient. The so-called return electrode monitoring (CQM) system (safety system) was developed to avoid burns under the return electrodes. This system measures the contact quality of the surface between the return electrode and the patient all the time, also while the generator is activated, and monitors every change during the entire surgical procedure.

- Anaesthesia equipment
  For preoperative monitoring, only ECG cables with high-resistance inputs or HF choke may be used. Before the operation, it is important to ensure that the current from the active electrode to the return electrode is not conducted through the heart area or that any such conduction is minimised.

Table 10.1 Differences between the monopolar and bipolar configuration in electrosurgery

	Monopolar	Bipolar
Poles	Electrodes with small surface area in operating region, return via large-area neutral electrode	Both poles are held directly over the tissue with forceps whose tines are insulated against each other. Current flows between the two poles only
Action	Strong local heating of the tissue at the electrode-tissue junction (coagulation) and sparking and fulguration at high voltages	Local heating of the tissue only between the electrodes; coagulation as a result
Uses	Coagulation, desiccation, fulguration, tissue cutting, sometimes with sloughing/scab formation, blood vessel closure	Coagulation, good closure of blood vessels
Advantages	Many different applications possible with change of electrodes; rapid haemostasis	Small currents required (only about 20–30% of that needed for monopolar HF), route followed by current can be calculated, risk of burns
Disadvantages	Neutral electrode needs to be fixed, risk of burns if neutral electrode comes unstuck, current flow through the body cannot be precisely controlled, short circuiting possible via contact with earthed metal items	Tissue cutting, fulguration

10.9 Tips and Tricks

- Correct positioning (dry and insulated)
- No contact with grounded objects
- No skin-to-skin contact (between individual parts of the patient's body)
- Short cables, no contact to grounded metal parts
- No looping of cables and no fixation with metal brackets
- Cautious handling of disinfectants (the alcohol contained can be ignited by electric sparks)
- Return electrode monitoring (CQM) system (safety system)

10.10 Current Trends

Further developments in electrosurgery involve the use of helium gas (cold plasma coagulation) or ionised argon gas (argon plasma coagulation) which allows current flow without contact between electrode and tissue. Both plasma coagulation techniques require no return electrode and do not involve current flow through the body or areas of vaporisation within the tissue. It therefore permits rapid and controlled haemostasis without major tissue damage.

References

1. Ainer BL (1991) Fundamentals of electrosurgery. J Am Board Fam Pract 4:419–426
2. Arnold P, Advincula WK (2008) The evolutionary state of electrosurgery: where are we now? Curr Opin Obstet Gynecol 20:353–358
3. Boughton RS, Spencer SK (1987) Electrosurgical fundamentals. J Am Acad Dermatol 16:862–867
4. Elliott-Lewis EW, Mason AM, Barrow DL (2009) Evaluation of a new bipolar coagulation forceps in a new bipolar coagulation forceps in a thermal damage assessment. Neurosurgery 65(6):1182–1187
5. Hainer BL (1991) Fundamentals of electrosurgery. J Am Board Fam Pract 4:419–426
6. Hausmann V (2006) High-frequency surgery. In: Krettek C, Aschemann D (eds) Positioning techniques in surgical applications. Springer, Heidelberg, pp 41–54
7. Reidenbach HD (1993) Fundamentals of bipolar high-frequency surgery. Endosc Surg Allied Technol 1:85–90
8. Vellimana AK, Sciubba DM, Noggle JC et al (2009) Current technological advantages of bipolar coagulation. Neurosurgery 64:11–19

Surgical Motor Systems in Spinal Surgery

Frank Grochulla and Uwe Vieweg

11.1 Introduction and Core Message

Surgical motor systems are important power tools in microsurgical procedures at the cervical, thoracic and lumbar spine, whenever preparation and removal of bone become necessary.

Motor systems are surgical instruments, which are divided in high- and low-speed systems. The motor systems are operating with electrical, pneumatic or akku power source controlled by foot pedal or hand tip. Common power tools in spinal surgery are: drill systems, bone saws and burrs. Especially high-speed drill systems are important tools for opening procedures of the spinal canal.

11.2 History

Important milestones were the invention of the first electric surgical motor in 1935 by Aesculap, the introduction of pneumatic power systems in the 1960s, pioneering work with flexible cable motors in the 1970s, battery-powered motor systems in the 1980s and the incorporation of pneumatic and electric high-speed systems in the 1990s. Power tools have undergone many improvisations and modifications in the past two decades and have improved tremendously in their functionality and versatility [1–4].

F. Grochulla, M.D. (✉)
Department for Spinal Surgery, Hospital for Orthopaedics, Trauma Surgery and Spinal Surgery, Euromed Clinic, Europa-Allee 1, 90763 Fürth, Germany
e-mail: frank.grochulla@euromed.de

U. Vieweg, M.D., Ph.D.
Clinic for Spinal Surgery, Sana Hospital Rummelsberg, 90593 Schwarzenbruck, Germany
e-mail: uwe.vieweg@yahoo.de

11.3 Components and Technical Details

There are a number of surgical motor systems on the market. Differences exist in the source of power, the revolutions per minute (rpm) ranging from 10,000 rpm up to 90,000 rpm and more and the activation of the motor system (by hand or by foot).

11.3.1 Power Systems

- *Pneumatic high-speed power system* (HiLAN® XS, ComPact Air Drive II, Air Pen Drive, Synthes).
  The sterilizable coaxial flexible hose connects the pneumatic motor with a foot pedal.
- *Electric power system* (microspeed® uni Aesculap; Servotonic EC I/II 100, Medicon Instruments; Linotec E9000, Stryker; Zimmer surgical motor systems, ElectricPen Drive, Synthes) (Fig. 11.1).
  The differences between an electric and pneumatic power systems are in respect to personal preference electric instead of pressure air.

Personal preference	Electric instead of pressured air
Noise level	Pneumatic systems generate a higher noise level than electric motor systems.
Handling	Electric systems is easier to set up (no need for pressured air). Cable is more flexible and lighter than air hoses.
Versatility	Electric system can usually cover more indication fields (low speed, high speed, pistol, shave in one system).
Individuality	Individual settings and acceleration/stopping characteristics. Oscillation angle, etc., can be adjusted via the control unit to individual preferences.
Price	Electric systems tend to be more expensive than pneumatic ones.

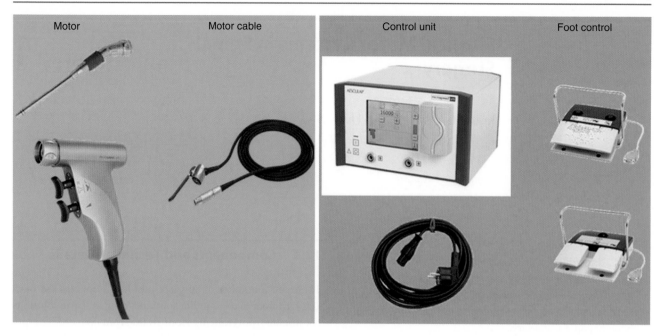

Fig. 11.1 Components of surgical motor systems (motor unit, handpiece, control unit, connecting cable, foot control) (With permission of Aesculap AG, Tuttlingen, Germany)

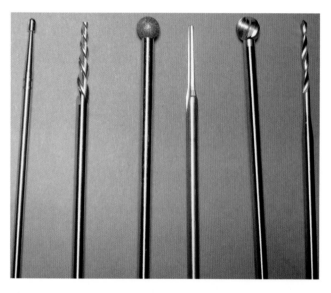

Fig. 11.2 Cutting and diamond burrs, Rosen burr and diamond burr

11.3.2 Accessories

The motor systems consist of various *attachments* (burrs, drills, saws). Burrs and drills are available in different sizes and shapes (Fig. 11.2). The more aggressive cutting burrs (cylindrical burr, Rosen burr) are applicable to remove hard cortical and cancellous bone. These cutting burrs should not be used in the spinal canal because of the risk of tearing soft tissue (dura, neural structures). Less aggressive burrs such as diamond burrs are more applicable for preparing in the near of important soft tissue structures such as vessels, nerves and dura.

The *handpieces* are available in angulated or straight designed shape. Angulated handpieces are more useful in microsurgical procedures. *Irrigation* is always necessary when using a high-speed motor system in order to avoid local hyperthermic reactions. Continuous irrigation should

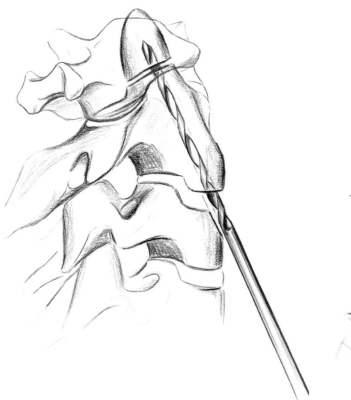

Fig. 11.3 Pre-drilling for osteosynthesis screws (With permission of Aesculap AG, Tuttlingen, Germany)

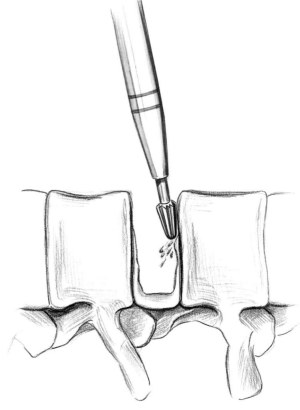

Fig. 11.5 Preparation of implant bed for corpectomies or interbody fusions (With permission of Aesculap AG, Tuttlingen, Germany)

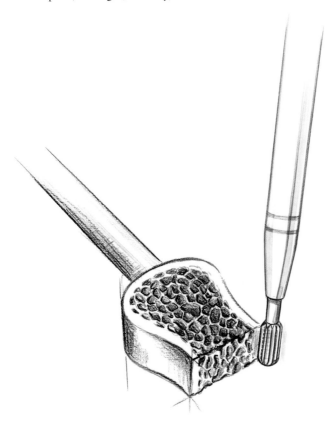

Fig. 11.4 Decortications/pre-drilling for distraction, pedicle or osteosynthesis screws with a high-speed burr or high-speed drill (With permission of Aesculap AG, Tuttlingen, Germany)

be used with an integrated irrigation system which provides an electronically controlled permanent irrigation. If not available, a simple irrigation by using a syringe is possible.

11.4 Indications

All the different systems available for varied indications on the spine.

- Decortications/pre-drilling for distraction, pedicle or osteosynthesis screws with a high-speed burr or high-speed drill (see Figs. 11.2 and 11.3)
- Preparation of implant bed for corpectomies or interbody fusions (see Fig. 11.4)
- Harvesting and modelling of autologous bone graft with a saws/high-speed or low-speed burrs (see Figs. 11.5 and 11.6)
- Decompression/access preparation (laminoplasty, laminotomy, laminectomy, facetectomy, foraminotomy) with a high-speed or low-speed burr or laminectomy drill/craniectomy (see Figs. 11.7, 11.8, 11.9, 11.10 and 11.11).

Figs. 11.6 and 11.7 Harvesting and modelling of autologous bone graft with a saws/high-speed or low-speed burrs (With permission of Aesculap AG, Tuttlingen, Germany)

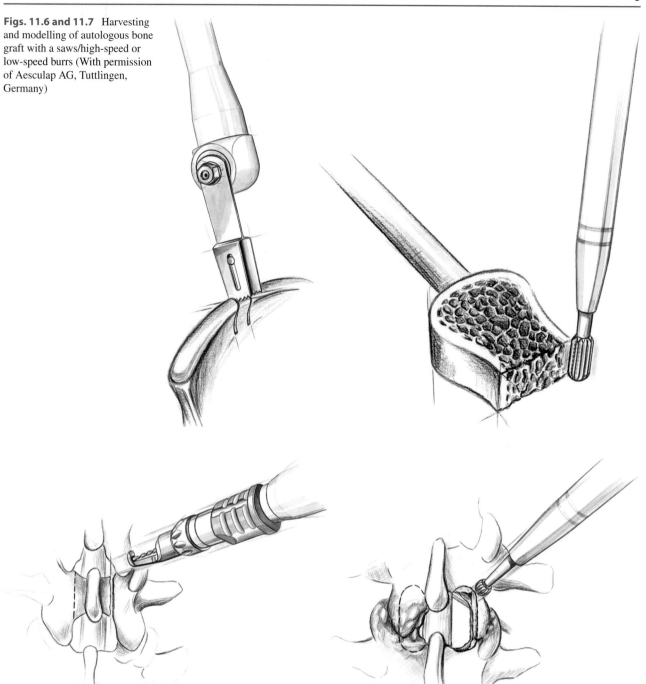

Figs. 11.8 and 11.9 Access preparation (laminoplasty, laminotomy, laminectomy facetectomy, foraminotomy) with a high-speed or low-speed burr or laminectomy craniectomy drill (With permission of Aesculap AG, Tuttlingen, Germany)

Fig. 11.10 Vertebral body resection with a long handpiece over a mini-thoracotomy (With permission of Aesculap AG, Tuttlingen. Germany)

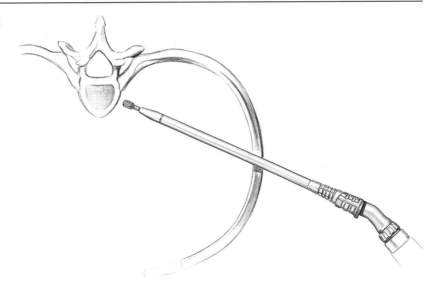

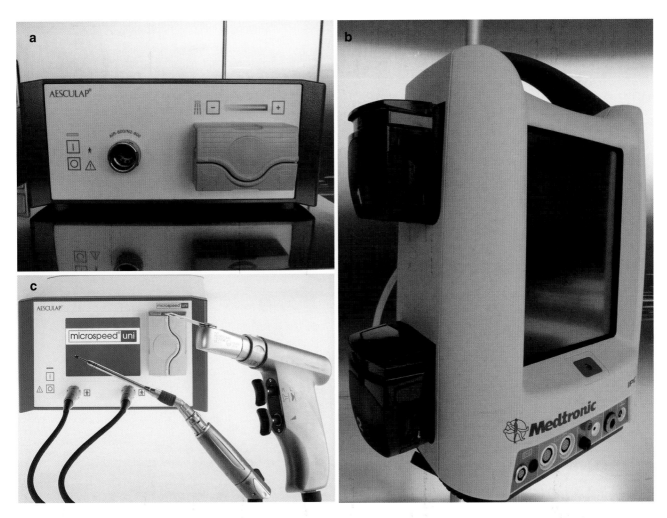

Fig. 11.11 (**a**) Pneumatic motor (HiLAN, Aesculap), (**b**) electric motor system (Midas Rex Legend, Medtronic) and (**c**) electric motor system with different handpiece (HiLAN, Aesculap) (With permission Aesculap AG, Tuttlingen, Germany)

11.5 Tips and Tricks

- Lubricating the power systems is a simple and safe affair. The motor and handpieces are sprayed with special oil spray before sterilization cycle.
- Complete lubrication of the motor and handpieces is ensured, making permanent intraoperative lubrication unnecessary.
- Before use, the instrument should be completely checked by the surgeon.
- A high-speed burr with foot pedal should be controlled by the surgeon only.
- Always work with intact and sharp tools (drills) to avoid damage or overheating of the motor system.

References

1. Albee FH (1929) Some scientific aspects of orthopaedic surgery. J Bone Joint Surg Am XI:696
2. Beer RR et al (1998) Biorobotic approaches to the study of motor systems. Curr Opin Neurobiol 8(6):777–782
3. Dyas FG (1914) The treatment of acute osteomyelitis of the long bones by means of the dental engine and a large burr: preliminary report. JAMA LXII(1):216
4. Kale S (2008) Power tools in orthopaedic surgery – an update. Orthop Prod News 48:56–62
5. Kurtz AD (1930) Chronic osteomyelitis: operation with large drill and high-speed motor. J Bone Joint Surg Am 12:182–183

Bone Grafts and Bone-Graft Substitutes

12

Robert Morrison

12.1 Introduction and Core Messages

Bone grafts or substitutes are used in spinal surgery to fill defects, bridge defects or to promote spondylodesis. The physiological process is similar to that of fracture healing and incorporates the same spatial and temporal factors. The ideal material should provide osteogenetic, osteoinductive and osteoconductive properties. The traditional autologous bone grafts are probably still considered the "golden standard", but the problems associated with them bring up the need for substitutes. One alternative is the acquirance of allogenic or xenogenic bone grafts, which have specific problems of their own, which limit their use. The other aspect is the use of bone substitutes, which come in a growing variety of materials, shapes and application forms. Currently, none of these substitutes unite all of the prerequisites shown above, but they have the advantage of unlimited supply without causing additional problems such as donor site morbidity. And the combination of such substitutes as scaffold with the utilization of growth factors and mesenchymal stem cells bring with them a completely new array of possibilities.

12.2 Definition

12.2.1 Bone Graft

Bone grafts are harvested from different parts of the patient. It is most commonly from the iliac crest, but can also be taken from the vertebral structures, the ribs, the tibia as well as the fibula [12].

12

12.2.2 Bone-Graft Substitute

It replaces autologous bone in order to achieve defect filling and bridging and also fusion [13]. It provides unlimited supply and eliminates donor site morbidity. But no substitute provides the combination of osteoinductive, osteoconductive and osteogenetic properties [12].

12.3 Physiology of Bone Regeneration

Bone is one of the few organs that retains the potential for regeneration throughout life. In contrast to other organs, bone does not repair defects with scar material of poor quality, but rather reinstates its original values. But fracture healing, and therefore also bone regeneration, is a complex physiological process.

Two basic principles of bone healing are described in literature [10]:
- Primary bone healing ("direct healing") is very rare and not the usual form of healing achieved in spinal surgery.
- Secondary bone healing involves intramembranous and endochondral ossification and leads to callus formation. Callus formation is achieved through undifferentiated multipotent mesenchymal stem cells (MSCs) and requires cell vitality and blood supply.

In this cascade of bone regeneration, certain prerequisites are known. Most importantly, a vital cell population has to be present. MSCs have to be either present or transferred to the site via blood supply. These cells are transferred to a cell population with osteoblastic phenotypes.

In addition, the fracture haematoma offers a vast supply of signalling molecules (ILs, TNFs, TGFs, VEGF) to induce healing. Within the group of TGFs, the so-called bone morphogenetic proteins (BMP-2, BMP-7) have been extensively studied and shown to play a decisive role in the healing process [8]. The third important element is the extracellular matrix, providing a natural scaffold for the cellular interactions. This can be replaced by an immense number of osteoconductive materials such as allografts, demineralized bone

12

12

R. Morrison, M.D.
Department of Spine Surgery,
Sana Rummelsberg Hospital,
Rummelsberg 1, Schwarzenbruck, Germany
e-mail: dr.r.morrison@googlemail.com

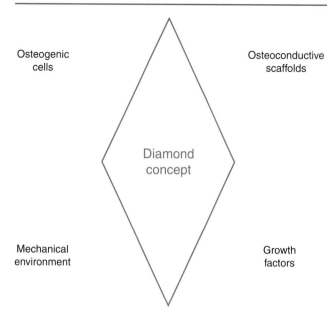

Fig. 12.1 Diamond concept fur ideal fracture healing constellation [5]

Advantages

- Osteogenetic
- Osteoconductive
- Osteoinductive

Disadvantages

- Limited supply.
- High failure rate is reported.
- Risk of iliac crest fracture (Fig. 12.4).
- Correctional loss due to remodelling [7].
- Donor site morbidity (limited with correct utilization).
- Additional operation time.

12.5.1 Harvest Sites

- Iliac crest (anterior, posterior)
- Locally (vertebral body, spinous process, lamina)
- Rib portion (in transthoracic approaches)
- Tibia/fibula

matrix (DBM), hydroxyapatite- and calcium-based ceramics, among others. These scaffolds have been shown to have an optimal pore size of 150–500 μm. The last important factor, important for fracture healing and bone formation, is the mechanical stability. All four components combined are described as the "diamond concept" (Fig. 12.1). It is well described in extremity fractures and of equal importance in spinal surgery [5].

12.4 Clinical Application

Therefore, bone or bone substitutes should preferably have the three properties mentioned above. *Osteogenicity* refers to the fact that they contain osteoblastic cells and are thereby capable of directly forming bone. *Osteoconductivity* refers to the situation in which they provide a structure along which osteoblasts can attach and thereby bone can grow. *Osteoinductivity* is the ability to induce non-differentiated stem cells or osteoprogenitor cells to differentiate into osteoblasts. A "perfect" bone-graft substitute would incorporate all three characteristics.

12.5 Autologous Bone Grafts

The "golden standard" of bone grafts is the autologous bone, although it is an area of growing controversy [12]. It is mostly harvested from the iliac crest, depending upon positioning of the patient. This donor site has the advantage of having a supply of cancellous as well as cortical bone (tricortical graft) (Figs. 12.2 and 12.3).

12.6 Surgical Technique of Iliac Crest Graft Harvesting

The bone from the iliac crest can be easily harvested. When choosing the anterior crest, one must be aware of the lateral femoral cutaneous nerve. On the other hand, a safety margin of at least 3 cm should be left from the anterior superior crest, where the hip flexion muscles derive from. We recommend harvesting the graft using a double-blade oscillating saw. The desired depth can also be harvested using a "graft cutter". This way, a defined cortical graft is obtained, leaving room for additional harvesting of cancellous bone chips using a spoon. The defect is filled using a haemostyptic pad, the fascia is closed, and a drain should be placed to prevent a painful haematoma. Alternatively, according to the clinical application, "bone plugs" can also be harvested using special instruments (Fig. 12.5). This leaves less defect and can also be harvested in other locations.

12.7 Bone-Graft Substitutes

These materials should ideally have the osteogenetic, osteoconductive and osteoinductive characteristics of an autograft without the substantial side effects. Most of these materials only provide osteoconductivity. Their integration into the bone substance can take place in different ways [2]. One way is the direct integration or resorption followed by conversion into bone. The other way would be some kind of "graft versus

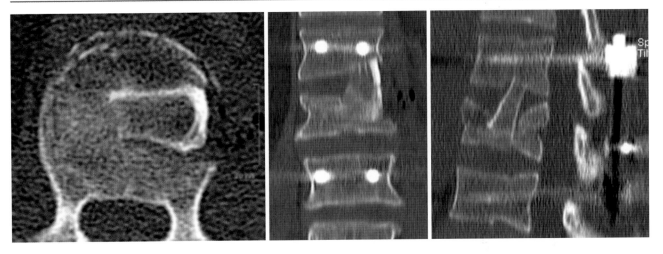

Fig. 12.2 CT scans in three planes documenting the correct size and positioning of a tricortical autograft

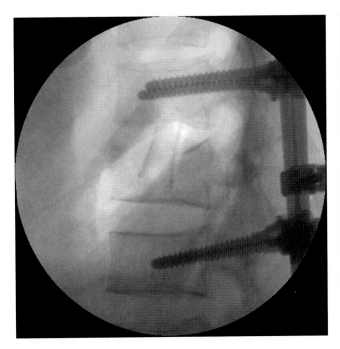

Fig. 12.3 Plain radiograph of a monosegmental, anterior spondylodesis with a tricortical iliac crest autograft following bisegmental, posterior stabilization

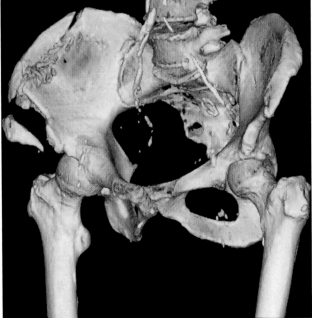

Fig. 12.4 Iliac crest fracture following bone harvest from the anterior iliac crest in the right side

host reaction", resulting in a self-contained graft or even a (partial) loss of graft substance without integration [11].

12.8 Allografts

This relates to tissue taken from one person for transplantation into another. This type of treatment has spread due to recent improvements in procurement, preparation and storage. Clinics with a high turnover of allografts have their own storage areas. This concept of bone banking is connected to a great deal of legal issues, showing great variations in different countries [3].

Advantages
- Osteoconductive
- Unlimited supply
- Multiple shapes and sizes
- No donor site morbidity

Disadvantages
- Not osteogenic (due to chemical processes in the making)
- Weak osteoinductive properties
- Possibility of infectious disease transmission

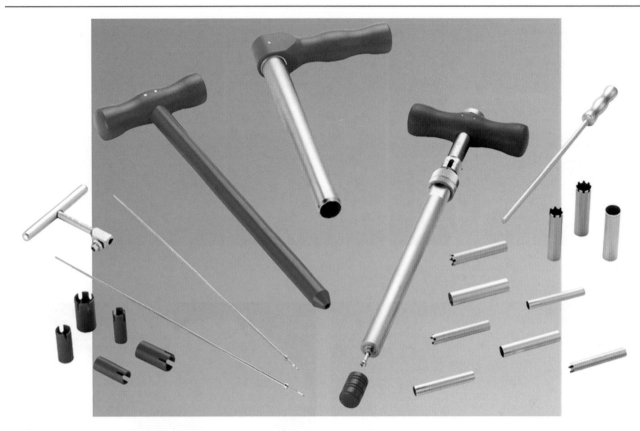

Fig. 12.5 Bone-graft harvesting set (Synthes) used for different sizes of "plugs" (© by Synthes)

12.9 Demineralized Bone Matrix (DBM) and Bone Morphogenetic Protein (BMP)

DBM is a demineralized allograft bone with osteoinductive activity [9]. Demineralized bone matrixes are prepared by acid extraction of allograft bone, resulting in loss of most of the mineralized components but retention of collagen and non-collagenous proteins, including growth factors. The efficacy of a demineralized bone matrix (DBM) as a bone-graft substitute or extender may be related to the total amount of bone morphogenetic protein (BMP) present and the ratios of the different BMPs present. The multitude of different BMPs are all capable of recruiting bone-forming cells and encouraging local cells to aid in the bone formation process. There are up to now over 20 different BMPs known, but the clinical research is currently limited to BMP 2 and BMP 7. The different types of BMPs seem to show substantial variations in their osteogenetic potency.

Advantages
- Osteoinductive with promoted bone formation [6].
- Osteoinductive potency is very variable in different products [8].
- Graft extender (in combination with autografts).

Disadvantages
- Poor structural integrity
- BMP alone not osteoconductive

12.10 Hydroxyapatite ($Ca_{10}(PO_4)_6(OH)_2$) and Tricalcium Phosphate ($Ca_3(PO_4)_2$)

These substitutes are mainly known as bone void fillers. Taking into account their specific strengths (e.g., fast curing, fluid injection) and their weaknesses (low shear stress, poor biodegradability), new applications have arisen. These materials come in a wide array of different application forms (Fig. 12.6, Table 12.1).

Advantages
- Osteoconductive (Fig. 12.7)
- Lasting stability
- Availability

Disadvantages
- Not osteoinductive
- Not osteogenic

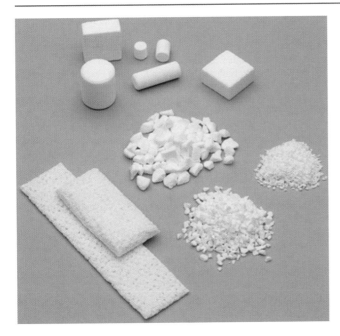

Fig. 12.6 An array of different forms and shapes used in calcium phosphate bone substitutes (© by Synthes)

Table 12.1 Exemplary list of calcium phosphate products on the market (among others)

Product	Company	Type
NanoStim	Medtronic	Synthetic tricalcium
BoneSource	Howmedica	CaP cement
Alpha-BSM	DePuy	CaP cement
Calcibon	Biomet/Merck	CaP putty
Mimix	Biomet	Synthetic tricalcium phosphate
Cerasorb	Curasan	Beta-tricalcium phosphate
ChronOS	Synthes	Beta-tricalcium phosphate
Vitoss	Orthovita	Beta-tricalcium phosphate
Pro Osteon	Interpore Cross	Coralline hydroxyapatite
Endobon	Biomet/Merck	Cancellous hydroxyapatite
BioFuse	Corin	Hydroxyapatite/CaP
Actifuse	Baxter	Silicated calcium phosphate

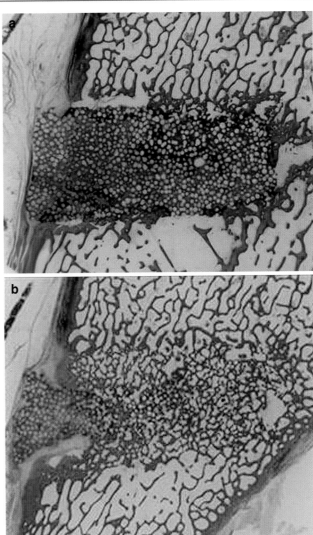

Fig. 12.7 (**a**, **b**) Histological findings using chronOS mixed with blood 6 weeks (**a**) and 12 weeks postoperatively (© by Synthes)

12.11 Clinical Application

Current evolutions within this field, such as biphasic, injectable CaP, calcium sulfate and silicated CaP, widen the array of applications, offering a good supplement in achieving spinal fusion [1] (filling cages, lining cages, extending grafts). These substances should be rehydrated using the patients' blood before applying (Fig. 12.8).

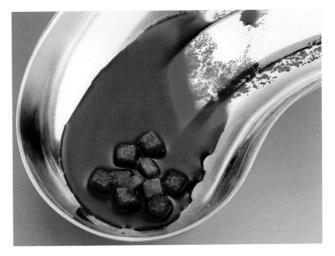

Fig. 12.8 ChronsOS blocs mixed with blood (© by Synthes)

12.12 Other Ceramics (Sea Corals, Calcium Sulphate)

These substances are currently researched to evaluate their usefulness to supplement or even replace the ceramics in use today.

12.13 Outlook

Tissue engineering and the further development of growth factors offer great potential for the future of fusion and bone substitutes. Materials will evolve and offer "ideal" and individual solutions for specific indications [4].

References

1. Becker S, Maissen O, Ponomarev I et al (2006) Osteopromotion by a beta-tricalcium phosphate/bone marrow hybrid implant for use in spine surgery. Spine 31(1):11–17
2. Berven S, Tay BK, Kleinstueck FS et al (2001) Clinical applications of bone graft substitutes in spine surgery: consideration of mineralized and demineralized preparations and growth factor supplementation. Eur Spine J 10(Suppl 2):S169–S177
3. Friedlaender GE (1982) Bone-banking. J Bone Joint Surg Am 64:307–311
4. Giannoudis PV, Tzioupis CC, Tsirids E (2006) Gene therapy in orthopaedics. Injury 37(Supp 1):S30–S40
5. Giannoudis PV, Einhorn TA, Marsh D (2007) Fracture healing: the diamond concept. Injury 38(Supp 4):S3–S6
6. Kwong FN, Harris MB (2008) Recent developments in the biology of fracture repair. J Am Acad Orthop Surg 16(11):619–625
7. Morrison RH, Thierolf A, Weckbach A (2007) Volumetric changes of iliac crest autografts used to reconstruct the anterior column in thoracolumbar fractures: a follow-up using CT scans. Spine 32(26):3030–3035
8. Papakostidis C, Kontakis D, Bhandari M et al (2008) Efficiency of autologous iliac crest bone graft and bone morphogenetic proteins for posterolateral fusion of lumbar spine – A meta-analysis of the results. Spine 33(19):E680–E692
9. Petersen B, Whang PG, Iglesias R et al (2004) Osteoinductivity of commercially available demineralized bone matrix. Preparations in a spine fusion model. J Bone Joint Surg Am 86-A(10):2243–2250
10. Phillips AM (2005) Overview of the fracture healing cascade. Injury 36(Supp 3):S5–S7
11. Schimandle JH, Boden SD (1997) Bone substitutes for lumbar fusion: present and future. Oper Tech Orthop 7:60–67
12. Sen MK, Miclau T (2007) Autologous iliac crest bone graft: should it still be the gold standard for treating nonunions? Injury 38(Supp 1):S75–S80
13. Bone Graft Alternatives (according to the North American Spine Society). http://www.spine.org/Documents/bone_grafts_2006.pdf

On- and Offline Documentation of Spine Procedures: Spine Tango

13

Christoph Röder and Thomas Zweig

13.1 Introduction and Core Messages

The mainstays of patient care throughout the ages used to be intuition, psychology and charisma. In this environment, which was characterized by trust on the part of the patients and society and self-confidence and dedication to the cause on the part of the clinician, considerable advances in medical therapy were made. Only a few players in the medical arena made initiatives for a systematic assessment of what was done and what the result of those treatments were. Among them was Florence Nightingale, a nurse, who applied statistical methods for analyzing preventable deaths in the British military during the Crimean War as early as 1854. Ernest Codman, a US physician and the father of what is today considered as outcomes management in patient care, became famous in the early 1900s for his "end results system" which stated that every patient needed to be followed up to assess the benefits and complications of the received treatment. Finally, Maurice E. Müller, cofounder of AO/ASIF (Arbeitsgemeinschaft Osteosynthese/Association for the Study of Internal Fixation), published his concept of a multisite trauma registry with centralized database for assessment of surgeon performance, efficacy of surgical techniques, and postmarket surveillance of implants in 1963 [11]. Even today, quality assurance and systematic data collections are mostly still isolated and independent undertakings of surgeons or hospitals. Using different terminologies, content, and separate databases makes data pooling and harmonization difficult and impedes benchmarking. EuroSpine, the Spine Society of Europe, developed Spine Tango, an on- and offline registry of spinal interventions for assuring outcome quality and enabling benchmarking. Spine Tango can also be used for outcome research and implant postmarket surveillance. Information and the battery of recommended physician and patient-based instruments can be found under www.eurospine.org – Spine Tango.

13.2 Definition of Quality in Health Care

To those not involved in quality improvement in a professional capacity, it might appear relatively simple to define quality; however, more than 2,000 years after Plato invented this term, there is still great debate regarding the meaning of the word [14]. The American Society for Quality (ASQ) defines quality as "a subjective term for which each person has his or her own definition" [1]. According to a user-based approach, quality can be defined as "meeting or exceeding customer satisfaction" [6]. Quality is a multidimensional construct, and the dimensions are specific for each category. The US Agency for Healthcare Research and Quality defines quality in health care as "doing the right thing, at the right time, in the right way, for the right person, and having the best possible results" [15].

The quality measures in health care assess three components:
- Structure (resources such as staff, equipment)
- Process (therapeutic interventions, prescribing, interactions with patients)
- Outcomes (end results of health care such as mortality and patient satisfaction) [3, 15]

The measures used to obtain the patients' view can be classified into three categories:
- Preferences
- Evaluations
- Reports

Wensing and Elwyn defined preferences as patient ideas about what should occur in health-care systems. Evaluations are patient "reactions" to their experience of health care, and reports are objective observations (e.g., how long the patients had to

C. Röder, M.D., Ph.D., M.P.H. (✉) • T. Zweig, M.D.
Institute for Evaluative Research in Orthopaedic Surgery, University of Bern, Stauffacherstrasse 78, 3014 Bern, Switzerland
e-mail: christoph.roeder@memcenter.unibe.ch

U. Vieweg, F. Grochulla (eds.), *Manual of Spine Surgery*,
DOI 10.1007/978-3-642-22682-3_13, © Springer-Verlag Berlin Heidelberg 2012

spend in the waiting room). The choice of the type of measure depends on the aspect being assessed and the purpose of the evaluation (educational, certification, accreditation, quality control, or quality improvement) [16]. One of the most widespread means of measuring processes and outcomes is the assessment of patient satisfaction (evaluation category). Outcome satisfaction is also one of the criteria for assessing the validity of process measures. Indeed, according to Chassin [4], a measure of process is valid when it is related to health outcomes (mortality, patient satisfaction, etc.). Hence, the responses to questions concerning satisfaction with treatment, typically used in treatment outcome studies, can also be seen as outcome measures in the quality control and improvement context.

13.2.1 Overlap of Outcome Research and Quality Control

Quality control in a more formal sense is meanwhile of much higher topicality in all medical disciplines, but a factual implementation and application in a stringent and meaningful way is still lacking in many cases. The growing emphasis on an evidence-based approach in the medical setting has led to a corresponding increase in the number and quality of studies in the twenty-first century, examining the efficacy of surgical and nonsurgical treatments. These studies are usually conducted in university hospitals and clinics that have an in-house research staff or that cooperate with academic research institutions. The studies are not commonly perceived by the care provider (hospitals and clinics) as being something from which they can benefit from an economical point of view; in contrast, carrying out such research can sometimes be seen as a drain on resources. The research activities on treatment outcomes are merely seen as something that may indirectly benefit the institution in terms of prestige and corporate social responsibility. However, the possibility of economic benefit from corporate social responsibility activities is not a sufficiently persuasive argument for increasing investment in research – otherwise, all the public and private hospital and clinics would likely have their own research departments or research staff. Significantly, in all of this, one important factor is typically overlooked: research projects in the field of treatment outcomes and their predictors can be useful to the provider in a much more direct way in terms of quality improvement and the control of service performance [7].

13.3 Eurospine "Spine Tango": An International Spine Registry for Quality Assurance, Outcome Research, and Postmarket Surveillance of Implants

13.3.1 History and Objectives

All over the world, efforts are being made to set up orthopedic registries on regional, state, or even national levels. Spine surgery represents a challenge for all registry endeavors. The variety of levels, pathologies, accesses, and surgical techniques confounds all attempts to invent a short yet comprehensive questionnaire. Under the auspices of EuroSpine, the Spine Society of Europe, a project was launched for the design and implementation of a documentation system for spinal surgery in 2000. This effort was introduced as "Spine Tango" and was conducted in collaboration with the Institute for Evaluative Research in Orthopaedic Surgery at the University of Bern, Switzerland.

Goals of the spine tango are:

- Presentation of the *state-of-the-art* European spine surgery, including all pathologies, levels, accesses, and single, as well as two-staged surgeries
- *Outcome research* and *prospective observational evaluation* of different surgical techniques as an alternative to randomized controlled trials
- *Benchmarking* on national and international levels
- *Quality assurance and quality improvement*

Spine Tango is probably the first spine registry initiative to face the challenge of developing a comprehensive questionnaire covering all major spine pathologies and interventions, as well as spanning all anatomical levels. To accomplish this task, a technically demanding computer application was a prerequisite. The consensus and piloting process for the Spine Tango surgical questionnaires "surgery," "staged surgery," and "follow-up" took about 5 years and needed around 4,000 completed forms. The result are two double-sided A4 questionnaires (surgery, staged surgery) and one single-sided questionnaire for follow-up that can all be completed online or using scannable paper questionnaires. At the same time that the physician-based content was finalized, a working group at the Schulthess Hospital in Zurich, Switzerland, had developed and validated the COMI (Core Outcome Measures Index) instruments for neck and low back pain (two instruments) which became the officially recommended patient-based documentation instruments in the framework of the Spine Tango registry [9]. Until today, the Spine Tango database has grown to over 30,000 nearly cases, and currently, about 40 hospitals participate worldwide [12].

13.3.2 Content: Physician Based

The refined set of questions still allows documentation of the broad spectrum of pathologies and treatments in spine surgery. This is made possible by means of a list of main pathologies and their specifications and the so-called surgical matrix, a terminology system reducing the interventions to their basic principles – decompression, fusion, stabilization rigid, stabilization motion preserving, percutaneous procedures, and others. The duplication and, hence, separation of these principles into anterior and posterior ones complete the matrix.

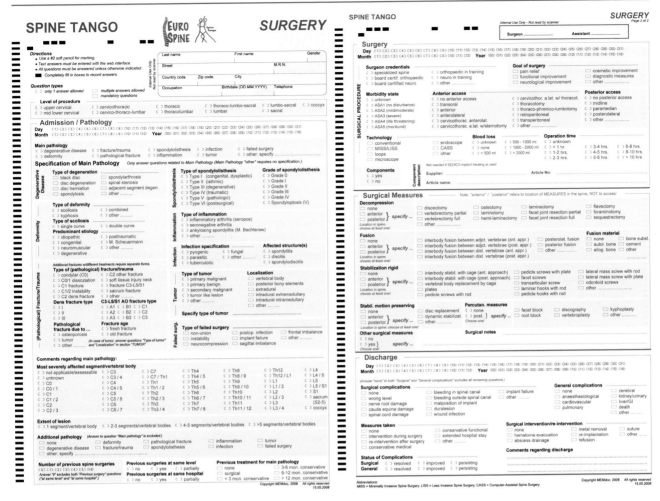

Fig. 13.1 SSE Spine Tango surgery form (front and back side). All questions with *blue* background are mandatory

13.3.3 Surgery Form

The first half of the front page of the "surgery" form serves to specify the level of the procedure, admission date, case history (previous conservative and surgical treatments), main and additional pathology, most severely affected segment, and extent of lesion. This information is grouped into the "admission" subform. The "specification of main pathology" subform makes up the second part of page one and comprises 1–3 questions per "main pathology" category. These serve to provide more information about the main pathology. On the reverse side of the sheet are the "surgery," "surgical measures," and "discharge" subforms. The "surgery" subform is the largest (12 questions) and inquires about surgery date, implants used, goals of surgery, the surgical matrix, surgeon credentials, access and technology, operation time, morbidity state, and blood loss. The "surgical measures" subform applies the same principle as the "specification of main pathology" subform – only the items relevant to the information given for the matrix questions need to be completed. Typically, this can be done with two

to four questions. Finally, the "discharge" subform inquires about the discharge date, surgical and general complications, measures taken, and the status of complications upon discharge. It makes up between 3 and 7 questions (Fig. 13.1).

13.3.4 Staged Surgery Form

In addition to the surgery form, there is also a so-called staged form and a follow-up form. The staged form serves to document the second part of planned two-stage procedures, i.e., procedures where the patient remains in the hospital between the first and the second intervention. If the patient is discharged, a new surgery form must be completed. Also, if an early revision is carried out, the correct way to document this is with a new surgery form with the diagnosis "failed surgery." The staged form is identical to the surgery form but without the anamnestic questions about previous surgeries and the discharge date.

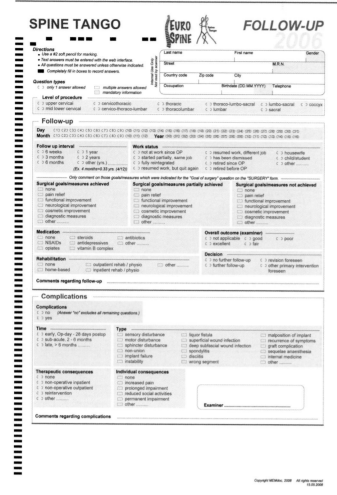

Fig. 13.2 SSE Spine Tango follow-up form (one page only)

13.3.5 Follow-up Form

The follow-up form is just one side of the A4 sheet and consists of a "follow-up" subform and a "complications" subform. In its paper format, it can be completed in less than a minute. After the date of follow-up and the follow-up interval have been completed, the patient's work status is documented, and the surgical goals that were achieved, partially achieved, or not achieved at all are indicated. Only the surgical goals that are indicated on the surgery form are to be considered. Current medication, rehabilitation, and the surgeon's rating of the outcome are then recorded. The last question in the "follow-up" subform inquires about the need (or not) for further follow-up, revision surgery, or another primary intervention.

In the absence of complications, the "complications" subform can be completed with just one answer "no" to the "complications" question. Where complications have arisen, the point of time at which they occurred, the type of complications, and therapeutic and individual consequences are inquired about (Fig. 13.2). All forms can be found as PDF files under www.eurospine.org – Spine Tango – forms.

13.3.6 Content: Patient Based

The proportion of positive outcomes after spinal surgery depends to a large extent on the manner in which outcome is assessed [8], and there is no single, universally accepted method. In the past, clinicians typically judged the outcome from their own perspective, using simple rating schemes such as "excellent, good, moderate, and poor." The technical success of the operation also lent itself to evaluation by means of sophisticated imaging at follow-up. However, most of the time, these measures proved to be only weakly associated with outcomes of relevance to the patient and to society [5]. It is now accepted that the focus should be placed on patient-orientated measures and that the patient should be the main judge of outcome, with the result that clinician-based methods have been superseded by a diverse range of patient self-assessment questionnaires. A standardized set of outcome measures for use with back patients were proposed in 1998 by a multinational group of experts [5]. There was general consensus that the most appropriate core outcome measures should include the domains pain, back specific function, generic health status (well-being), work disability, social disability, and patient satisfaction [2, 5]. Accordingly, the group proposed a parsimonious set of seven preoperative questions that would cover each of these domains, yet be brief enough to alleviate respondent burden, and hence be practical for routine clinical use and quality management. At the time of follow-up, information about occurrence of complications and their bothersomeness from the patient's perspective, reoperations, satisfaction with overall medical care in the hospital, and extent to which the surgery helped are inquired with four additional questions. The satisfaction question can, for example, be used to evaluate the patient perception of the "process performance" in a six-sigma quality improvement initiative [4, 7]. Sufficient clinical research has meanwhile been conducted with the COMIs for providing details about its application and administration and about clinically and statistically important facts like the minimum clinically relevant score improvement, standardized response mean values (effect sizes), and dichotomization of outcomes into "good" and "poor" results [10] (Fig. 13.3). All COMI forms can be found as PDF files under www.eurospine. org – Spine Tango – forms.

13.3.7 Technology

Spine Tango has long left the early stage of a simple web page for data entry and has grown into an international project with a sophisticated IT (information technology) structure and a multitude of clinical and scientific experts serving the user community and developing the registry further. The central database is part of a powerful scientific documentation portal hosted by the University of Bern; it offers various methods

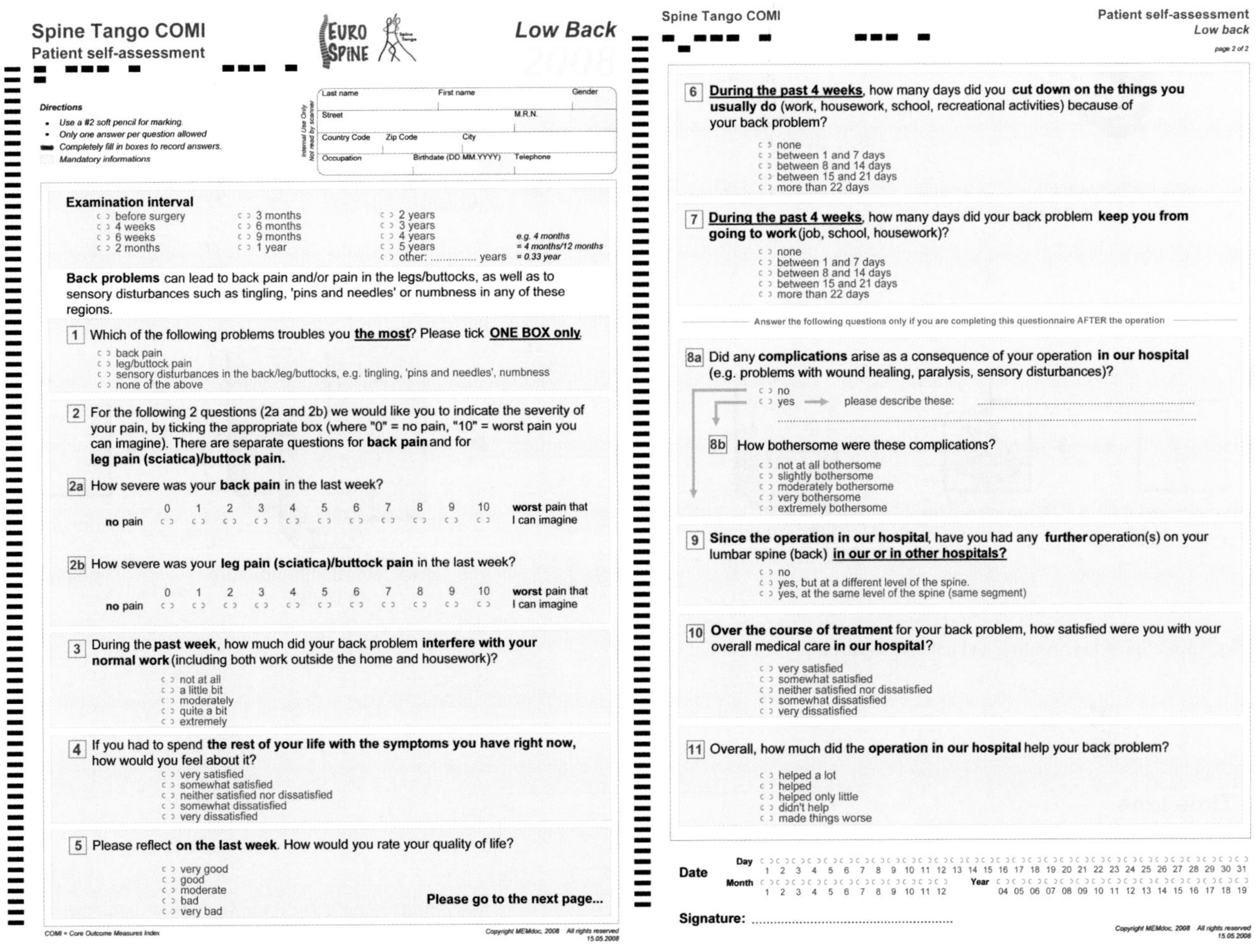
Spine Tango COMI
Patient self-assessment
Low Back

Directions
- Use a #2 soft pencil for marking.
- Only one answer per question allowed
- Completely fill in boxes to record answers.
- Mandatory informations

Last name | First name | Gender
Street | M.R.N.
Country Code | Zip Code | City
Occupation | Birthdate (DD.MM.YYYY) | Telephone

Internal Use Only
Not read by scanner

Examination interval
- before surgery
- 4 weeks
- 6 weeks
- 2 months
- 3 months
- 6 months
- 9 months
- 1 year
- 2 years
- 3 years
- 4 years
- 5 years
- other: .... years

e.g. 4 months = 4 months/12 months = 0.33 year

Back problems can lead to back pain and/or pain in the legs/buttocks, as well as to sensory disturbances such as tingling, 'pins and needles' or numbness in any of these regions.

1 Which of the following problems troubles you **the most**? Please tick **ONE BOX only**.
- back pain
- leg/buttock pain
- sensory disturbances in the back/leg/buttocks, e.g. tingling, 'pins and needles', numbness
- none of the above

2 For the following 2 questions (2a and 2b) we would like you to indicate the severity of your pain, by ticking the appropriate box (where "0" = no pain, "10" = worst pain you can imagine). There are separate questions for **back pain** and for **leg pain (sciatica)/buttock pain.**

2a How severe was your **back pain** in the last week?
no pain 0 1 2 3 4 5 6 7 8 9 10 worst pain that I can imagine

2b How severe was your **leg pain (sciatica)/buttock pain** in the last week?
no pain 0 1 2 3 4 5 6 7 8 9 10 worst pain that I can imagine

3 During the **past week**, how much did your back problem **interfere with your normal work** (including both work outside the home and housework)?
- not at all
- a little bit
- moderately
- quite a bit
- extremely

4 If you had to spend **the rest of your life with the symptoms you have right now**, how would you feel about it?
- very satisfied
- somewhat satisfied
- neither satisfied nor dissatisfied
- somewhat dissatisfied
- very dissatisfied

5 Please reflect **on the last week**. How would you rate your quality of life?
- very good
- good
- moderate
- bad
- very bad

Please go to the next page...

COMI = Core Outcome Measures Index
Copyright MEMdoc, 2008 All rights reserved 15.05.2008

Spine Tango COMI
Patient self-assessment
Low back
page 2 of 2

6 **During the past 4 weeks**, how many days did you **cut down on the things you usually do** (work, housework, school, recreational activities) because of your back problem?
- none
- between 1 and 7 days
- between 8 and 14 days
- between 15 and 21 days
- more than 22 days

7 **During the past 4 weeks**, how many days did your back problem **keep you from going to work** (job, school, housework)?
- none
- between 1 and 7 days
- between 8 and 14 days
- between 15 and 21 days
- more than 22 days

Answer the following questions only if you are completing this questionnaire AFTER the operation

8a Did any **complications** arise as a consequence of your operation **in our hospital** (e.g. problems with wound healing, paralysis, sensory disturbances)?
- no
- yes → please describe these: ....

8b How bothersome were these complications?
- not at all bothersome
- slightly bothersome
- moderately bothersome
- very bothersome
- extremely bothersome

9 **Since the operation in our hospital**, have you had any **further** operation(s) on your lumbar spine (back) **in our or in other hospitals?**
- no
- yes, but at a different level of the spine.
- yes, at the same level of the spine (same segment)

10 **Over the course of treatment** for your back problem, how satisfied were you with your overall medical care **in our hospital**?
- very satisfied
- somewhat satisfied
- neither satisfied nor dissatisfied
- somewhat dissatisfied
- very dissatisfied

11 Overall, how much did the **operation in our hospital** help your back problem?
- helped a lot
- helped
- helped only little
- didn't help
- made things worse

Date Day 1 2 3 4 5 6 7 8 9 10 11 12 13 14 15 16 17 18 19 20 21 22 23 24 25 26 27 28 29 30 31
Month 1 2 3 4 5 6 7 8 9 10 11 12
Year 04 05 06 07 08 09 10 11 12 13 14 15 16 17 18 19

Signature: ....

Copyright MEMdoc, 2008 All rights reserved 15.05.2008

Fig. 13.3 COMI patient assessment form for low back pain

for clinical, implant and radiographic data collection, and a multitude of possibilities for data downloads and online statistical queries. An important step was the implementation of so-called modules, national satellite servers that anonymize data for protecting user and patient privacy in the respective country before sending the clinical data set to the central server in Switzerland (Fig. 13.4). Such modules are meanwhile installed in Germany, Austria, Italy, Great Britain, Australia, USA, Mexico, and Brazil. Users whose country does not yet have such a national filter server may use the Swiss/International module under www.spinetango.org. Access to the servers is centrally routed via the EuroSpine home page under www.eurospine.org – Spine Tango – modules. The Spine Tango Pathways user manual is available for download in English on all module front pages [13].

13.3.8 Workflow

A generic application which serves a multitude of hospitals with different sizes, structures, and staff coverage can only be customized to a certain extent to the individual expectations and needs of a user, i.e., a single surgeon or a department. Therefore, an intelligent and creative integration of the Tango project and its processes into the day-to-day workflows is key for success and a sustainable future of the data collection efforts. Direct online data entry, paper-based data collection with OMR (optical mark reader) compatible paper forms, or simple PDFs for later data punching are options which mainly depend on factors like web access and number of web terminals in the OR, wards, and outpatient clinic; pre- and postoperative administration of patient questionnaires by face-to-face interview, mail, or telephone interview in addition to the surgeon-based data collection represent additional efforts that need the respective financial and human resources (Fig. 13.5). There are currently five possible ways that forms and questionnaires can be transferred to the database (Fig. 13.6). Online data entry (a), paper-based data capture with OMR scanner-assisted entry of data (b), paper-based data capture with data punching using the online interface (c), paper-based data capture with mailing of the forms to the IEFO or other partner institutions for OMR scanner-assisted

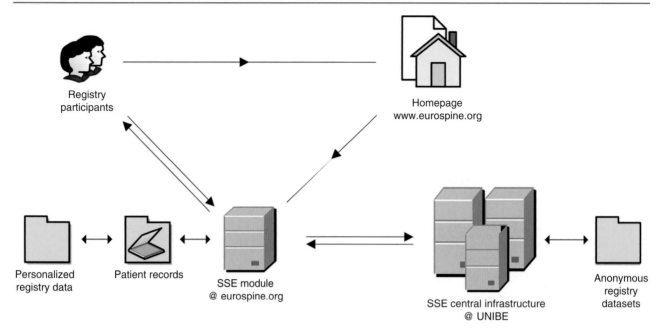

Fig. 13.4 Spine user routing and data segregation in the national modules

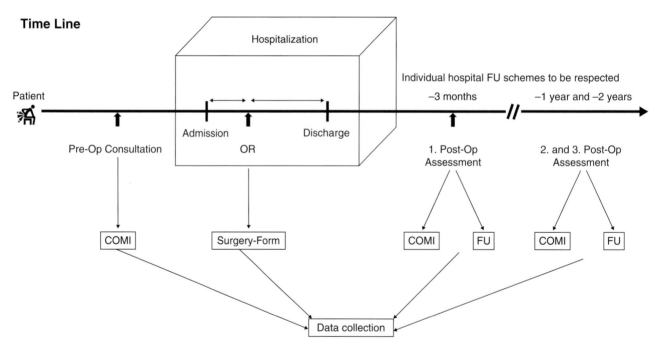

Fig. 13.5 Spine Tango pre- and postoperative physician- and patient-based data collection

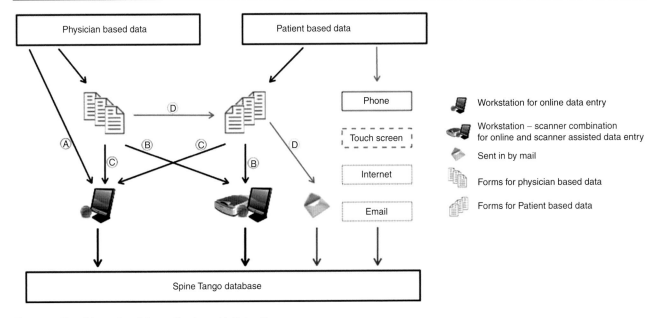

Fig. 13.6 Possible modes of data collection with Spine Tango

entry of data (d), and finally, a hybrid method of direct online entry of surgical data (a) and OMR scanner-assisted entry of patient questionnaires (b) or direct online entry of surgical data (a) and delayed online entry of questionnaires that were completed on paper by the patients (c). Some solutions seem to work better than others. They were summarized in a review article, and it is highly recommended to study the various suggestions for Spine Tango workflow integration for planning its implementation in the own institution [17].

References

1. American Society for Quality (2002) Quality glossary. Qual Prog 35:43–61. http://www.ncbi.nlm.nih.gov/pmc/articles/PMC2899321/, Ref 17
2. Bombardier C (2000) Outcome assessments in the evaluation of treatment of spinal disorders: summary and general recommendations. Spine 25:3100–3103
3. Campbell SM, Braspenning J, Hutchinson A et al (2003) Research methods used in developing and applying quality indicators in primary care. BMJ 326:816–819
4. Chassin MR (1998) Is health care ready for Six Sigma quality? Milbank Q 76:565–591
5. Deyo RA, Battie M, Boerskens AJ et al (1998) Outcome measures for low back pain research. A proposal for standardized use. Spine 23(2):003–013
6. Garvin D (1984) What does product quality really mean? Sloan Manage Rev 26:25–43
7. Impellizzeri FM, Bizini M, Leunig M et al (2009) Money matters: exploiting the data from outcomes research for quality improvement initiatives. Eur Spine J 3:348–359
8. Mannion AF, Elfering A (2006) Predictors of surgical outcome and their assessment. Eur Spine J 1:93–108
9. Mannion AF, Elfering A, Staerkle AR et al (2005) Outcome assessment in low back pain: how low can you go? Eur Spine J 14: 1014–1026
10. Mannion AF, Porchet F, Kleinstück FS et al (2009) The quality of spine surgery from the patient's perspective. Part 1: the core outcome measures index in clinical practice. Eur Spine J 3: 367–373
11. Müller ME, Allgöwer M, Willenegger H (1963) Die Gemeinschaftserhebung der Arbeitsgemeinschaft für Osteosynthesefragen. Arch klin Chir 304:808–817
12. Röder C, El-Kerdi A, Grob D et al (2002) A European spine registry. Eur Spine J 11:303–307
13. Röder C, Chavanne A, Mannion AF et al (2005) SSE Spine Tango–content, workflow, set-up. www.eurospine.org-Spine Tango. Eur Spine J 14:920–924
14. Sower S, Fair F (2005) There is more to quality than continuous improvement: listening to Plato. Qual Manag J 12:8–20
15. Varkey P, Reller MK, Resar RK (2007) Basics of quality improvement in health care. Mayo Clin Proc 82:735–739
16. Wensing M, Elwyn G (2003) Methods for incorporating patients' views in health care. BMJ 326:877–879
17. Zweig T, Mannion AF, Grob D et al (2009) How to Tango: a manual for implementing Spine Tango. Eur Spine J 3:312–320

Part II

Anterior Upper Cervical Spine

Overview of Surgical Techniques and Implants for the Anterior Upper Cervical Spine

14

Meic H. Schmidt

14.1 Introduction and Core Messages

The upper cervical spine represents a unique biomechanical and anatomic region that requires specialized surgical techniques and implants. Most commonly, the upper cervical spine is affected by trauma (odontoid fractures and nonunions), occipital-cervical dislocations, or degenerative processes, particularly rheumatoid arthritis, which result in atlantoaxial instability. Trauma indications include Jefferson fractures with instability and disruption of the transverse ligament, odontoid fractures that are mobile in flexion and extension, and C1–2 dislocations. In rheumatoid degenerative instability of the C1–2 joints, the indications are also decompression of the spinal cord and then subsequent stabilization. The four most common surgical techniques for the region are anterior odontoid screw fixation, transoral resection of the odontoid process, posterior C1–2 fixation, and anterior transarticular screw fixation [1–4].

14.2 Approaches

Approaches and implants for the anterior upper cervical spine are complex, corresponding to the unusual biomechanical and anatomic arrangement of that part of the spine. Some of them are not recommended as a stand-alone technique. Frequently, for example, a transoral resection of the odontoid is performed in conjunction with a posterior cervical fusion. Anterior approaches to the upper cervical spine are frequently based on modifications of the standard approach for anterior cervical discectomy and fusion, which is extended toward the head (cephalad).

14.2.1 Transoral Approach

There are two common transoral approaches for the treatment of rheumatoid arthritis or fracture/instability. The transoral resection is more commonly performed in rheumatoid disease for decompression of the spinal cord. This is frequently done through the mouth if the patient is able to open the mouth widely enough (Fig. 14.1). It requires a specialized retractor system, as described in Chap. 17. We do not usually place instrumentation using this approach.

14.2.2 Extraoral Ventral Retropharyngeal Approach

On rare occasions, a similar approach can be used for the placement of anterior transarticular screws (see Chap. 16). This can be done when there is C1–2 instability or an odontoid fracture (Fig. 14.2). The retropharyngeal approach is used, and then bilateral transarticular screws are passed from an anterior approach using a K-wire system. This can be done in combination with an odontoid screw. Typically, this procedure can also be done with K-wires and cannulated screws, but the K-wires must be carefully monitored so they do not migrate after insertion of the screws.

M.H. Schmidt, M.D., FACS
Division of Spine Surgery, Department of Neurosurgery,
Clinical Neurosciences Center, University of Utah,
175 N. Medical Drive East, Bldg 550, Salt Lake City,
UT 84132-2303, USA
e-mail: meic.schmidt@hsc.utah.edu

U. Vieweg, F. Grochulla (eds.), *Manual of Spine Surgery*,
DOI 10.1007/978-3-642-22682-3_14, © Springer-Verlag Berlin Heidelberg 2012

Fig. 14.1 Photograph
showing transoral exposure
using the Spetzler-Sonntag
retractor

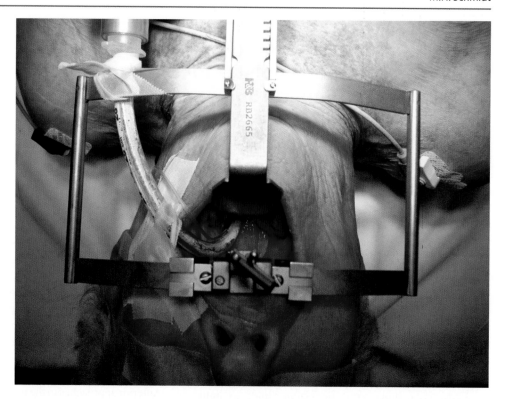

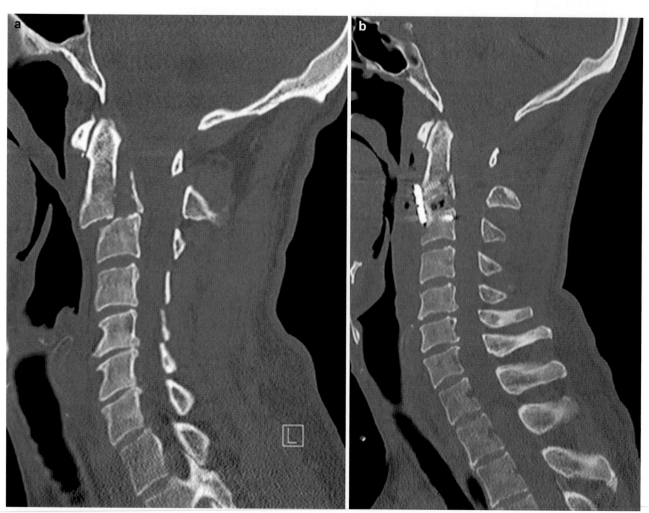

Fig. 14.2 Computed tomography scans showing C2/3 fracture dislocation (**a**) and C2/3 anterior cervical discectomy and fusion (**b**) using a retropharyngeal submandibular approach

14.3 Implants

14.3.1 Screws

The screws used for fixation in anterior approaches to the upper cervical spine are varied and depend on the approach used. With odontoid screw fixation, we use noncannulated screws, although others advise against their use. For the retropharyngeal approach, bilateral transarticular screws are typically used, sometimes in combination with an odontoid screw. Cannulated screws can be used. Anterior transarticular screws should be lag screws since this will "lag" together the C1/2 joint for fusion.

14.3.2 Plating

Anterior plating has been described but is rarely used. The predominant indication is traumatic instability after C1 fracture or resection of the odontoid. The Harms plating system has been described by Ruf et al. [1].

References

1. Ruf M, Melcher R, Harms J (2004) Transoral reduction and osteosynthesis C1 as a function-preserving option in the treatment of unstable Jefferson fractures. Spine 29:823–827
2. Russo A, Albanese E, Quiroga M, Ulm AJ (2009) Submandibular approach to the C2–3 disc level: microsurgical anatomy with clinical application. J Neurosurg Spine 10:380–389
3. Schmelzle R, Harms J (1987) Craniocervical junction–diseases, diagnostic application of imaging procedures, surgical techniques. Fortschr Kiefer Gesichtschir 32:206–208
4. Vender JR, Harrison SJ, McDonnell DE (2000) Fusion and instrumentation at C1–3 via the high anterior cervical approach. J Neurosurg 92:24–29

Odontoid Screw Fixation

15

Meic H. Schmidt

15.1 Introduction and Core Messages

Anterior odontoid screw fixation is ideal for fixation of unstable odontoid fractures and is superior to posterior C1–2 arthrodesis as it preserves C1–2 rotational movement and obviates the need for autograft bone harvest. This method has become increasingly popular since the time it was introduced by Bohler [4], and it is now widely used to treat unstable type II and shallow type III odontoid fractures [1–3, 5–9]. The goals of odontoid screw fixation are immediate stabilization of type II odontoid fractures or shallow type III odontoid fractures with no need for external orthosis.

15.2 Indications

- Type II odontoid fractures
- Shallow type III odontoid fractures that have failed non-operative treatment
- Elderly patients who have failed halo fixation and external orthosis
- Patients that do not want to use halo fixation or external orthosis

M.H. Schmidt, M.D., FACS
Department of Neurosurgery, Division of Spine Surgery,
Clinical Neurosciences Center, University of Utah,
175 N. Medical Drive East, Bldg 550, Salt Lake City,
UT 84132-2303, USA
e-mail: meic.schmidt@hsc.utah.edu

15.3 Contraindications

- Severe associated C1 and C2 fractures
- Occipital cervical instability associated with type II odontoid fractures
- Fractures that are older than 18 months
- Patients that have excessive cervical kyphosis
- Patients with a large chest (barrel chest)
- Anterior oblique fracture (see Fig. 15.1a)

15.4 Technical Prerequisites

It is essential that the patient can be intubated fiberoptically by an experienced anesthesiologist. Neuromonitoring, including somatosensory evoked potentials (SSEPs) and motor evoked potentials (MEPs), can be performed.

Awake nasotracheal or fiberoptic intubation is used if there is instability in extension. Traditional laryngoscopic intubation is safe if the fracture reduces in extension. We highly recommend using two fluoroscopy machines for bilateral views simultaneously of the anterior-posterior (AP) upper cervical spine and the lateral upper cervical spine. Because we use the Aesculap anterior odontoid screw fixation system, which allows for intraoperative reduction of the odontoid fracture, we do not require complete preoperative reduction of the fracture.

15.5 Planning, Preparation, and Positioning

We routinely include the upper sternum and the neck in the sterile preparation. The patient is placed in the supine position with head immobilized with 10 lb of traction via a halter device. Alternatively, Gardner-Wells tongs can be used or halo traction can be used if the patient has already been in the

U. Vieweg, F. Grochulla (eds.), *Manual of Spine Surgery*,
DOI 10.1007/978-3-642-22682-3_15, © Springer-Verlag Berlin Heidelberg 2012

a

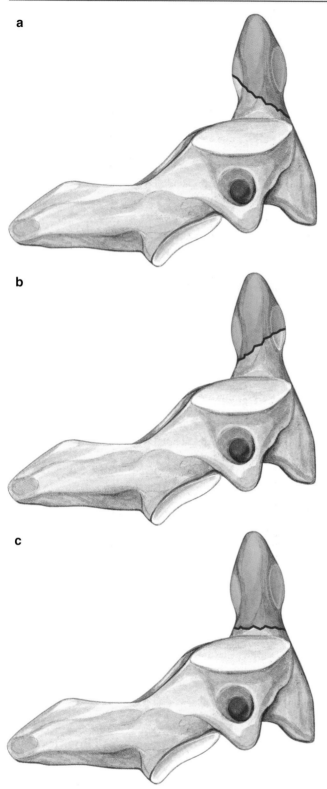

b

c

Fig. 15.1 Classification based on the direction of the slope of the fracture: anterior oblique (**a**), posterior oblique (**b**), and horizontal (**c**)

halo. We always place a shoulder roll between the shoulder blades to maximally extend the neck. To get a good AP view of the odontoid process, a radiolucent mouth gag is frequently used (a wine bottle cork can be notched into the teeth).

15.6 Operating Technique

15.6.1 Approach

- Lateral fluoroscopy is used to ensure the proper trajectory; we place a K-wire along the neck of the patient to ensure that the sternum does not interfere with the screw placement.
- Once this is done, we infiltrate the skin with epinephrine and perform a standard Cloward approach to the anterior spine (see Fig. 15.2).
- At the C5 level, we place a small unilateral midcervical incision in the skin crease. Then the platysma muscle is divided horizontally, and the plane between the pharynx and esophagus medially and the carotid sheath laterally is developed.
- We use blunt finger dissection to expose the cervical spine.
- The longus colli muscle is then incised and bilaterally elevated, and sharp-tooth cervical retractor blades are inserted firmly under these muscles and attached to a special retractor blade.
- Firm fixation is important because a fair amount of tension is placed on the retractor during the drilling and screw placement. After this retractor is placed, we use a Kittner dissector to sweep up the anterior cervical spine to approximately the level of C1.
- Once this dissection is completed, we place a superior angled retractor blade (see Fig. 15.2). This blade should reach up approximately to C1. A choice of six different blades is available.
- This retractor blade is then connected via a special retractor system to the lateral retractor blades. Once the retractor is in place, a working tunnel is created for the drilling and placement of the odontoid screws.

15.6.2 Instrumentation

- Using a sharp K-wire, we find the entry site at the inferior anterior edge of C2 on the lateral and AP fluoroscopy (see Fig. 15.3a). The entry point location is chosen based on whether one or two screws will be placed: If only one

Fig. 15.2 The C5 skin incision and the position of the soft tissue retractors (With permission of Aesculap AG, Tuttlingen, Germany)

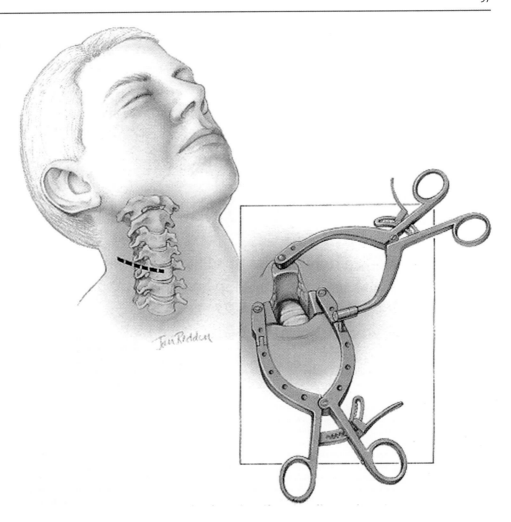

screw is placed, the entry point should be at the anterior inferior edge of C2 at the midline. We place the entry point slightly laterally about 2–3 mm off the midline if two screws are to be placed.

- The K-wire is then manipulated under biplanar fluoroscopy and impacted approximately 5 mm into the C2 vertebral body (see Fig. 15.3a).
- Once the K-wire is impacted, we use a hollow cord drill that is passed over the K-wire, and a shallow groove is cut into the anterior face of C3 and the C2–3 annulus (Fig. 15.3).
- We then put together the inner and outer drill guides and pass them over the K-wire. The outer drill guide has spikes (see Fig. 15.4), which are carefully maneuvered over the C3 vertebral body under fluoroscopy.
- At this point, the K-wire frequently needs to be shortened with a wire cutter since it protrudes over the inner tube guide. It is important to leave at least 1 cm of the K-wire protruding beyond the inner tube guide in order to be able to remove it.

- The plastic impact sleeve is then fitted over the guide wire assembly, and a mallet is used to impact the spikes into the C3 vertebral body (see Fig. 15.5).
- The inner tube guide is then advanced until it contacts the inferior edge of C2. The surgeon at this point can manipulate the handle and adjust the cervical spine to the appropriate trajectory (see Fig. 15.6).
- The K-wire then can be removed without loss of alignment and positional stability. By lifting and depressing the guide tube assembly that is impacted into C3, the alignment between C1 and C2 can be carefully manipulated. If the odontoid process is retrolisthesed, the guide tube assembly can be depressed to get the optimal angle for drilling. This is monitored under fluoroscopy.
- Next, the drill is inserted through the drill guide and through the C2 odontoid process under AP and lateral fluoroscopy. The drill guide can be adjusted before the fracture site is crossed by depressing or elevating the C2–3 complex (see Fig. 15.7).

Fig. 15.3 After dissection of the retropharyngeal space, the K-wire is placed (**a**) and the entry site at C2/3 is drilled (**b**, **c**, **d**) (With permission of Aesculap AG, Tuttlingen, Germany)

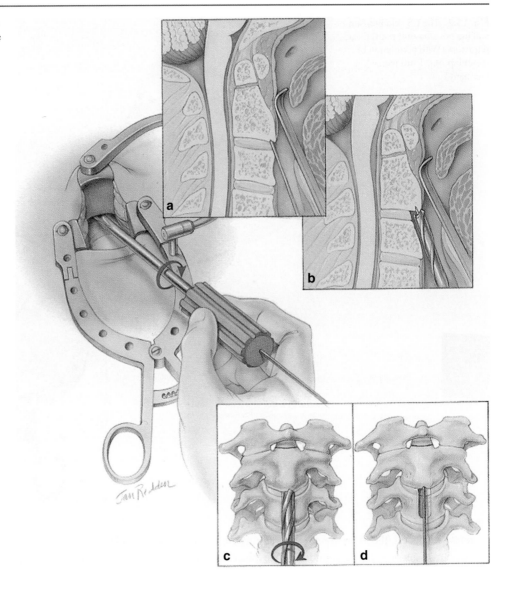

Fig. 15.4 Inner and outer drill guide assembly (With permission of Aesculap AG, Tuttlingen, Germany)

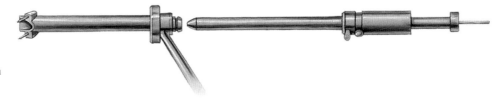

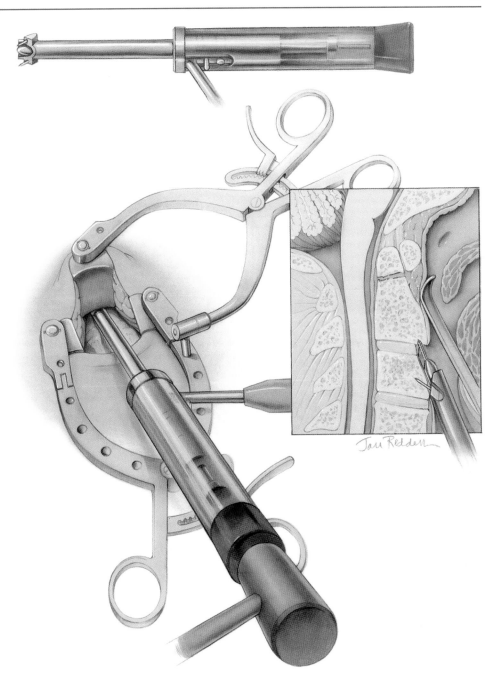

Fig. 15.5 Advancing the inner drill guide in the previously created C2/3 groove (With permission of Aesculap AG, Tuttlingen, Germany)

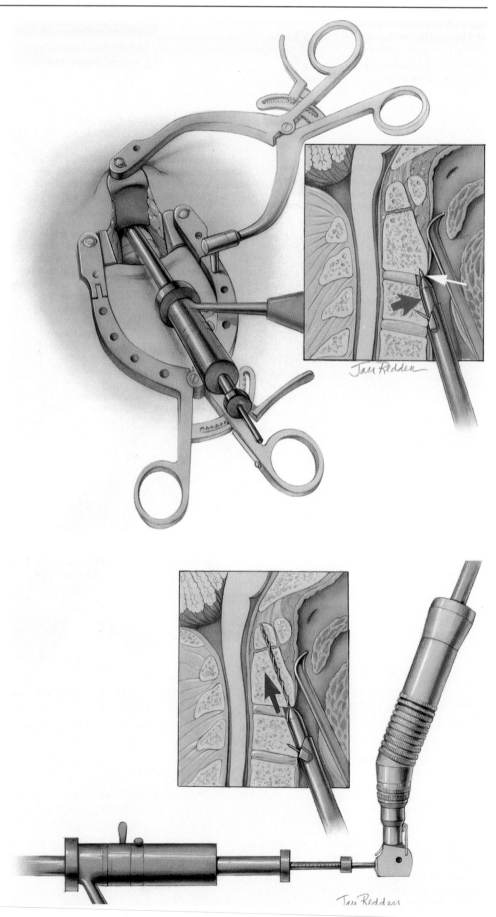

Fig. 15.6 Securing of the teeth of the guide tube to C3 with impactor (With permission of Aesculap AG, Tuttlingen, Germany)

Fig. 15.7 The guide tube is secured into the C3 vertebral body to drill through C2 into the apex of the odontoid tip (With permission of Aesculap AG, Tuttlingen, Germany)

Fig. 15.8 After the drill is withdrawn, the hole is tapped, and the length of the screw is determined (With permission of Aesculap AG, Tuttlingen, Germany)

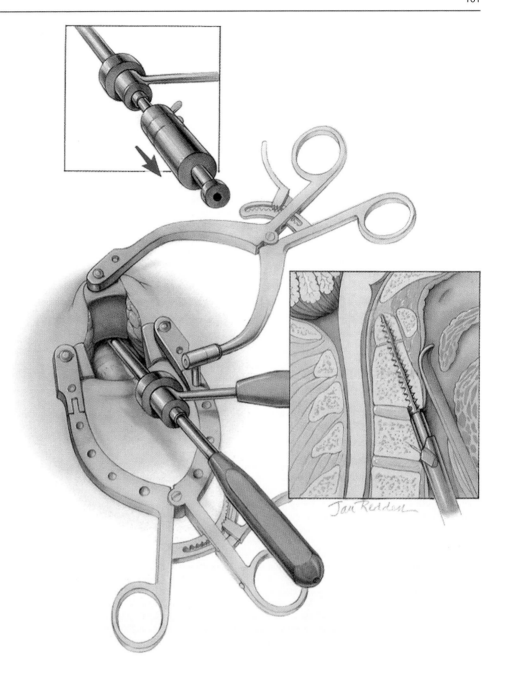

- Once the desired alignment has been achieved, the drill can be advanced through the tip of the odontoid process. In osteoporotic bone in particular, it is important that the drill is placed bicortically through the apical cortex, which will prevent back out of the screw.
- The appropriate screw length is determined from the calibrated marks at the proximal end of the drill. A partially threaded screw is initially selected. Then, the drill is withdrawn, and a tap is inserted. In general, we tap the entire drill path bicortically through the tip of the odontoid process. The length of the screw can then be confirmed with the tap (see Fig. 15.8).

- After the tap is removed, we place the titanium screw under bilateral fluoroscopy until the distal cortex of the odontoid is fully engaged and sometimes draws back slightly to pull together the bone fragments. The "lag effect" assists with closing the fracture gap and the healing process (see Fig. 15.9).
- If a second screw is to be placed, the same process is repeated (see Fig. 15.10).
- Then, the retractors are removed, and the muscle is lightly approximated with 3.0 absorbable stitches, and the skin is closed. We generally do not place drains. The immediate stability can be confirmed by extending and flexing the neck under lateral fluoroscopy.

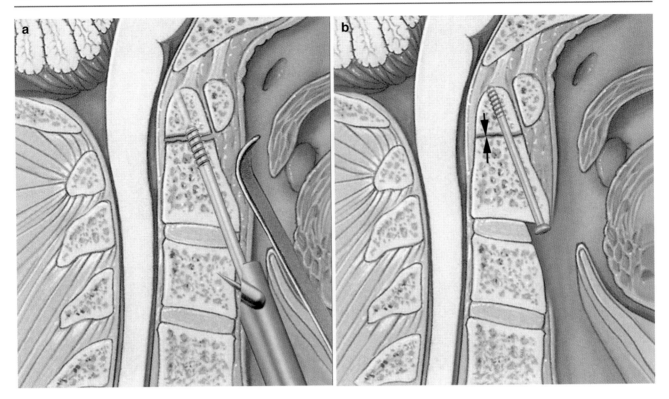

Fig. 15.9 Illustration of screw insertion (**a**) and the lag effect (*arrows*, **b**) (With permission of Aesculap AG, Tuttlingen, Germany)

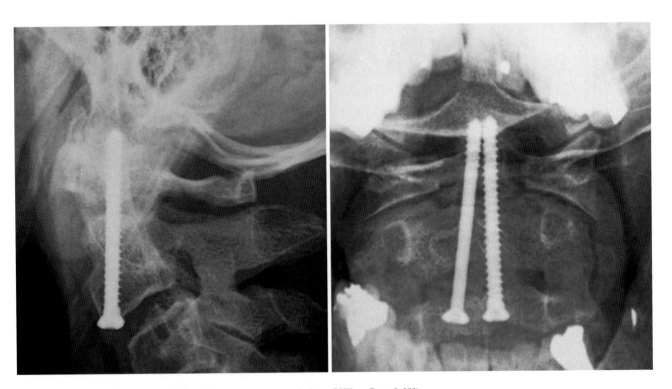

Fig. 15.10 Postoperative x-rays of odontoid screws (With permission of Kilmo P et al. [8])

References

1. Aebi M, Etter C, Coscia M (1989) Fractures of the odontoid process. Treatment with anterior screw fixation. Spine 14:1065–1070
2. Apfelbaum RI (1992) Anterior screw fixation for odontoid fractures. In: Rengachary SS, Wilkins RH (eds) Neurosurgery operative atlas, vol 2, 3rd edn. American Association of Neurological Surgeons, Park Ridge, pp 189–199
3. Apfelbaum RI, Lonser RR, Veres R, Casey A (2000) Direct anterior screw fixation for recent and remote odontoid fractures. J Neurosurg 93:227–236
4. Bohler J (1982) Anterior stabilization for acute fractures and nonunions of the dens. J Bone Joint Surg Am 64:18–27
5. Dunn ME, Seljeskog EL (1986) Experience in the management of odontoid process injuries: an analysis of 128 cases. Neurosurgery 18:306–310
6. Etter C, Coscia M, Jaberg H et al (1991) Direct anterior fixation of dens fractures with a cannulated screw system. Spine 16:S25–S32
7. Jenkins JD, Coric D, Branch CL Jr (1998) A clinical comparison of one- and two-screw odontoid fixation. J Neurosurg 89:366–370
8. Klimo P, Rao G, Apfelbaum RI (2005) Microsurgical treatment of odontoid fractures. In: Mayer HM (ed) Minimally Invasive Spinal Surgery. Springer, New York
9. Montesano PX, Anderson PA, Schlehr F et al (1991) Odontoid fractures treated by anterior odontoid screw fixation. Spine 16:S33–S37
10. Subach BR, Morone MA, Haid RW Jr, McLaughlin MR, Rodts GR, Comey CH (1999) Management of acute odontoid fractures with single-screw anterior fixation. Neurosurgery 45:812–819; discussion 819–820

Anterior Transarticular Screw Fixation C1/C2

16

Uwe Vieweg and Meic H. Schmidt

16.1 Introduction and Core Messages

Anterior transarticular screw fixation is a useful minimally invasive technique for achieving C1–2 stabilization. This chapter describes the anterior transarticular screw fixation of the atlantoaxial joints using an anterior (Smith-Robinson) approach to the cervical spine. Cannulated or noncannulated screws can be inserted with a lateral angulation of 20° relative to the sagittal plane and a posterior angulation of 30° relative to the coronal plane. The advantages of this method are immediate stability, the elimination of external orthosis, and cost-effectiveness. This form of anterior transarticular screw fixation is as stable and rigid as posterior transarticular screw fixation [3–6].

16.2 Indications [1, 2, 8, 9]

- Atlantoaxial instabilities (acute and chronic)
- C1–2 instability in cases where a posterior approach is impossible
- Failure of previous posterior treatment
- C1 type II odontoid combination fracture [1]

16.3 Contraindications

- Fracture of the C1–2 joint complex
- Vertebral artery with atypical course
- Some cases where neck is very short or thick
- Some cases with high barrel-shaped thorax

16.4 Equipment

Two C-arms for simultaneous anteroposterior and lateral fluoroscopy are essential for this technique. The settings and other equipment, and the operative approach, are the same as those for osteosynthesis using expansion screws (e.g., positioning device, rechargeable drill, appropriate screws for small fragments, Synthes odontoid screw system).

16.5 Planning, Preparation, and Positioning

The planning of the operation requires a CT to ensure that the C1–2 joint complex is intact (look out for rotational malalignment). The patient is put in a supine position, and the head is stabilized using a Mayfield headholder. Two C-arms are necessary to identify the anatomical structures of the upper cervical spine in the anteroposterior and lateral projections

U. Vieweg, M.D., Ph.D. (✉)
Clinic for Spinal Surgery, Sana Hospital Rummelsberg,
90593 Schwarzenbruck, Germany
e-mail: uwe.vieweg@yahoo.de

M.H. Schmidt, M.D., FACS
Division of Spine Surgery, Department of Neurosurgery,
Clinical Neurosciences Center, University of Utah,
175 N. Medical Drive East, Bldg 550, Salt Lake City,
UT 84132-2303, USA
e-mail: meic.schmidt@hsc.utah.edu

U. Vieweg, F. Grochulla (eds.), *Manual of Spine Surgery*,
DOI 10.1007/978-3-642-22682-3_16, © Springer-Verlag Berlin Heidelberg 2012

Fig. 16.1 (**a**) Patient positioned on operating table. (**b**) Note the placement of two C-arm fluoroscopic units for anteroposterior (transoral) and lateral fluoroscopic control

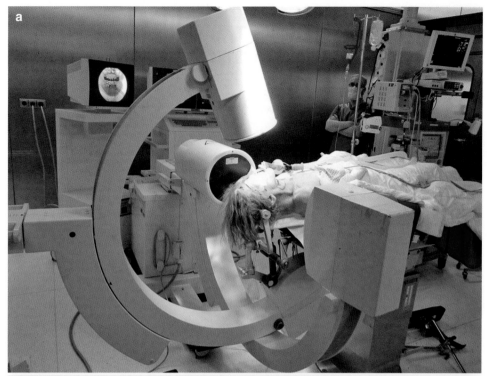

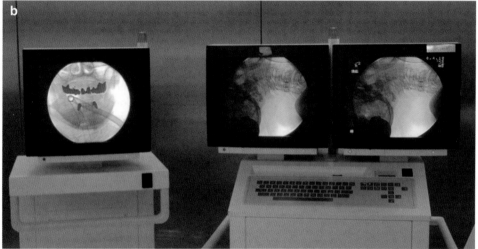

(see Fig. 16.1a, b). The site of the incision (usually at the C4/C5 level) is determined by placing a K-wire along the side of the neck in the intended direction of the screw and viewing it with the image intensifier (see Fig. 16.2).

16.6 Surgical Technique

16.6.1 Approach

- A transverse skin incision is recommended as, in most cases, only one segment is involved (for C3/C4, two

fingerbreadths caudal to the mandible at the level of the lingual bone; for C4/C5, at the level of the Adam's apple).

- Using a routine anterior approach to the cervical spine at the C4–5 level, the anterior side of the C2 vertebral body is exposed.
- The platysma is cut, and the superficial nuchal fascia is exposed. This is then cut longitudinally at the anterior edge of the sternocleidomastoid muscle.
- The sternocleidomastoid muscle is then moved to the side, exposing the two longus colli muscles beneath.
- Blunt dissection is carried out in the prevertebral facial plane using a side sweeping motion with a small gauze pad. Exposure of the upper half of C3 and the lower half

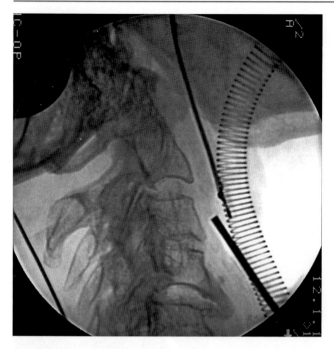

Fig. 16.2 K-wire along the side of the neck in the intended direction of the screws and viewed on the image intensifier

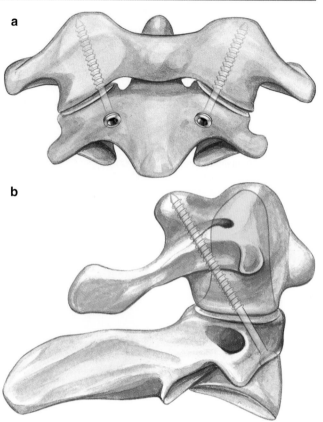

Fig. 16.3 Orientation of anterior transarticular screws relative to C1–2. (**a**) anteroposterior view (20°). (**b**) lateral view (30°)

of C2 is usually sufficient. Preparation can often be carried out with the fingers.

16.6.2 Instrumentation

- The insertion point for the screws is at the midpoint of the C2 vertebral body in the medial third of the C1–2 articulation, just below the sulcus on the anterior side [7].
- After drilling and tapping, 3.5-mm or 4-mm small fragment screws are placed across the joint in the C1 massa lateralis, diverging about 20° and inclined upwards about 30° (standard lag screw technique).
- It is absolutely essential that tissue protectors are used when drilling and tapping.
- Note: The use of cannulated screws and predrilling with a K-wire make instrumentation much easier. The cannulated screw technique can be used for this (see Fig. 16.3).
- A threaded K-wire of 1.2-mm diameter and 20-cm length is advanced into the body of C2 in a posterior and superior direction at an angle of 20° to the coronal plane and 30° to the sagittal plane (see Fig. 16.3a, b).
- The length of the K-wire in the bone is measured with the ruler, indicating the length of screw required.
- The screw length is 20–25 mm. When odontoid screws is used, only the 28-mm screws may be readily available. It is possible to place these screws safely (see Fig. 16.4a–f).

- 3.5-mm cannulated fully threaded and short-thread screws can be used.
- Cannulated screws are inserted after predrilling of the subchondral bone of the joint surface of the lateral mass of C2 and C1.
- The screws are inserted using a cannulated screwdriver. Note: Observe the insertion of the cannulated screws on the lateral image intensifier to ensure that the K-wire does not advance in an anterior direction.
- The ventral portions of the C1–2 joint are decorticated, and spongiosa is applied (arthrodesis).

16.7   Tips and Tricks

- Do not go too far in a cranial direction and cross into the occipitoatlantal joint. If the screw trajectory is too lateral, there is a risk of injuring the vertebral artery.
- Odontoid and bilateral C1–2 transarticular screw fixation through a small anterior skin incision is an alternative

Fig. 16.4 Different CT images of the transarticular screws at C1–2 and the odontoid screw of a 82-year-old woman show an odontoid type II and C1 arc fracture. (**a**) screws in the of base of C2, (**b**) in the middle of the corpus C2, (**c**) the tip of the screws in the odontoid process and in the joint C1/C2, (**d**) lateral view of the screw in the right joint C1/C2, (**e**) odontoid screw, and (**f**) lateral view of the screw in the right joint C1/C2

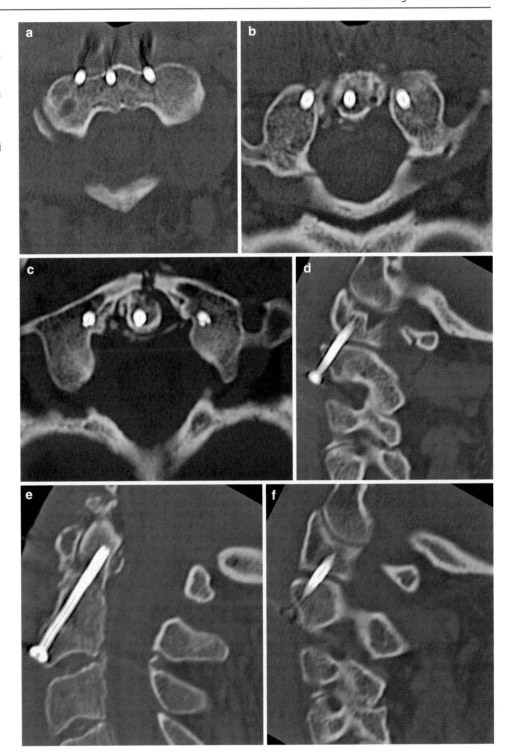

option for patients with odontoid fracture, worsened clinical state, and poor bone quality.

• This procedure is helpful in polytraumatized or elderly patients where surgery needs to be limited, but stability of the C1/C2 complex is absolutely essential.

References

1. Dean Q, Jiefu S, Jie W, Yunxing S (2009) Minimally invasive technique of triple anterior screw fixation for an acute combination atlas axis fracture: case report and literature review. Spinal Cord 48(2):174–177
2. Kim SM, Lim TJ, Paterno J, Hwang TJ et al (2004) Biomechanical comparison of anterior and posterior stabilization methods in atlantoaxial instability. J Neurosurg 100(3 suppl):277–283
3. Koller H, Kammermeier V, Ulbricht D, Assuncao A, Karolus S, van den Berg B, Holz U (2006) Anterior retropharyngeal fixation C1–2 for stabilization of atlantoaxial instabilities: study of feasibility, technical description and preliminary results. Eur Spine J 15:1326–1338
4. Lu J, Ebrahim NA, Yonk H et al (1998) Anatomic considerations of anterior transarticular screw fixation for atlantoaxial instability. Point of view. Spine 23:1229–1236
5. Pepin JW, Boune RB, Hawkins RJ (1985) Odontoid fractures with special references to the elderly patients. Clin Orthop Relat Res 193:178–183
6. Reindl R, Sen M, Aebi M (2003) Anterior instrumentation for traumatic C1-C2 instability. Spine 28:E329–E333
7. Sen MK, Steffen T, Beckman L et al (2005) Atlantoaxial fusion using anterior transarticular screw fixation of C1-C2: technical innovation and biomechanical study. Eur Spine J 14:512–518
8. Six E, Kelly DL (1981) Technique for C1, C2 and C3 fixation in cases of odontoid fractures. Neurosurgery 8:374–377
9. Vaccaro AR, Lehman AP, Ahlgren BD, Garfin SR (1999) Anterior C1-C2 screw fixation and bony fusion through an anterior retropharyngeal approach. Orthopedics 22:1165–1170

Transoral Resection of the Odontoid Process

17

Meic H. Schmidt and Uwe Vieweg

17.1 Introduction and Core Messages

The transoral approach to anteriorly placed lesions at the craniocervical junction is not new [1] but is still infrequently used by neurosurgeons for tumors in this region [4]. The anterior inferior aspect of the craniocervical junction constitutes the upper posterior wall of the oral cavity. The open oral cavity can therefore be used to access this region without disturbing the medulla.

17.2 Indications

- Spinal column tumor with neural compression
- Extradural metastatic tumor
- Irreducible subluxations
- Os odontoideum
- Rheumatoid pannus

17.3 Contraindications

- Inability to open the mouth widely for the transoral approach, i.e., severe arthritis of the temporomandibular joints (TMJ)
- Intradural pathologies

M.H. Schmidt, M.D., FACS (✉)
Division of Spine Surgery, Department of Neurosurgery,
Clinical Neurosciences Center, University of Utah,
175 N. Medical Drive East, Bldg 550, Salt Lake City,
UT 84132-2303, USA
e-mail: meic.schmidt@hsc.utah.edu

U. Vieweg, M.D., Ph.D.
Clinic for Spinal Surgery, Sana Hospital Rummelsberg,
90593 Schwarzenbruck, Germany
e-mail: uwe.vieweg@yahoo.de

17.4 Technical Prerequisites

Fluoroscope, retractor system, long forceps, dissectors, and burrs. In general, any resection of the odontoid process results in instability. It is therefore most often performed in conjunction with posterior C1–2 fusion. Alternatively, the use of various screw systems and plating systems for anterior plating has been described [6].

17.5 Planning, Preparation, and Positioning

The transoral exposure of the clivus, atlas, and ventral aspect of C2 is commonly performed in our practice. After induction of general anesthesia, the patient is placed with the neck extended in the supine position. For the transoral approach, it is important to ensure that the patient can open his or her mouth sufficiently. This can frequently be a problem in patients with arthritic temporomandibular joints, which are common in rheumatoid patients. In such cases, the procedure can be modified to include transmandibular splitting, but this is not common. Regular intubation is performed, and we use the Spetzler-Sonntag retraction system to allow exposure of the oral cavity (Fig. 17.1). It is important to protect the teeth during the placement of this retractor. It is also important to protect the tongue since significant tongue swelling can occur if retraction is performed against the teeth. Some authors advocate nasal intubation, but we have found this unnecessary. Once the retractors are placed, the posterior pharynx is sufficiently exposed, and the C1 tubercle is palpated.

17.6 Operating Technique

17.6.1 Approach

- The surgical site is infiltrated with lidocaine and epinephrine, and the midline is incised with a monopolar cautery,

U. Vieweg, F. Grochulla (eds.), *Manual of Spine Surgery*,
DOI 10.1007/978-3-642-22682-3_17, © Springer-Verlag Berlin Heidelberg 2012

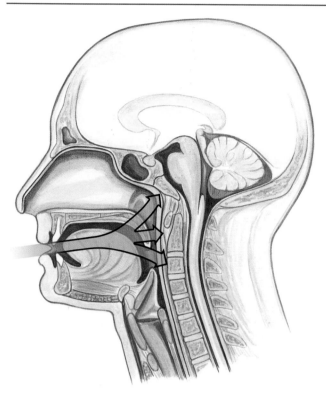

Fig. 17.1 Diagram of the upper cervical resections that can be performed cranially and caudally from a transoral approach

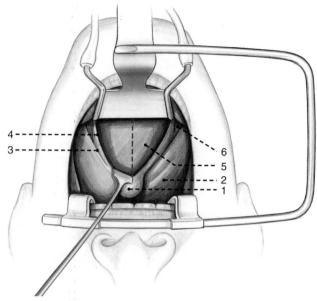

Fig. 17.2 Retraction of the soft palate with subsequent longitudinal incision of the dorsal wall of the pharynx (*1* Uvula, *2* palatum molle, *3* arcus palatoglossus, *4* arcus palatopharyngeus, *5* dorsal wall of pharynx with mucosa, *6* tonsilla palatina)

with the incision extending approximately 2–3 cm from the anterior arch of C1 to the bottom of C2.

- With this dissection, the bone is exposed, and the pharyngeal tissues are retracted laterally. This is greatly facilitated by placement of the retractor plate (see Figs. 17.2 and 17.3).
- Once the retractors are placed, we use the Midas Rex drill or remove the anterior aspect of the arch of C1.
- We then proceed with drilling of the C2 dens. It is important initially to preserve the outer shell of the C2 dens to prevent the soft tissues from falling into the surgical site.
- Once the C2 dens is eggshell thin, we remove the remaining tissues. This allows access for removal of the pannus in rheumatoid patients and decompression of the upper cervical canal.

17.6.2 Instrumentation (Additional)

- The transoral exposure of the posterior pharynx has been described by Schmelzle and Harms [5] for treatment of unstable Jefferson fractures.
- Reduction is achieved by placing the patient in traction. C1 and C2 are then exposed anteriorly (Fig. 17.4).
- Osteosynthesis is performed with a compression plate or a screw/rod system.

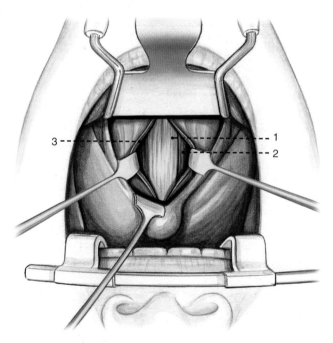

Fig. 17.3 After incision has been made in dorsal wall of pharynx (*1* longus colli muscle, *2* longus capitis muscle, *3* superior constrictor pharyngis muscle)

- Polyaxial screws are placed into both C1 lateral masses and then connected with a rod. This allows for preservation of the C1–2 motion segment in cases with Jefferson fractures [3].

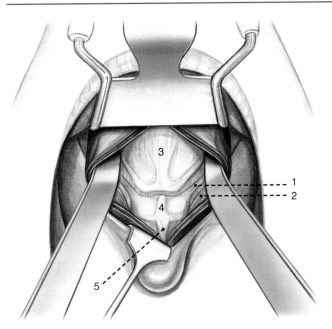

Fig. 17.4 Atlas and axis (*1* longus colli muscle, *2* longus capitis muscle, *3* corpus axis, *4* tuberculum anterius atlantis, *5* membrana atlantooccipitalis anterior)

17.7   Tips and Tricks

- Reconstruction of the dens using a C2 prosthesis, as described by Jeszenszky et al. [2].
- Additional dorsal instrumentation and fusion of C1–C3.
- Primary dorsal instrumentation with decompression may also be considered for patients with rheumatoid arthritis.

References

1. Hall JE, Dennis F, Murray J (1977) Exposure of the upper cervical spine for spinal decompression by mandible and tongue-splitting approach. J Bone Joint Surg Am 59A:121
2. Jeszenszky D, Harms J, Hadasch R et al (1999) C2 Prosthesis allowing optimal stabilisation after C2 resection following destructive lesions. Eur Spine J 8(Suppl 1):S40
3. Ruf M, Melcher R, Harms J (2004) Transoral reduction and osteosynthesis C1 as a function-preserving option in the treatment of unstable Jefferson fractures. Spine 29:823–827
4. Russo A, Albanese E, Quiroga M et al (2009) Submandibular approach to the C2–3 disc level: microsurgical anatomy with clinical application. J Neurosurg Spine 10:380–389
5. Schmelzle R, Harms J (1987) Craniocervical junction-diseases, diagnostic application of imaging procedures, surgical techniques. Fortschr Kiefer Gesichtschir 32:206–208
6. Vender JR, Harrison SJ, McDonnell DE (2000) Fusion and instrumentation at C1–3 via the high anterior cervical approach. J Neurosurg 92:24–29

Part III

Anterior Cervical Spine C3–C8 (T1)

Overview of Surgical Techniques and Implants

18

Tobias Pitzen

18.1 Introduction and Core Messages

Short overview on different techniques and implants for anterior decompression, fixation, and realignment within the cervical spine. Degenerative disc diseases, ossifications of the posterior longitudinal ligament, vertebral body tumours, spondylodiscitis, and vertebral body compression fractures are among the most frequent cervical spine pathologies a spine surgeon has to deal with. All these are located within the anterior aspect of the cervical spine – which are the vertebral bodies and the discs. Thus, anterior cervical spine techniques (including anterior decompression, fixation, and realignment) are among the most popular and necessary ones within the armamentarium of a spine surgeon. Within this chapter, we will give a short overview on different techniques for anterior decompression, fixation, and realignment within the cervical spine. Moreover, different anterior implants for dynamic and permanent osseous fixation, distributed by different companies, are presented.

18.2 Approaches

18.2.1 Anterolateral Approach

The standard approach for anterior cervical spine procedures – by which almost all regions may be exposed easily – is an anterolateral as described by Cloward [6, 7]. Take care that the incision usually crosses the midline by 1 cm and reaches the medial edge of the sternocleidomastoid muscle. The incision should be placed above the centre of the lesion.

18.2.2 Anterolateral Approach with Partial Split of the Sternum

If the first or second thoracic vertebral body is involved, it is beneficial to split at least the cranial part of the sternum. In this case, ask for help by a thoracic surgeon. The standard approach is medial to the carotid artery to the anterior aspect of the spine. Self holding sharp retractors are placed under the longus colli muscles; blunt retractors are used to spread the wound in cranio-caudal direction.

18.3 Techniques for Decompression

18.3.1 Uncoforaminotomy

This is a technique that may be used for anterior lateral decompression within the cervical spine for the indication of soft disc prolapse or spondylosis that compresses a root. The main advantage of this is that the main parts of the disc are spared, range of motion is probably not affected significantly, and no implants are necessary. However, the technique is not

T. Pitzen, M.D., Ph.D.
Department of Spine Surgery, SRH Klinikum Karlsbad-Langensteinbach, Guttmannstrasse 1, 76307 Karlsbad, Germany
e-mail: tobias.pitzen@kkl.srh.de

U. Vieweg, F. Grochulla (eds.), *Manual of Spine Surgery*,
DOI 10.1007/978-3-642-22682-3_18, © Springer-Verlag Berlin Heidelberg 2012

very easy to learn and take care of the vertebral artery that is pretty close to your high-speed drill. For detailed information about this, look at Chap. 20.

18.3.2 Discectomy

The technique of cervical spine discectomy is the basic one for anterior cervical spine decompression. No matter, if a one or more level discectomy or a one or more level vertebral body resection, you usually start by performing a cervical spine discectomy via anterior approach. Following anterior approach and placing of the retractor and spreading system, the anterior longitudinal ligament must be incised and removed with the disc by means of curettes and rongeurs. I prefer to remove the lateral aspects of the disc towards the uncus using a 4-mm Kerrison (Take care: the vertebral artery is very close here!). I usually remove the anterior rim of the superior vertebra using the size 4 Kerrison. The bone chips taken this way are used to fill a cage. A cylindrical burr is used to perform a rectangular shape of the disc space. A round burr is used to remove posterior osteophytes in the presence of an intact posterior ligament. Alternatively; these spurs may be removed after resection of the posterior longitudinal ligament. Again, these bone chips may or even should be taken to fill a cervical spine fusion cage.

18.3.3 Vertebral Body Resection

Before a vertebral body resection is performed, all discs adjacent to the vertebral body should be removed as described above. The thecal sac should be exposed within the segment where spinal encroachment is least. Vertebral body resection starts using big size rongeurs. Again, the bone is taken to fill a cage; 8 mm of the vertebral body at each side of the midline is removed for median resection of a vertebral body – which is sufficient for placing a cage for vertebral body replacement. Use sharp drills to remove the posterior cortical shell down to the soft parts of the posterior longitudinal ligament. Resection of this may be performed finally using a size 2 Kerrison; the cuts are performed at the most lateral parts of the ligament. Finally, the ligament may be removed en bloc.

18.3.4 Spondylectomy

Spondylectomy is usually indicated in case of primary bone tumours or single metastasis. Spondylectomy first requires a complete removal of the posterior structures. Via anterior approach, the discs are excised, and lateral circumferential dissection is performed until the vertebra can be removed

"en bloc". If this procedure has to be performed between C1 and C6, think about asking a vascular bypass surgeon for help.

18.4 Techniques for Interbody Fixation

18.4.1 Cages

Cages are among the most successful implants within spine surgery and especially within cervical spine surgery within the last years. Obviously, these implants helped to solve the problem of graft site morbidity, which was mainly but not only a problem of long-lasting donor site pain. Using cages in (cervical) spine surgery does not only reduce but eliminate the problem of donor site morbidity. Cages usually consist of titanium, PEEK, or carbon fibre composit. They usually have one or more perforations to allow bony ingrowth for long-term stability and teeth/fins or similar for secure fixation after insertion until bony ingrowth is completed. It is believed that cages made from titanium have a greater tendency for settling, but the main disadvantage of these is that bony fusion is difficult to judge via x-ray or CAT scan, and visualization of soft tissue (tumour cases) is difficult if not impossible via MRI. Cages can be used to replace one single or more discs or to replace one or even more vertebral bodies. There is a huge variety of cages available on the market; Table 18.1 gives a short overview on cervical cages for disc replacement (see additionally Chap. 22). Although I do not recommend (too expensive, too technical), I would like to mention cages for vertebral body replacement that include mechanisms to distract and screws to fix the cage into the adjacent vertebral body cages that can be stabled.

18.4.2 Disc Prostheses

Disc protheses have been introduced into surgical treatment of the degenerative disc disease of the lumbar spine as early as in 1960s but disappeared from the market due to major problems until they had a second peak in the early 2000. Within the cervical spine, they became more popular when Hilibrand in 1999 reported that more than 25.6% of all patients having received an ACDF will receive an adjacent level disease within 10 years. Today, these values are known to be probably overestimated, but meanwhile, cervical disc prostheses became a popular – and efficient – tool to deal with the problem of degenerative disc disease within the cervical spine. The clinical results are good, and there is some evidence that segmental motility may be preserved at least for a certain time. If however, disc prosthesis will reduce the problem of ALD or if this is a natural history is still unclear. Moreover, we face another problem in cervical spine disc

Table 18.1 Some current cages for C-Spine surgery

	Stryker	Synthes	Ulrich	Zimmer	Signus medical	Medtronic	Scientx	DePuy	Spineart	AMT
PEEK	Solis cage	Cervios		Fidji	Nubic/Rabea		PCB evolution		Tryptik	Shell
Titanium		Syncage-C	Mini disc spacer	BAK/C	Rabea	Affinity	PCB cage			
Other				TM-100		Cornerstone		Bengal		

replacement using prosthesis, that is, heterotopic ossification. The problem of revision surgery, however, is not as pronounced as it is (no big vessels) within the lumbar spine. Thus, insertion of disc prosthesis became a useful technique within cervical spine surgery. Table 18.2 gives an overview on current implants designed and distributed by several companies.

18.4.3 Anterior Cervical Plating

Anterior cervical plating has been introduced into routine cervical spine surgery by Caspar in the 1980s to reduce graft-related complications [3, 4]. In fact, there is some evidence that anterior cervical plating may reduce complications such as graft compression fracture, graft dislocation, or pseudarthrotic healing. Every anterior cervical plate will add stability to a cervical spine segment in flexion – extension, axial rotation, and lateral bending. However, complications such as screw loosening or even plate loosening as a consequence of screw loosening occurred in the presence of this plate. Thus, more recently, plating concepts in which the screws are connected to the plate – thus secured against screw back out – have been developed.

Among these, rigid plate designs and dynamic plate designs will be discussed a little more in detail here. Rigid plates do not allow any screw motility within the plate. Thus, they are believed to give more stability especially in trauma cases. There is, however, some evidence that this is not the case. Loading of the interbody cage or graft is less pronounced when compared to dynamic plates. Dynamic plates allow some screw motility within the plate, with the consequence of graft or cage loading, thus resulting in higher speed of fusion and lower incidence of implant complications. Table 18.3 gives a short overview on different implants, supplied by different companies. To supply quick information to the reader, they are listed here according to their mechanical basic principle:

- Unrestricted back out devices (Caspar and Orozco plate systems)
- Restricted, constrained devices (CSLP/Morscher plate (Synthes),Orion plate Atlantis ACP system)
- Semiconstrained, rotational devices (Codman plate system, Atlantis system)
- Semiconstrained, translational devices (DOC anterior cervical stabilization system (Acromed's), ABC plating system (Aesculap))
- Multiconstruct system (Atlantis ACP system) [1–5, 8–11]

Table 18.2 Overview about different artificial disc implants for the cervical spine

Features	Activ C (Aesculap)	Prodisc C (Synthes)	Bryan (SDGI)	Prestige ST (SDGI)	Prestige LP (SDGI)	PCM (Cervi-tech/link)	Cervidisc (Scient'x)	Discocerv (Scient'x)
Picture								
Biomechanics	• Ball and socket • Fixed post. COR • Motion limitation	• Ball and socket • Fixed central COR • Forced translation	• Biconvex core • Floating central COR • Forced translation	• Ball and socket • Elongated socket • Free translation	• Ball and socket • Elongated socket • Free translation	• Ball and socket • Fixed central COR	• Ball and socket • Fixed central COR • Forced translation	• Ball and socket
Material	• CoCr/PE	• CoCr/PE	• Ti/PU	• SS/SS • Ti/Ti	• Ti/Ti	• CoCr/PE	• Ce/Ce in Ti	• Titanium endplates • Ce/Ce bearing
Fixation	• Sup: spikes/grooves • Inf: keel • Plasmapore	• Keel • Porous coating	• Press-fit • Porous coating	• Screws	• Keels • Porous coating	• Press-fit • Porous coating • Grooves	• Sup: grooves • Inf: teeth	• Anatomic endplate design leading to excellent prim.stab.
Endplate design	• Trapezoidal • Sup: convex • Inf: flat	• Rectangular • Flat	• Circular • Convex	• Long rectangular • Flat	•	• Long rectangular • Flat	• Rectangular • Sup: convex • Inf: flat	• Trapezoidal • Convex inferior surface in frontal plane
Sizes (ml x ap)	• 16 x 13, 16 x 14 • 17 x 15, 18 x 16 • 19 x 17, 19 x 18	• M: 15 x 12, 15 x 14 • L: 17 x 14, 17 x 16 • XL: 19 x 16, 19 x 18	• Ø14/15/16/17/18	• Ap: 12/14	• Ap: 12/14/16/18	• S/M/L	• 17 x 13	• 17 x 13 • 20 x 15
Heights	• 5/6/7	• 5/6/7	• 6,5/8,5	• 8	• 6/7/8	• 6,5/8	• 7/8/9	• 17 x 13 5,25/6,75/7,5 • 20 x 15 6,75/7,5/8,25
Flexion/extension	• 24°	• 17,2°						• 18°
Lateral bending	• 24°	• 17,2°						• 18°
Lordosis	• 3°	• 0°	• 0°	• 0°			• 4°	
Surgical techn./ instrumentation	• Easy • Safe	• Easy	• Difficult	• Easy			• Easy	
Keel preparation	• Motor system	• Chiseling • Motor system						
Problems		• Bone bridges	• Bone bridges • Kyphotic segments	• Breaking screws		• Anterior migration • Bone bridges	• Subsidence • Migration (displacement)	

(continued)

Table 18.2 (continued)

Features	Activ C (Aesculap)	CerviCore (Stryker) Developed by Spinecore	CMP (Vertebron)	Kineflex C (Spinalmotion)	M6 (Spinal kinetics)	Mobi C LDR spine	Secrue C (Globus medical)
Picture					M6-c Artificial Cervical Disc / polymer sheath / keels / polymer Nucleus / Fiber Annulus		
Biomechanics	• Ball and socket • Fixed post. COR • Motion limitation	• Saddle joint • Central COR (min. movement due to saddle)	•	• Biconvex core	• Elastomer core	• Ball and socket • Movable insert	
Material	• CoCr/PE	• CoCr/CoCr	• CoCr/CoCr	• Metal/metal	• Elstomer • Ti-endplates	• CoCr/PE • Porous coating	• Porous coating
Fixation	• Sup: spikes/grooves • Inf: keel • Plasmapore	• Screws • Spikes	• Keel • Screws	• Keel • Rough surface	• Keel • Porous coating	• Spikes in line	• Keel
Endplate design	• Trapezoidal • Sup: convex • Inf: flat	• Round • Flat		• Rectangular	• Rectangular	• Rectangular	
Sizes (ml x ap)	• 16 x 13, 16 x 14 • 17 x 15, 18 x 16 • 19 x 17, 19 x 18	• S: 12 x 12 • M: 14 x 12 • L: 16 x 14			• M: 15 x 12,5 • ML: 15 x 15 • L: 17 x 14 • LL: 17 x 16	• 13 x 15 • 13 x 17 • 15 x 17 • 15 x 20	
Heights	• 5/6/7	• 6–12 mm			• 6/7	• 4.5/5/6/7	
Flexion/extension	• 24°				• 13,5°	• 20°	
Lateral bending	• 24°					• 20°	
Lordosis	• 3°						
Surgical techn./instrumentation	• Easy • Safe						
Keel preparation	• Motor system					• No keel preparation	
Problems							

Features	Activ C (Aesculap)	Altia (?) (Amedica)	Discove (DePuy)	Physio-C (Nexgen spine)	Neo Disc (NuVasive)	CAdisc-C (Rainer)	NuNec (Pioneer)
Picture							
Biomechanics	• Ball and socket • Fixed post. COR • Motion limitation		• Ball and socket	• Elastomer core	• Elastomer core	• Elastomer core	
Material	• CoCr/PE	• Ceramic					• PEEK/PEEK
Fixation	• Sup: spikes/grooves • Inf: keel • Plasmapore			• Keel	• Screws		• Cam locking mechanism
Endplate design	• Trapezoidal • Sup: convex • Inf: flat			• Rectangular			
Sizes (ml x ap)	• 16 x 13, 16 x 14 • 17 x 15, 18 x 16 • 19 x 17, 19 x 18			• 14 x 12 • 16 x 12 • 16 x 14 • 18 x 14 • 18 x 16 • 20 x 16			• 14 x 12 • 14 x 14,5 • 17 x 14,5 • 17 x 17
Heights	• 5/6/7			• 8			• 5/6/7
Flexion/extension	• 24°			• 30			
Lateral bending	• 24°			• 20			
Lordosis	• 3°						
Surgical techn./instrumentation	• Easy • Safe						
Keel preparation	• Motor system						
Problems							

Table 18.3 Some current anterior cervical plate design

	Dynamic	Semiconstrained	Constrained	Hybrid
Aesculap	ABC	Caspar	Ø	Ø
Synthes	Vectra T	CSLP Variable	CSLP	Vectra / ACC
Medtronic	Premier	Venture/Zephir	Atlantis	Atlantis S
DePuy	Swift	Eagle SlimLoc Uniplate	Ø	Skyline

References

1. Bohler J, Gaudernak T (1980) Anterior plate stabilization for fracture dislocations of the lower cervical spine. J Trauma 20:203–205

2. Bose B (1998) Anterior cervical fusion using Caspar plating: analysis of results and review of the literature. Surg Neurol 49:25–31

3. Caspar W, Barbier DD, Klara PM (1989) Anterior cervical fusion and Caspar plate stabilization for cervical trauma. Neurosurgery 25:491–502

4. Caspar W, Geisler FH, Pitzen T et al (1998) Anterior cervical plate stabilization in one- and two-level degenerative disease: overtreatment or benefit? J Spinal Disord 11:1–11

5. Chen IH (1996) Biomechanical evaluation of subcortical versus bicortical screw purchase in anterior cervical plating. Acta Neurochir 138:167–173

6. Cloward RB (1958) The anterior approach for removal of ruptured cervical discs. J Neurosurg 15:602–617

7. Cloward RB (1961) Treatment of acute fractures and fracture-dislocations of the cervical spine by vertebral-body fusion. J Neurosurg 18:201–209

8. Haid RW, Foley KT, Rodts GE et al (2002) The cervical spine study group anterior cervical plate nomenclature. Neurosurg Focus 12(1):Article 15

9. Morscher E, Sutter F, Jenny H et al (1986) Die vordere Verplattung der Halswirbelsaule mit dem Hohlschrauben-Plattensystem aus Titanium. Chirurg 57:702–707

10. Orozco DR, Llovet TR (1971) Osteosintesis en las lesions traumaticas y degeneratives de la columna vertebral. Revista Traumatol Cirurg Rehabil 1:45–52

11. Rengachary SS, Sanan A (1996) Anterior stabilization of the cervical spine using locking plate systems. In: Wilkins RH, Rengachary SS (eds) Neurosurgery. McGraw-Hill, New York, pp 2983–2986

Anterior Cervical Discectomy and Fusion

19

Frank Grochulla

19.1 Introduction and Core Messages

Anterior cervical discectomy and fusion (ACDF) is a widely used technique and has become the gold standard for the treatment of cervical radiculopathy. The surgical principles of the surgical treatment are the decompression of neurostructures, the restoration of the cervical lordosis, and the stabilization. The surgical outcome is mainly dependent on the decompression effect. Fusion rates are dependent on the number of levels treated. Actually, there is no evidence for the superiority of cage fusions compared to fusions with autologous bone graft from the iliac crest, except of iliac crest donor site pain. In the 1950s, the first reports of anterior approaches to cervical disc pathology appeared. The two most common methods for ACDF were described by Robinson and Smith in 1955 [7] and by Cloward in 1958 [4]. Robinson and Smith did not decompress the neural structures and believed that osteophytes and herniated discs would be reabsorbed during immobilizing the segment.

19.2 Indications

- Single or multiple level soft disc herniation
- Single or multiple level spondylosis
- Ossification of the posterior longitudinal ligament (OPLL)
- Trauma (vertebral body fractures, subluxations, luxations)
- Tumors (vertebral body tumors or metastases)
- Infectious diseases

F. Grochulla, M.D.
Department for Spinal Surgery, Hospital for Orthopaedics,
Trauma Surgery and Spinal Surgery, Euromed Clinic,
Europa-Allee 1, 90763 Fürth, Germany
e-mail: frank.grochulla@euromed.de

19.3 Contraindications

- Predominant posterior compression of the neural structures
- Isolated traumatic disruption of the posterior elements

19.4 Technical Prerequisites

The technical prerequisites are the microscope, different microsurgical instruments, retractor systems for ventral approach to the cervical spine (e.g., Caspar retractor system), high-speed drill, and the intraoperative fluoroscopy.

19.5 Planning, Preparation, and Positioning

ACDF is usually performed under general anesthesia with optimum muscle relaxation.

The patient is positioned supine on the operating table. A rolled towel or sandbag is placed under the cervicothoracic junction between the shoulders for head and neck extension. Head traction device incases with instability. Shoulder countertraction may be necessary, particularly in patients with short necks and for approaches to the lower cervical spine and the cervicothoracic junction. A right-sided approach is generally recommended because it is easier for the right-handed surgeon. Some authors recommend a left-side approach to reduce the risk of injury to the recurrent laryngeal nerve. However, a review of 328 cases [3] showed no association between the side of the approach and the incidence of recurrent laryngeal nerve symptoms. The location of the skin incision is estimated with a lateral fluoroscopic image.

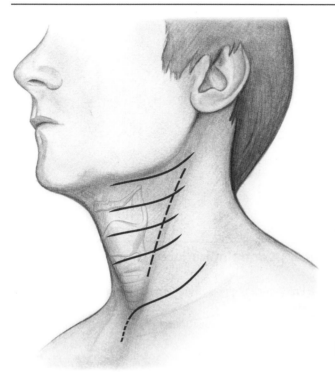

Fig. 19.1 Skin incision

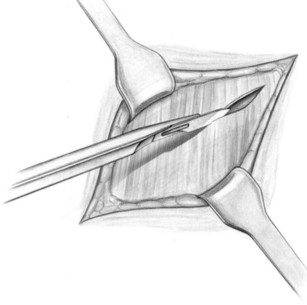

Fig. 19.2 Incision of the platysma muscle

19.6 Surgical Technique

19.6.1 Approach

- The skin incision (3–4 cm) is usually slightly oblique along Langer's lines; this provides the best possible cosmetic result (Fig. 19.1). A skin incision along the medial border of the sternocleidomastoid muscle may be used for multilevel disease.
- Dissection is carried sharply through the subcutaneous tissue. The platysma muscle may be sharply divided transverse or split longitudinally (Fig. 19.2).
- After subplatysmal dissection, the superficial fascia overlying the medial border of the sternocleidomastoid muscle is sharply divided.
- The following deep dissection between sternocleidomastoid muscle and carotid sheath laterally and trachea, esophagus, and strap muscles of the neck medially is performed careful with blunt finger dissection. In patients without previous ventral cervical surgery, blunt dissection is easily and safely accomplished. In patients with previous ventral cervical surgery, sharp dissection may be necessary. In this case, it is important to confirm that the sharp dissection remains dorsal to the esophagus and the hypopharynx. A placed nasogastric tube may be helpful to confirm the location of esophagus and hypopharynx by palpation.
- After entering the prevertebral space, the correct intervertebral disc is marked by fluoroscopy.

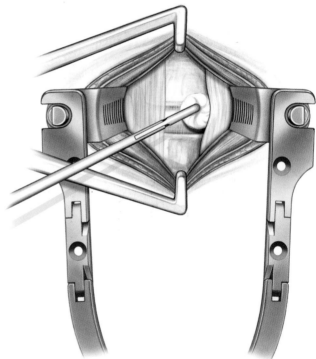

Fig. 19.3 The longus colli muscles are elevated from the vertebral bodies

- The longus colli muscles are elevated from the vertebral bodies (Fig. 19.3) and discs bilaterally, and self-retaining retractors are placed under the longus colli muscle (Fig. 19.4).
- A drill guide is used to position the drill hole for the first distraction screw in the middle third of the inferior vertebral body (Fig. 19.5a). The drilling direction is orientated approximately parallel to the index disc space.

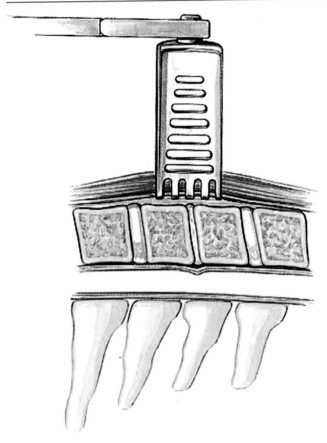

Fig. 19.4 Self-retaining retractors are placed under the longus colli muscle (With permission Aesculap AG, Tuttlingen, Germany)

19.6.2 Discectomy and Fusion

- The distraction screw is inserted through the drill guide with the screwdriver. The screw should not penetrate the posterior cortex of the vertebral body.
- After drilling the hole, the second distraction screw is placed into the middle third of the superior vertebral body parallel to the first screw (Fig. 19.5b).
- The distractor is pushed onto the distraction screws as far as possible up to the screw base plates.
- After distraction, an operating microscope with powerful illumination should be used to improve the magnification and lighting.
- Discectomy: following the incision of the anterior annulus (Fig. 19.6a), the disc is completely removed from the cranial and caudal end plates and in between the medial borders of the uncinate processes (Fig. 19.6b). Adequate posterior disc removal is accomplished when the white, vertically organized fibers of the posterior longitudinal ligament are well visualized.
- In the case of extruded and sequestered disc fragments (Fig. 19.6c), perforations of the posterior longitudinal ligament (OPLL) can be identified under microscopical view. It is important to open the OPLL to explore all sequestered epidural disc fragments. In most cases, it is not necessary to remove all portions of the OPLL, unless fragments have migrated bilaterally and extensively [6].
- If spondylosis/osteophytes are present, it is necessary to recreate an interspace height with parallel preparation of the end plates with cylindrical or coronial burrs and to remove posterior osteophytes with drills and Kerrison rongeurs.
- The complete resection of osteophytes is checked with a blunt hook under fluoroscopic control (Fig. 19.7).

19.6.3 Preparation of Bone Graft Side: Bone Graft Harvesting and Impacting of the Bone

- The bone graft site is prepared with curettes and burrs, as far as possible plane parallel.
- The height and a.p. depth of the intervertebral space are measured with a gauge (Fig. 19.8).
- Graft harvesting: the most commonly used area to harvest tricortical grafts for ACDF is the anterior iliac crest.
- A skin incision and muscular detachment with monopolar is performed over the anterior iliac crest.
- A tricortical bone graft with parallel cut edges is prepared (oscillating saw with appropriate size for the graft) (Fig. 19.9a). A graft cutter is set to the measured depth of the intervertebral space, and the correctly sized bone graft is then cut from the iliac crest (Fig. 19.9b).
- The bone graft is drilled and then screwed onto the graft holder (Fig. 19.10).
- The graft is impacted with slight press fit under image intensifier guidance.

19.6.4 Cages

- The use of structural autografts for ACDF is related to a relatively high rate of morbidity at the donor site in the range of 10–25%.
- As an alternative, a variety of interbody cages are now available for use in the cervical spine. The materials used are carbon fiber, polyether ether ketone (PEEK), titanium, or bioabsorbable implants. The cages can be classified into screw-in, box-type, and cylindrical design categories.
- Interbody cages should provide the immediate load-bearing capacity while allowing bony fusion.

19.6.5 Plating

- Indications and techniques for the use of anterior cervical plates are described in detail in Chap. 21

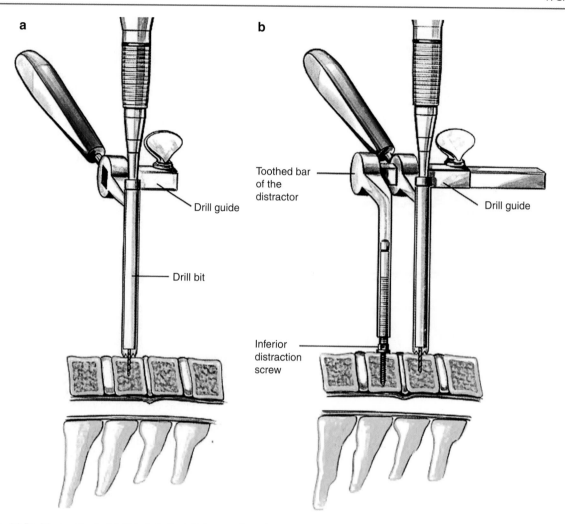

Fig. 19.5 (**a**) Positioning the first drill hole in the inferior vertebra with the drill guide. (**b**) Sitting the second (superior) distraction screw (With permission Aesculap AG, Tuttlingen, Germany)

19.7   Postoperative Care

Patients can be mobilized on the day of surgery approximately 4–6 h after surgery.

Soft drain for 24 h. In the case of ACDF, a soft collar is applied for 6–8 weeks postoperatively.

19.8   Tips and Tricks

- Monitoring of the endotracheal cuff pressure and its release after retractor placement can decrease the rate of recurrent laryngeal nerve temporary paralysis [1].
- Excessively, longus colli dissection can cause Horner's syndrome. The incidence varies from 0.2% to 2% [2, 5]. Therefore, longus colli dissection should be limited to 4 mm of the muscle.

- Each of the surgical steps must be monitored and performed individually using an image intensifier.
- Adequate visualization is essential for performing the decompression procedure safely. A microscope with powerful illumination should be used to improve the magnification and lighting.
- Width of decompression of the spinal canal: for an adequate decompression, an approximately 15-mm bony dissection centered over the midline is necessary. If nerve root decompression is part of the surgical procedure, a wider discectomy/decompression on one or both sides may be necessary.
- Manipulation of the nerve root is particularly problematic with the C5 nerve root, which appears to be more vulnerable to injury. Therefore, extreme care should be taken during performing discectomies in the level C4/5. C5 palsy is more common in posterior approaches.

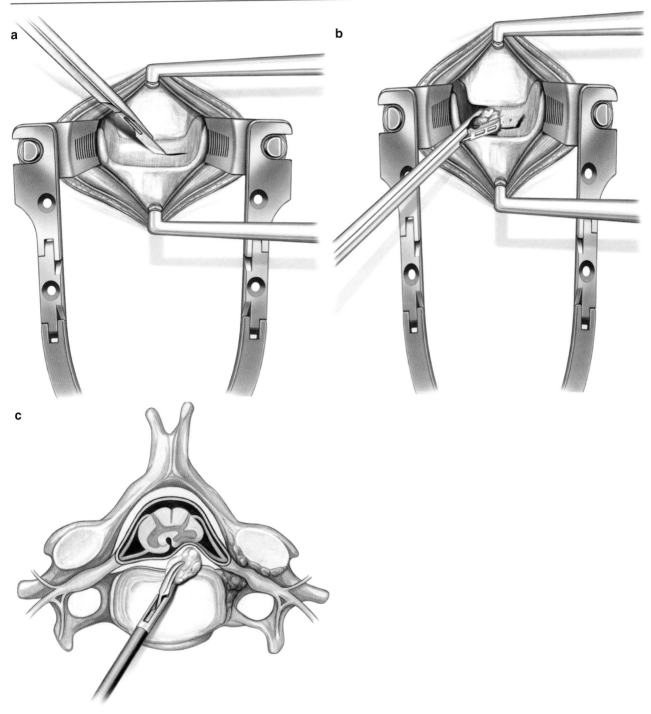

Fig. 19.6 (**a**) Incision of the anterior annulus. (**b**) The disc is completely removed. (**c**) Removal of sequestrates disc fragments

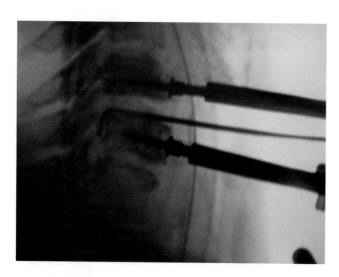

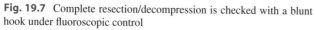

Fig. 19.7 Complete resection/decompression is checked with a blunt hook under fluoroscopic control

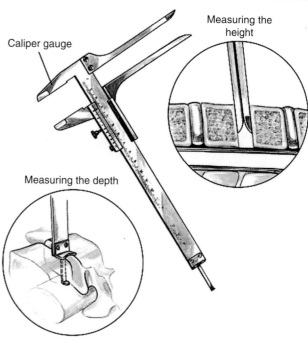

Fig. 19.8 Measuring the height and the depth of the intervertebral space (With permission of Aesculap AG, Tuttlingen, Germany)

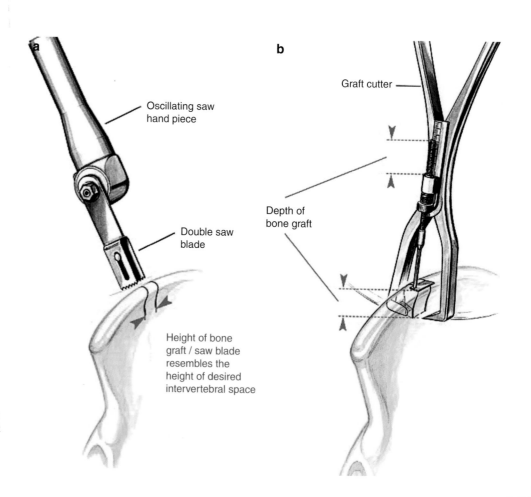

Fig. 19.9 (**a**) Bone graft harvesting from the iliac crest with oscillating saw. (**b**) Graft cutter (With permission Aesculap AG, Tuttlingen, Germany)

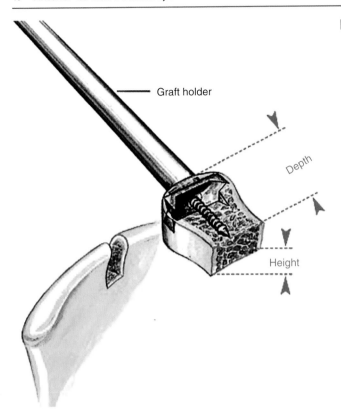

Fig. 19.10 The bone graft is drilled and screwed onto the graft holder (With permission Aesculap AG, Tuttlingen, Germany)

References

1. Apfelbaum RI, Kriskovich MD, Haller JR (2000) On the incidence, cause, and prevention of recurrent laryngeal nerve palsies during anterior cervical spine surgery. Spine 25:2906–2912
2. Bertalanffy H, Eggert HR (1989) Complications of anterior cervical discectomy without fusion in 450 consecutive patients. Acta Neurochir (Wien) 99:41–50
3. Beutler WJ, Sweeney CA, Conolly PJ (2001) Recurrent laryngeal nerve injury with anterior cervical spine surgery risk with laterally of surgical approach. Spine 26:1337–1342
4. Cloward RB (1958) The anterior approach for removal of ruptured discs. J Neurosurg 15:602–614
5. DePalma A, Rothmann R, Lewinnek G et al (1972) Anterior interbody fusion for severe cervical disc degeneration. Surg Gyecol Obstet 134:755–758
6. McCulloch JA, Young PH (eds) (1998) Essentials of spinal microsurgery. Raven Lippincott, Philadelphia
7. Robinson RA, Smith GW (1955) Anterolateral cervical disc removal and interbody fusion for cervical disc syndrome (abstract). Bull John Hopkins Hosp 96:223–224

Uncoforaminotomy

Kirsten Schmieder

20.1 Introduction and Core Message

In carefully selected cases and in experienced hands, this surgical method provides good clinical results and preserves motion in the affected segment [8, 9]. Uncoforaminotomy is a minimally invasive surgical technique. The approach uses the uncovertebral joint to create direct access to the neuroforamen. Within the bony canal, there is a close proximity between the bony borders and the nerve root. In cases of an additional hard or soft disc disease, a significant narrowing or obstruction is present. Via a ventral route on the side of the symptoms, the offending lesion is removed resulting in a decompression of the nerve root in its neuroforaminal segment. Since the disc itself is left in place, motion of the segment can be preserved [5, 6].

20.2 Indications

- Unilateral disc herniation
- Unilateral osseous foraminal stenosis
- Unilevel hard or soft disc disease
- Bisegmental foraminal obstruction
- Failed conservative treatment
- Neurological deficit correlating with the radiological finding

20.3 Contraindications

- Cervical myelopathy
- Multilevel hard or soft disc pathology
- Ossification of the posterior ligament
- Bilateral foraminal obstruction
- Segmental instability
- Kyphotic malalignment of the cervical spine

20.4 Technical Prerequisites

Fluoroscopy, operation microscope, adequate instrumentation for ventral discectomy (punches, forceps, ball piler), and drill (rosen und diamant, preferable high-speed drilling system).

- Caspar retractor system or similar retractor for ventral approach to the cervical spine
- No additional implantation system required

K. Schmieder, M.D., Ph.D.
Department of Neurosurgery, University Hospital Mannheim,
University of Heidelberg, Theodor-Kutzer-Ufer 1-3, 68167
Mannheim, Germany
e-mail: kirsten.schmieder@umm.de,
kirsten.schmieder@nch.ma.uni-heidelberg.de

U. Vieweg, F. Grochulla (eds.), *Manual of Spine Surgery*,
DOI 10.1007/978-3-642-22682-3_20, © Springer-Verlag Berlin Heidelberg 2012

Fig. 20.1 Anterior approach to the cervical spine on the side of the offending lesion and the symptomatology

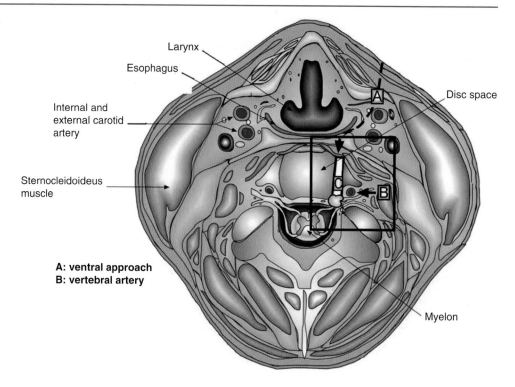

Larynx

Esophagus

Internal and external carotid artery

Sternocleidoideus muscle

Disc space

A: ventral approach
B: vertebral artery

Myelon

20.5   Planning, Preparation and Positioning

Prior to surgery, MRI or CT scans are reviewed to see where exactly within the neuroforamen the offending process is located. Vertebral artery on the side of the approach has to be localized. Knowledge of normal anatomy of the uncovertebral joint and the surrounding structures is essential. The patient is placed on its back, and the head is on a horseshoe-like positioning device. The fluoroscopy is draped sterile.

20.6   Surgical Technique

20.6.1 Approach

An anterior approach to the cervical spine is performed on the side of the patient's complaints (Fig. 20.1). The skin incision is placed in relation to the affected segment on the anterior border of the sternocleidomastoid muscle about 3 cm long (same incision used for ACDF). At the ventral surface of the cervical spine, the self-retaining retractor is inserted and placed above the longus colli muscle (Figs. 20.2 and 20.3). No Caspar pins are placed in the adjacent vertebral bodies. After lateralization of the longus colli muscle at the level of the disc, the lateral border of the adjacent vertebral bodies is identified, and the uncovertebral joint is localized (Fig. 20.4).

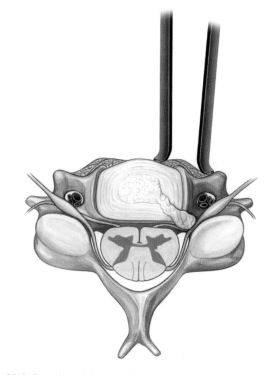

Fig. 20.2 Insertion of the retractor system

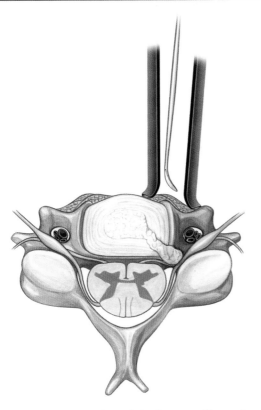

Fig. 20.3 Lateral mobilization of the longus colli muscle with a dissector

20.6.2 Microsurgical Decompression

- Drill an upper uncoforaminotomy down to the neuroforamen (Fig. 20.5) [3, 7].
- Prevent a too lateral drilling (vertebral artery!) [1, 2].
- Control the direction and depth with fluoroscopy [4].
- Beware that at level C6/7, the vertebral artery enters the cervical spine from lateral.
- Identify the neuroforamen after reaching the posterior border of the vertebral body (Fig. 20.6).
- Remove the longitudinal ligament above the nerve root.
- Remove offending disc material or osseous spurs.
- Identify the nerve root.
- Make sure that the lateral osseous portion of the neuroforamen is removed.
- Using a small dissector or nerve hook, the medial part of the foramen is checked (Fig. 20.7).
- Using a small punch, remaining parts of the longitudinal ligament are removed if necessary (Fig. 20.8a, b).
- Control the localization of the removed disc material with the morphology on the preoperative images.
- Follow the course of the nerve root into the neuroforamen (Figs. 20.9).

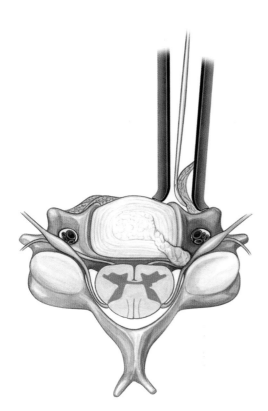

Fig. 20.4 Identification of the lateral border of the vertebral body and the uncus

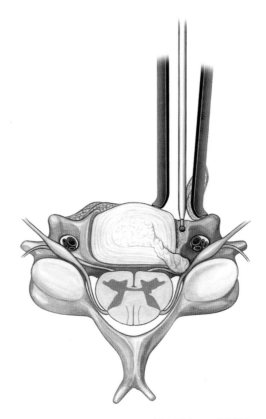

Fig. 20.5 Upper uncoforaminotomy with a high speed drill (cave: vertebral artery!)

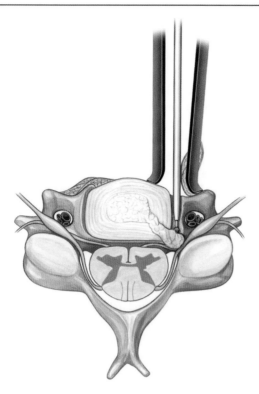

Fig. 20.6 Mobilization of the disc material with a nerve hook

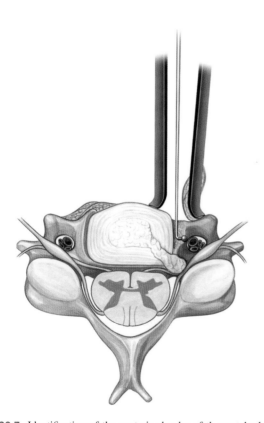

Fig. 20.7 Identification of the posterior border of the vertebral body and the neuroforamen

a

b

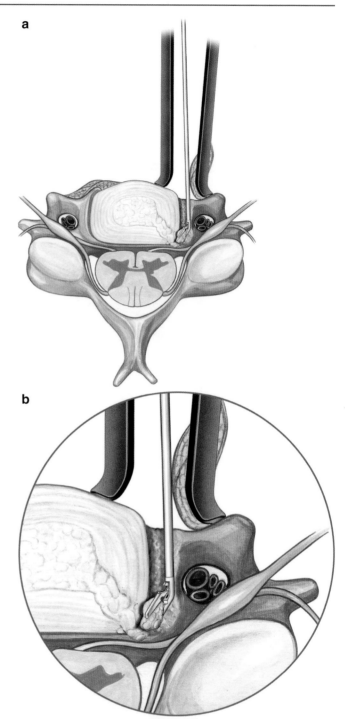

Fig. 20.8 (**a**, **b**) Removal of the disc material with a small punch

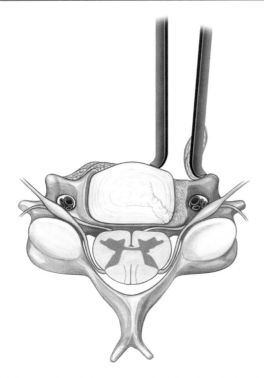

Fig. 20.9 Inspection of the nerve root in its intraforaminal part

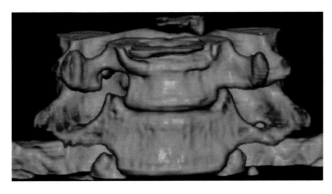

Fig. 20.10 Postoperative CT scan of the uncoforaminotomy

20.7 Tips and Tricks

- In the event of a venous bleeding from the epidural intraforaminal plexus, use a small collagen sponge and a cotton to apply gentle pressure and wait for some time. It will stop bleeding, and the removal of the material is possible. In some cases, a small piece of collagen sponge has to be left in place.
- If the insight into the neuroforamen is not sufficient, an enlargement of the uncoforaminotomy may be necessary. If so, drill away the adjacent part of the vertebral body offending the direct view into the neuroforamen.

References

1. Benazzo F, Alvarez AA, Nalli D et al (1994) Pathogenesis of uncus deformation and vertebral artery compression: histologic investigations of the uncus and dynamic angiography of the vertebral artery in the cadaveric spine. J Spinal Disord 7:111–119
2. Ebraheim NA, Lu J, Haman SP et al (1998) Anatomic basis of anterior surgery on the cervical spine: relationships between uncus-artery-root complex and vertebral artery injury. Surg Radiol Anat 20:389–392
3. Hayashi K, Yabuki T (1985) Origin of the uncus and of Luschka's Joint in the cervical spine. J Bone Joint Surg 67:788–791
4. Hirsch C, Schajowicz F, Galante J (1967) Structural changes in the cervical spine – a study on autopsy specimens in different age groups. Acta Orthop Scand 109(Suppl):34–41
5. Jho HD (1996) Microsurgical anterior cervical foraminotomy for radiculopathy: a new approach to cervical disc herniation. J Neurosurg 84:155–160
6. Jho HD (2003) Editorial: failed anterior cervical foraminotomy. J Neurosurg Spine 98:121–125
7. Orofino C, Sherman MS, Schlechter D (1960) Luschka's Joint – a degenerative phenomenon. J Bone Joint Surg 42:853–858
8. Pechlivanis I, Brenke C, Scholz M, Engelhardt M, Harders A, Schmieder K (2008) Treatment of degenerative cervical disc disease with uncoforaminotomy – intermediate clinical outcome. Minim Invasive Neurosurg 51:211–217
9. Schmieder K, Kettner A, Brenke C, Harders A, Pechlivanis I, Wilke HJ (2007) In vitro flexibility of the cervical spine after ventral uncoforaminotomy. Laboratory investigation. J Neurosurg Spine 7:537–541

Anterior Cervical Discectomy, Fusion, and Plating

21

Tobias Pitzen

21.1 Introduction and Core Message

Anterior cervical discectomy, fusion, and plating is a routine technique in both neurosurgical and orthopedic surgery. Here, indications, technical prerequisites, approach, and performance as well as tips and tricks to avoid complications are illuminated. Anterior cervical decompression and fusion using an autologous bone graft has been developed by Bailey and Badgley [1] and refined by Cloward [7], Smith and Robinson [18], and Verbiest [21]. Using this technique for fixation of traumatic instability of the cervical spine, it was shown that the treated segment was prone to displacement [20]. To avoid graft complications such as graft dislocation or graft settling and to avoid the necessity of an external orthosis – i.e., a halo body jacket – anterior cervical plating was first used by Hermann [9], who published his experiences in 1975. Several other authors already had reported their results [2, 8–12, 19, 21] when Caspar in 1989 [3] presented a standardized technique using a unique system of instruments for positioning, approach, decompression, fusion, and stabilization as well-suitable implants (bicortical screws and plates). Since then, the plate has been redesigned several times, and monocortical screws as well as thicker revision screws have been developed, and several other plate designs have been developed.

21.2 Indications

Any pathology of the anterior aspect within the subaxial cervical spine may be treated by anterior decompression and bone graft (or cage) insertion followed by stabilization using

the plate and screws. In particular, the main indications for this procedure include [3–6]:

- Degenerative disease of the cervical spine (with the clinical signs of radiculopathy and/or myelopathy)
- Trauma
- Tumor
- Rheumatoid instability
- Spondylodiscitis
- Failed surgery of the cervical spine

21.3 Contraindications

- Hypersensitivity to any of the implant materials

21.4 Technical Prerequisites

Adjustable head-neck rest according to Caspar (Aesculap, Tuttlingen, Germany), head fixed using a clamp according to Mayfield or Gardner-Wells, shoulders pulled down by tape. C-arm, microscope, high-speed drill.

21.5 Planning, Preparation, and Positioning

The patient is placed supine with the head on an adjustable head-neck rest and the head additionally fixed by an elastic band and a cervical traction (see Fig. 21.1). A c-arm is placed under the rest and used for intraoperative visualization. It is very helpful and time effective to have the c-arm permanently placed throughout the time of surgery within a lateral projection of the cervical spine.

21.6 Surgical Technique

21.6.1 Approach

- Perform standard anterolateral cervical approach, cross midline by 1 cm

T. Pitzen, M.D., Ph.D.
Department of Spine Surgery, SRH Klinikum Karlsbad-Langensteinbach,
Guttmannstrasse 1, 76307 Karlsbad, Germany
e-mail: tobias.pitzen@kkl.srh.de

U. Vieweg, F. Grochulla (eds.), *Manual of Spine Surgery*,
DOI 10.1007/978-3-642-22682-3_21, © Springer-Verlag Berlin Heidelberg 2012

Fig. 21.1 Schematic drawing of the patient positioned on the adjustable neck-head rest (With permission of Aesculap AG, Tuttlingen, Germany)

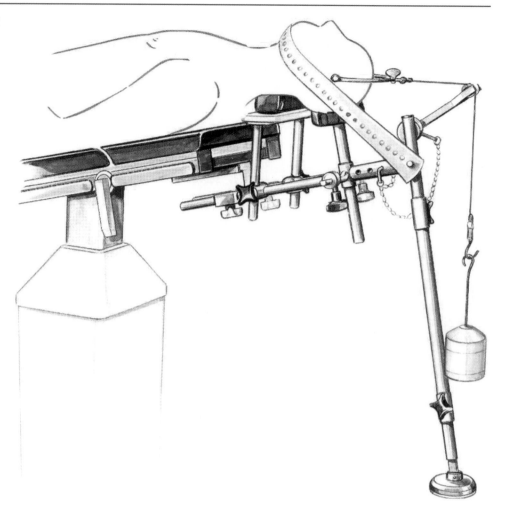

- Mark target level by needle insertion, not deeper than 2 mm into the disc, checked by fluoroscopy
- Mark the midline (diamond drill)
- Detach longus colli muscle
- Insert the sharp blades of the Caspar Cervical Retractor (CCR, Aesculap, Tuttlingen, Germany) under the detached areas of the longus colli muscle, connected to the self-holding spreader (see Fig. 21.2)
- Use blunt blades within another retractor of the CCR system (see Fig. 21.3). For longitudinal opening of the wound

21.6.2 Instrumentation

- Insert distraction screws within the vertebral bodies.
- Perform slight distraction via the vertebral body distractor (see Fig. 21.4).
- Remove the disc.
- Resect anterior osteophytes (shape the anterior aspect of the spine toward normal anatomic conditions).
- Keep these bone chips to fill a monosegmental cage (see Fig. 21.5).

- Remove posterior osteophytes using rongeurs or high-speed drills (see Fig. 21.6).
- Resect the posterior longitudinal ligament.
- Insert the cage under slight disc traction, remove distractor.
- Length of the plate is determined using lateral fluoroscopy (it should not touch the adjacent discs and should be adopted (using different bending forceps) to the patient's individual lordosis).
- Fix the plate temporarily by spikes in the upper and lower vertebral bodies exactly in the midline.
- Drill two burr holes into each vertebral body, insert the screws in a convergent angle. The screws should be as long as possible. However, perforation of the posterior cortical shell is not necessary (see Fig. 21.7): There is no proof that bicortical screw fixation is necessary to ensure tight fixation [13, 16].
- In case of bad bone quality resulting in a free spinning screw, there are two options: one may use a rescue screw or enlarge the burr hole, fill in bone cement, and insert the screw again. When using bone cement, we prefer to tighten the screw finally after hardening of the cement.

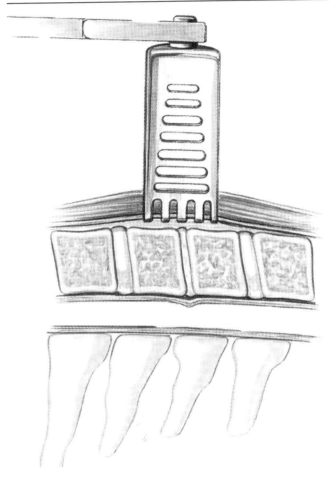

Fig. 21.2 Schematic drawing of the left-right (sharp) blades under the detached longus colli muscle (With permission of Aesculap AG, Tuttlingen, Germany)

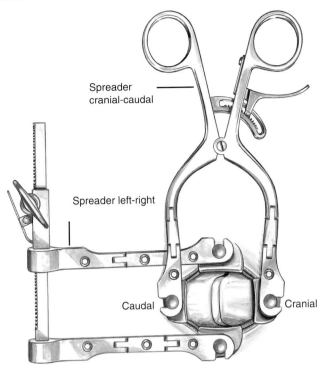

Fig. 21.3 Schematic drawing of the left-right and longitudinal blades in place (With permission of Aesculap AG, Tuttlingen, Germany)

Usually, this technique results in very high insertional screw torque.
- Check the final situation by fluoroscopy. Figures 21.8 and 21.9 give an example of a perfectly placed four-segmental ABC plate (Aesculap, Tuttlingen, Germany) in ap as well as lateral projection

Resection of One or More Vertebral Bodies

- Excise the corresponding discs
- Decompress the thecal sac where spinal encroachment is least
- Resect the vertebral body by rongeurs first – graft the bone for filling of the cage for vertebral body replacement (see Fig. 21.10)
- Resect the posterior wall by a sharp high-speed drill
- Resect the posterior longitudinal ligament by a 2-mm rongeur
- Insert the cage under slight disc traction, remove distractor
- Continue as described above.

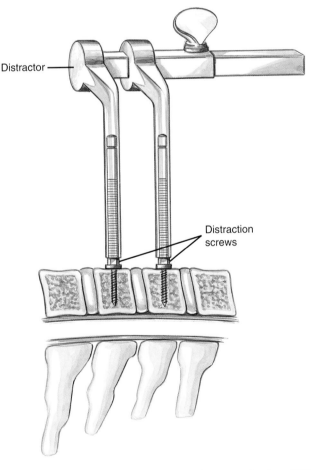

Fig. 21.4 Schematic drawing of the distraction screws in place (With permission of Aesculap AG, Tuttlingen, Germany)

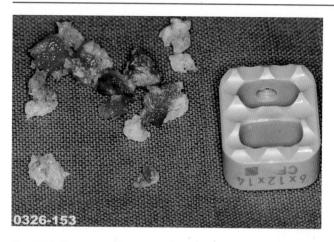

Fig. 21.5 Photograph of a cage and bone chips taken from the anterior rim of the target segment

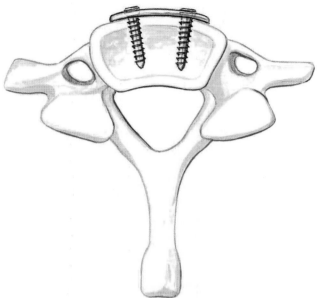

Fig. 21.7 Schematic drawing of the monocortical screws in place, axial view (With permission of Aesculap AG, Tuttlingen, Germany)

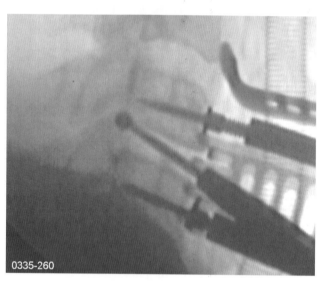

Fig. 21.6 Intraoperative x-ray, lateral projection. Posterior osteophytes are removed using a sharp drill

21.7   Tips and Tricks

- Note that any plate is designed to be fixed within the midline. Fixing the plate in the midline prevents screw malpositioning toward the roots. Therefore, it is of benefit to mark the midline (see above) before the longus colli muscle is detached. Using this technique, correct positioning of the plate is easy. The plate is temporarily fixed with two or more spikes. Also, try to adopt the contour of the plate to the anterior aspect of the spine using different bending forcepses. Removing anterior osteophytes facilitates adopting the plate.

- Although there is no evidence that filling the cervical spine cage is necessary for earlier fusion, it is easy to apply bone into the perforation of the cage used. To do so, grasp the bone from the adjacent anterior rims of the disc removed. This technique has been described and evaluated by the author [14].

- Next, the importance of lateral fluoroscopy cannot be overemphasized, check the direction as well as the position of the screw. Again, to my knowledge, there is no proof that engaging the screws into the posterior cortical shell does increase the initial postoperative stability or pullout force or screw torque [13, 16]. Note, however, that the screws should be as long as possible. Therefore, the author prefers to orient the screws toward the adjacent discs if possible.

- Insertional screw torque is important to obtain tight implant fixation [17]. Therefore, if the screw can just be inserted with very low torque or the screw is even free spinning, do not hesitate to use a thicker screw (revision or rescue screw) or to enlarge the burr hole, to fill the burr hole with bone cement (methylmethacrylate cement), and to insert the screw again. After hardening of the cement, the screw is finally tightened with usually very high torque. The authors never saw any implant loosening using this technique.

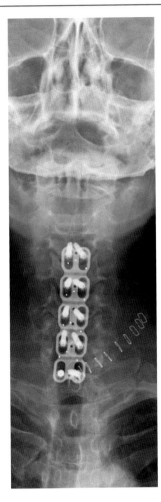

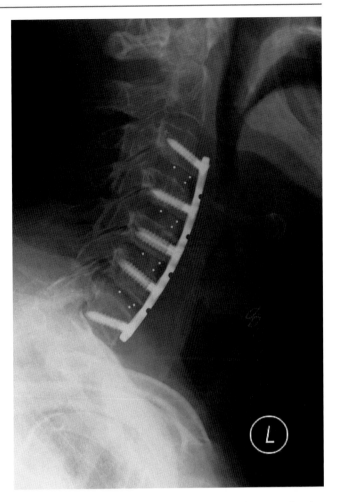

Fig. 21.8 AP and lateral projection of a cervical spine x-ray, showing a four-segmental plate in perfect position following four-segmental ACDF with bone-filled cage

Fig. 21.9 AP and lateral projection of a cervical spine x-ray, showing a four-segmental plate in perfect position following four-segmental ACDF with bone-filled cage

- An anterior cervical plate may be used for any kind of instability within the anterior part of the cervical spine as mentioned above. Even in case of limited posterior instability – that does not involve the capsular ligaments or the facets – anterior stabilization using this plate is sufficient [15]. The use of an anterior plate following monosegmental discectomy and fusion is usually not necessary. However, there are at least some clues that anterior additional plating reduces the rate of graft complications and pseudarthrosis. Resection of more than one vertebral body, however, or complete vertebrectomy or instability within the cervicothoracic junction usually calls for additional posterior instrumentation to avoid severe loss of correction or deformity.

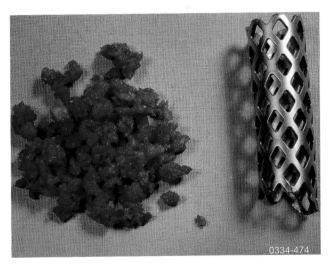

Fig. 21.10 Photograph of a Harms cage for vertebral body replacement and bone chips made from the resected vertebral body

References

1. Bailey RW, Badgley CE (1960) Stabilization of the cervical spine by anterior fusion. J Bone Joint Surg Am 42:565–594
2. Böhler J, Gaudernack T (1980) Anterior plate stabilization for fracture-dislocations of the lower cervical spine. J Trauma 20:203–205
3. Caspar W, Barbier D, Klara PM (1989) Anterior cervical fusion and Caspar plate stabilization for cervical trauma. Neurosurgery 25:491–502
4. Caspar W, Geisler F, Pitzen T et al (1998) Anterior cervical plate stabilization in one – and two – level degenerative disease: overtreatment or benefit? J Spinal Disord 11:1–11
5. Caspar W, Pitzen T (1999) Anterior cervical fusion and trapezoidal plate stabilization for re – do surgery. Surg Neuro 52:345–352
6. Caspar W, Pitzen T, Papavero L et al (1999) Anterior cervical plating for the treatment of neoplasms in the cervical spine. J Neurosurg Spine 1:27–34
7. Cloward RB (1998) The anterior approach for removal of ruptured discs. J Neurosurg 15:602–617
8. De Olivera JC (1987) Anterior plate fixation of traumatic lesions of the lower cervical spine. Spine 12:324–331
9. Hermann HD (1975) Metal plate fixation after anterior fusion of unstable fracture dislocation of the cervical spine. Acta Neurochir 32:101–111
10. Karasick D (1993) Anterior cervical spine fusion: struts, plugs and plates. Skeletal Radiol 22:85–94
11. Orozco DR, Llovet TR (1972) Osteosintesis en las lesiones traumaticas y degeneratives de la columna vertebral. Revista Traumatol Chirurg Rehabil 1:45–52
12. Papadopoulos MS (1993) Anterior cervical instrumentation. Clin Neurosurg 40:273–285
13. Pitzen T, Barbier D, Tintinger F et al (2002) Screw fixation to the posterior cortical shell does not influence peak torque and pullout in anterior cervical plating. Eur Spine J 11:494–499
14. Pitzen T, Kiefer R et al (2006) Filling a cervical spine cage with local autograft: change of bone density and assessment of bony fusion. Zentralbl Neurochir 67:8–13
15. Pitzen T, Lane C, Goertzen D, Dvorak M et al (2003) Anterior cervical plate fixation: biomechanical effectiveness as a function of posterior element injury. J Neurosurg 99:84–90
16. Pitzen T, Wilke HJ, Caspar W, Steudel WI, Claes L (1999) Evaluation of a new monocortical screw for anterior cervical fusion and plating by a combined biomechanical and clinical study. Eur Spine J 8:382–387
17. Ryken TC, Clausen JD, Traynelis VC, Goel VK (1995) Biomechanical analysis of bone mineral density, insertion technique, screw torque, and holding strength of anterior cervical plate screws. J Neurosurg 83:324–329
18. Smith GW, Robinson RA (1985) The treatment of cervical spine disorders by anterior removal of the intervertebral disc and interbody fusion. J Bone Joint Surg Am 40:607–624
19. Tippits R, Apfelbaum R (1998) Anterior cervical fusion with the Caspar instrumentation system. Neurosurgery 22:1008–1013
20. Van Petegham PK, Schweigel JF (1979) The fractured cervical spine rendered unstable by anterior cervical fusion. J Trauma 19:110–114
21. Verbiest H (1969) Antero-lateral operation for fractures and dislocations in the middle and lower parts of the cervical spine. J Bone Joint Surg Am 51:1489–1530

Uwe Vieweg

22.1 Introduction and Core Messages

Anterior cervical discectomy is the most common surgical procedure used to treat damaged cervical discs. Its goal is to relieve pressure on the nerve roots or on the spinal cord by removing the ruptured disc. In the operation, the soft tissues of the neck are separated and the disc is removed. In order to maintain the normal height of the disc space, the surgeon may choose to fill the space with a bone graft or cage. This chapter describes the implantation of a fusion cage.

22.2 Indications

- Degenerative disease of the cervical spine with clinical signs (radiculopathy, myelopathy) as described in Chap. 19
- Single or multilevel soft disc herniation
- Disc ligament injuries with additional plating [1–3]

22.3 Contraindications

- Predominant posterior compression of the neural structures

22.4 Technical Prerequisites

Fluoroscopy, operating microscope, adequate instrumentation for ventral discectomy (punches, forceps), high-speed drill (rose and diamond), Caspar retractor system (see

Fig. 22.8) or similar retractor for ventral approach to the cervical spine. A ring retractor system (Synthes Synframe) is an alternative. Different interbody fusion cages can be used (see Fig. 22.12a–f).

22.5 Planning, Preparation and Positioning

The patient is positioned supine on the operating table, and the head is supported on a Mayfield horseshoe headrest. General anaesthetic giving optimal muscle relaxation is administered. The neck is placed in a neutral position with the aid of fluoroscopy. Note: shoulder roll placed between scapulae to increase neck extension in this patient whose fracture reduced in extension (see Fig. 22.1). The arms are tucked to the side. Wrist restraints with long extensions or shoulder tape can be useful to enhance X-ray visualization (see Fig. 22.2a–c). The location of the incision is estimated

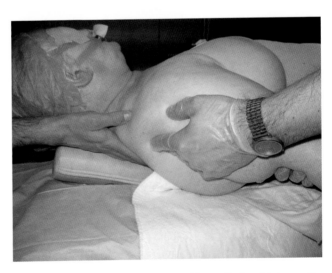

Fig. 22.1 Positioning of the patient with a roll placed between the shoulder blades. Padding is placed under the shoulders

U. Vieweg, M.D., Ph.D.
Clinic for Spinal Surgery, Sana Hospital Rummelsberg,
90593 Schwarzenbruck, Germany
e-mail: uwe.vieweg@yahoo.de

U. Vieweg, F. Grochulla (eds.), *Manual of Spine Surgery*,
DOI 10.1007/978-3-642-22682-3_22, © Springer-Verlag Berlin Heidelberg 2012

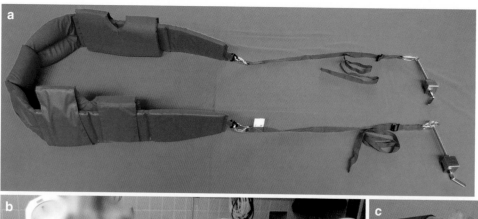

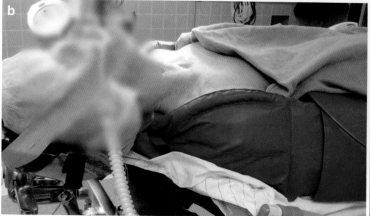

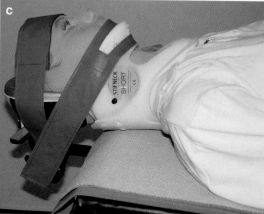

Fig. 22.2 (**a–c**) Special shoulder-, arm-, head-fixation systems

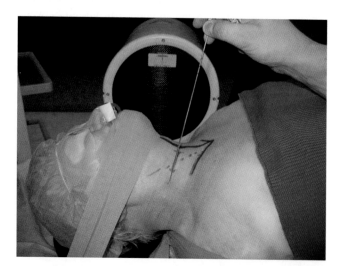

Fig. 22.3 Marking of the skin incision with the aid of the C-arm

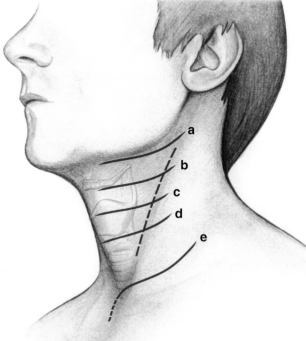

using the lateral fluoroscopic image (see Fig. 22.3). Localization of the skin incision to the level of pathology via external landmarks (see Fig. 22.4): hard palate – arch of atlas, lower border of mandible – C2/3, hyoid – C3, thyroid cartilage – C4/5, cricoid cartilage – C6 and carotid tubercle (anterior transverse process) – C6.

Fig. 22.4 (**a**) Skin incision in relation to the anatomical level. External landmarks are hard palate – arch of atlas, (**b**) lower border of mandible – C2/3, (**c**) hyoid – C3, thyroid cartilage – C4/5, (**d**) cricoid cartilage – C6, (**e**) carotid tubercle (anterior transverse process) – C6

22.6 Surgical Technique [1–3]

22.6.1 Approach

- The Cloward standard approach to the anterior cervical spine [2] is recommended (see Fig. 22.6).
- A transverse skin incision should be made on the left or right side for access. The author prefers access from the right. (see Fig. 22.4 demonstrated the incisions on the left side). The recurrent laryngeal nerve may be traumatized during the deepest layer of the approach. Many surgeons prefer a left side approach because the nerve takes a more predictable course on this side, descending into the thorax with the carotid sheath, curving around the aortic arch and ascending between the trachea and oesophagus to supply the larynx. On the other hand, a right side approach may be easier for a right-handed surgeon. Yet, the recurrent laryngeal nerve descends with the carotid sheath and curves around the subclavian artery to ascend into the neck at a higher level than on the left.
- The incision should be medial to the anterior border of the sternomastoid muscle and should extend to the midline. For cosmetic reasons, we recommend a diagonal incision along the Langer's line. Alternatively, a longitudinal incision can be made along the anterior edge of the sternocleidomastoid muscle.
- The skin is undermined in a cranial and caudal direction.
- Immediately following the incision, the platysmas muscle is identified and incised (see Fig. 22.5). Directly beneath the skin lies the platysma, which may be divided longitudinally (in line with the fibres) with the tip of the index

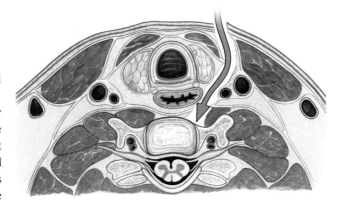

Fig. 22.6 Axial schematics of the Smith-Robinson approach (standard anterolateral approach) to the middle anterior cervical spine, trachea, strap muscle, longus coli muscle, pretracheal fascia, prevertebral fascia, superficial fascia

fingers. Alternatively, the platysma may be divided, without functional consequences, in line with a transverse incision.
- The deep cervical fascia is next identified as an investing layer that splits around the sternocleidomastoid. It is superficial to all of structures of the neck except the platysma and external jugular vein. The sternocleidomastoid may now be gently laterally retracted (see Fig. 22.5).
- Blunt dissection using scissors reveals the carotid sheath (carotid artery, internal jugular vein, vagus nerve).
- When the omohyoid muscle has been found, it should be passed either cranially (C2–5) or caudally (C5–T2) or should be severed.
- The trachea and oesophagus are moved towards the middle, and the carotid artery and jugular vein are moved to the side. Both are then protected with metal retractors which can occasionally cause a sore throat or hoarseness for a short time after surgery.
- The attachments of the longus colli muscle are separated on both sides by means of alternating use of scissors, bipolar forceps and swab (see Fig. 22.7).
- The relevant disc is localized using intraoperative fluoroscopy.
- Once the correct level has been identified, the longus colli muscles are moved away from the lateral edge of the anterior cervical vertebra so that retractors will be able to engage the tissue (see Fig. 22.8).
- Ventral spondylophytes are removed with a high-speed drill or Luer.
- After exposure of the anterior aspects of the spine and detachment of the medial insertion of the longus colli muscles on both sides, the soft tissue is retracted using the Caspar cervical retractor. Retractor valves are inserted under the belly of each muscle (see Fig. 22.8). The cervical ring of the Synframe retractor system can also be used as an alternative.

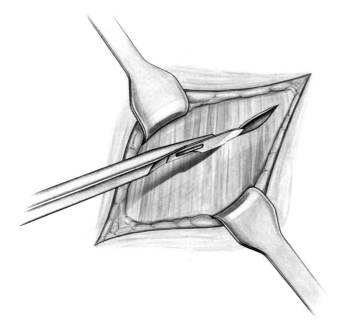

Fig. 22.5 Identification and incision of the platysmas muscle

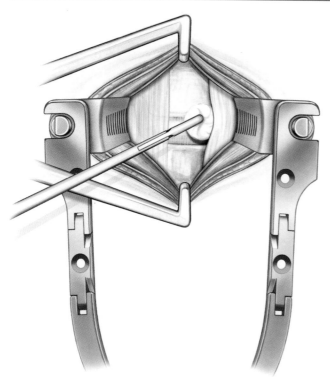

Fig. 22.7 Pushing the two longus colli muscles aside with small swabs

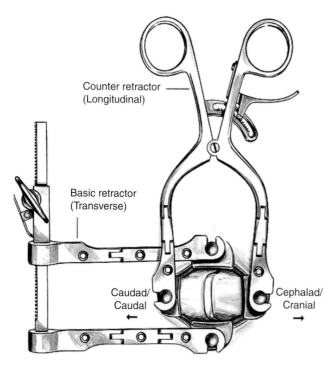

Counter retractor (Longitudinal)

Basic retractor (Transverse)

Caudad/ Caudal ←

Cephalad/ Cranial →

Fig. 22.8 Caspar cervical retractor system in position (With permission of Aesculap AG, Tuttlingen, Germany)

22.6.2 Discectomy and Decompression

- The midline between the two longus colli muscles is marked using a small diamond burr.
- The Caspar distraction screws are positioned. Note: they should be placed centrally in the midline of the vertebral body.
- A drill guide is used to position the drill hole for the first distraction screw in the middle of the inferior vertebral body. The drilling depth of the drill is fixed at 8 mm to exclude the possibility of inadvertent penetration into the spinal canal. The drilling direction is usually approximately parallel to the adjacent vertebral end plates. The screw should not penetrate the posterior cortex (see Chap. 19). Screws with self-cutting threads should be used. The correct choice of thread length is determined by the anteroposterior diameter of the vertebral body. The screw should not penetrate the posterior cortex.
- The distraction screw is inserted through the drill guide using the screwdriver. Care must be taken to screw in the distraction screw right up to its base plate in order to embed it firmly in the vertebral body. This prevents screw pullout during the distraction process.
- After removing the moveable distractor arm, the drill guide is fitted onto the toothed distractor bar, and this assembly is positioned over the distraction screw which is already in place.
- After drilling in the centre of the vertebral body, the second (superior) distraction screw is screwed in, and the drill guide assembly is removed. The drill guide is subsequently taken off the distractor bar and replaced by the moveable distractor arm.
- The disc is then excised near the anterior longitudinal ligament and detached using a sharp spoon and curette (Fig. 22.9).
- The disc should be completely removed from the cranial and caudal end plates and laterally from the uncovertebral joints, with Kerrison rongeurs and straight curettes (see Fig. 22.10a, b).
- Discectomy is completed under mild distraction, and decompression of the neural structures is then performed. The posterior longitudinal ligament is normally retrieved and detached as far as is necessary to remove osteophytes using the longitudinal ligament dissector.
- The dorsal spondylosis is ablated with a high-speed burr and punch, and the posterior longitudinal ligament is removed. Note: when the high-speed diamond burr is used to remove the dorsal edge or dorsal osteophytes, care should always be taken to ensure that the end plates remain undamaged.

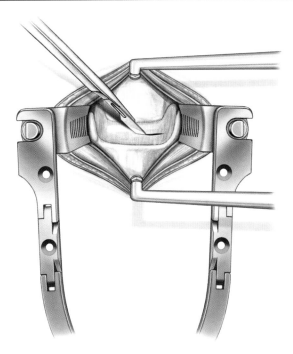

Fig. 22.9 Cutting into the disc with a microscapel

- After the disc has been removed, the posterior longitudinal ligament is also removed revealing the anterior aspect of the dura.

22.6.3 Cage Implantation

- Once the neural structures have been fully decompressed, the appropriate implant size can be determined with the aid of the trial implants (see Fig. 22.11a).
- Using the insertion instrument set, the cage is introduced into the intervertebral space (see Fig. 22.11b). The implant should usually lie centrally about 1–2 mm in front of the rear edge.
- By relaxing the Caspar retractor, the ligaments are reactivated so that the implant is held securely in the intervertebral space (see Fig. 22.11c). The cage must be firmly held and not easy to move!

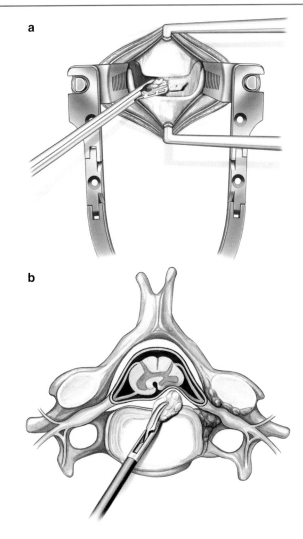

Fig. 22.10 (**a**, **b**) Removal of the disc with rongeurs

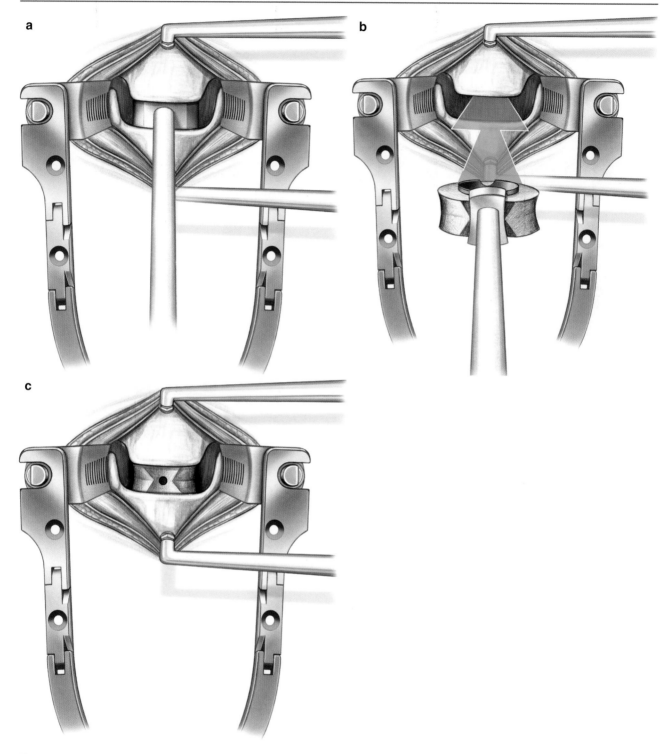

Fig. 22.11 (**a**) Determining implant size. (**b**) Cage implantation. (**c**) Cage in situ

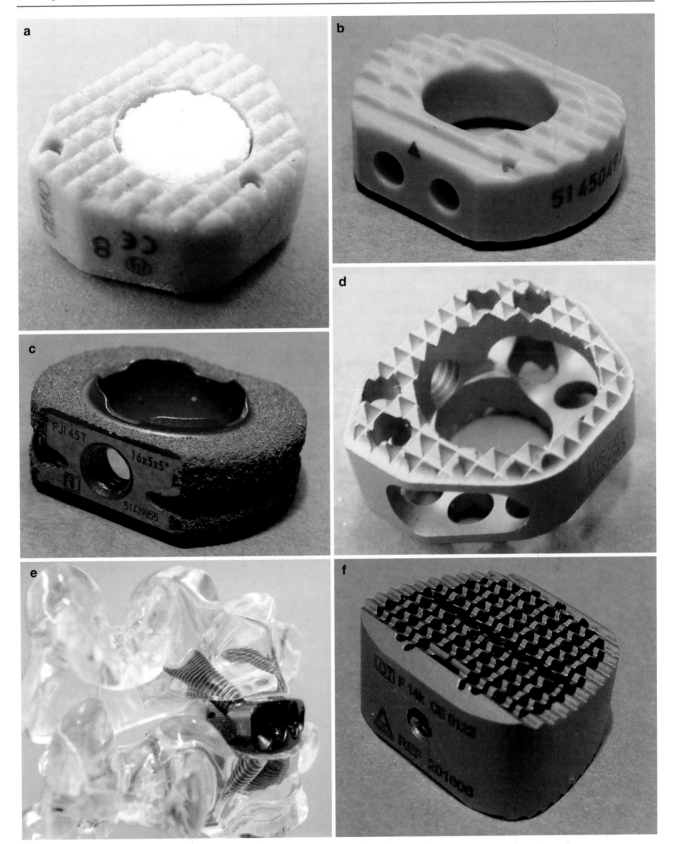

Fig. 22.12 Different interbody fusion cages. (**a**) Syncage with Chronos (Synthes). (**b**) C-Space PEEK (Aesculap). (**c**) C-Space Titan Plasmapore-coated (Aesculap). (**d**) Cervios Titan cage (Synthes). (**e**) Zero-P cage with integrated plate (Synthes). (**f**) Hydro Deltacor

References

1. Bailey RW, Badgley CE (1960) Stabilization of the cervical spine by anterior fusion. J Bone Joint Surg Am 42:565–594
2. Cloward RB (1958) The anterior approach for removal of ruptured discs. J Neurosurg 15:602–617
3. Smith GR, Robinson RA (1958) The treatment of certain cervical spine disorders by anterior removal of the intervertebral disc and interbody fusion. J Bone Joint Surg Am 40:607–624

Implantation of a Cervical Disc Prosthesis

23

Bernhard Bruns and Uwe Vieweg

23.1 Introduction and Core Messages

Anterior cervical decompression and interbody fusion with an internal fixation device (ACDF – anterior cervical decompression and fusion) has, for some time, been the classic treatment for cervical spondylosis, but this technique could result in accelerated degeneration of the adjacent level. It was hypothesised that this degeneration could be prevented or at least decelerated by replacing the diseased disc with a prosthesis and thus preserving motion. Over the last decades, numerous disc prostheses designs have been developed and have been approved for specific indications. The evidence available to date indicates that they help to prevent or slowdown degeneration of the adjacent disc and segment [4, 13]. Disc replacement can restore the physiological curvature and range of motion of the cervical vertebrae to a greater extent than other forms of treatment [1, 2, 5]. Implantation of a cervical disc prosthesis consists of two fundamental steps. The first is decompression of the neural structures, for which a conventional approach via the left or right blood vessel compartment is usually taken. The second step involves thorough preparation of the site followed by secure, central placement of the implant in the prepared space.

23.2 Indications

Clear

Clinically proofed and accepted
- Soft disc prolapse
- Symptomatic cervical discopathy with neck and/or arm pain with or without neurological deficit concordant with MRI of disc pathology

Questionable

- Preoperative segmental kyphosis or "straight neck"
- Narrow, hard disc
- Acute myelopathy with MRI signal changes
- Osteophytic and sclerotic changes of the vertebral bodies
- Anterior or posterior longitudinal ligament ossifications

B. Bruns, M.D. (✉)
Department of Neurosurgery,
Hospital Meiningen,
Bergstrasse 3, Meiningen, Germany
e-mail: bernhard.bruns@klinikum-meiningen.de

U. Vieweg, M.D., Ph.D.
Clinic for Spinal Surgery, Sana Hospital Rummelsberg,
90593 Schwarzenbruck, Germany
e-mail: uwe.vieweg@yahoo.de

U. Vieweg, F. Grochulla (eds.), *Manual of Spine Surgery*,
DOI 10.1007/978-3-642-22682-3_23, © Springer-Verlag Berlin Heidelberg 2012

23.3 Contraindications

- Spinal deformities following trauma and laminectomy
- Spondylarthrosis, facet joint degeneration
- Chronic degenerative spinal stenosis
- Segmental instability (more than 3 mm of translation)
- Segmental immobility (segmental mobility less than 2° in flexion and extension)
- Chronic myelopathy
- Osteoporosis
- Metal (CoCrMo) allergy
- Pregnancy, rheumatoid arthritis, systemic illness
- Deformation of the end plates

23.4 Technical Requirement

- Head fixed using a clamp according to Mayfield or Gardner-Wells
- C-arm
- Microscope
- High-speed drill

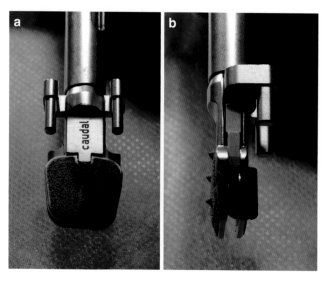

Fig. 23.1 (**a**, **b**) Activ C prosthesis in the implant holder

The primary goal of cervical arthroplasty is to remove the pathologically herniated disc while maintaining disc height and preserving motion. This chapter describes the implantation of the activ C prosthesis. The activ C intervertebral disc prosthesis is used to replace intervertebral discs in the cervical spine. The activ C intervertebral disc prosthesis consists of two components: superior prosthesis plate with spikes for anchoring in the vertebral body and inferior prosthesis plate with integrated polyethylene inlay and central anchoring fin for fixation in the vertebral body. The prosthesis plates and the polyethylene inlay together form a ball-and-socket joint. The polyethylene inlay is anchored to form-fit in the inferior prosthesis plate (see Fig. 23.1).

The activ C intervertebral disc prosthesis is available in six different sizes (XS, S, M, L, XL, and XXL) and up to three different heights (5, 6, and 7 mm). Activ C intervertebral disc prostheses are supplied fully pre-assembled.

- Many designs have been advocated as replacements for cervical discs. They consist of either articulating or non-articulating components constructed from various materials (see Table 23.1 and Fig. 23.2).

23.5 Planning, Preparation, and Positioning

- Patient's neck is placed in a neutral position – not in hyperlordosis which is routinely used for anterior fusion techniques (see Fig. 23.3b).
- If necessary, the operating position is adjusted according to a preoperative X-ray of the patient standing in a neutral position.
- Positions of the head, the cervical spine, and the patient are fixed.
- Radiographic visibility of the relevant segments (lateral and anteroposterior (AP) views) is ensured.

Note: Positioning of the patient's neck in hyperlordosis can result in inappropriate positioning of the prosthesis. During the operation, the alignment of the prosthesis and the spinal segment can wrongly appear as "correct." As soon as

Table 23.1 Different artificial disc prosthesis with different design details [1–3, 7–12]

Device	Prestige	Activ C	Bryan	ProDisc C	Cervicore	Porous coated motion
Company	Medtronic	Aesculap	Medtronic	Synthes	Stryker	
Articulating materials	Metal-metal	Metal-polyethylene	Metal-polyethylene	Metal-polyethylene	Metal-metal	Metal-polyethylene
Theoretical centre of rotation location	Superior vertebra	Directly below the inferior plate	Within implant	Inferior vertebra	Superior and inferior vertebra	Inferior vertebra
Initial fixation	Screws	Combination of spikes and keel	Milled bone	Keels	Screws and spikes	Ridges

Fig. 23.2 Classification of different designs for cervical arthroplasty by the Cervical Spine Study Group on "artificial cervical nomenclature" [6]

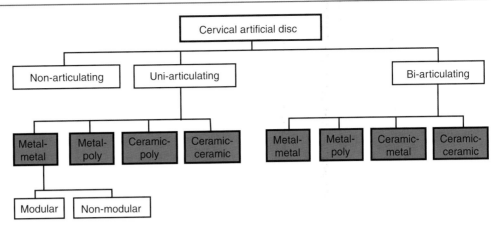

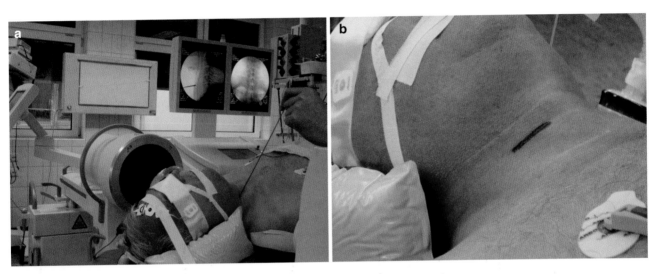

Fig. 23.3 Skin incision (**b**) and planning of the skin incision. A horizontal "cosmetic" skin incision targeted with fluoroscopy (**a**)

the spine returns to a neutral position in post-operative daily life, the segment and the prosthesis can fall into a kyphotic position.

23.6 Surgical Technique

23.6.1 Approach

- A standard anterolateral approach allows a precise view of all anterior parts of the cervical spine that are affected during a discectomy and the implantation of a disc prosthesis.
- Subaxial cervical spine can be approached from the right or left side depending on surgeon's preference.

- Most surgeons approach the upper part from the right and the lower part (C5/6 and C6/7) from the left side because of the anatomical positions of the recurrent nerves.
- A horizontal "cosmetic" skin incision, targeted using fluoroscopy, is currently preferred (see Fig. 23.3b).
- The medial sheet is sharply cut, and the anterior spine is accessed by approaching between the neuromuscular bundle (v. jugularis, a. carotis, vagus nerve) and the visceral organs (trachea and oesophagus).
- Cutting of the pre-vertebral lamina allows sharp dissection of the walls of the medial longus colli muscle. This step is important in order to anchor the wound distractor firmly and safely (regarding oesophagus) beneath the muscle bundles. Alternatively, a Synframe (Synthes) or Caspar retractor (Aesculap) (see Fig. 23.4) can be used.

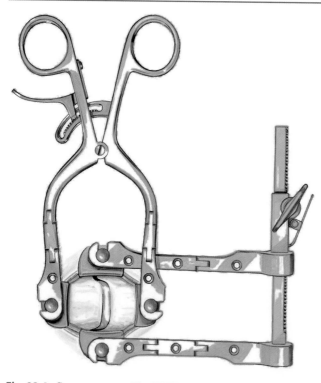

Fig. 23.4 Caspar retractor. The PEEK material provides enough biomechanical stability and, which feature of radiolucency excellent visibility in both lateral and AP fluoroscopic view (With permission of Aesculap AG, Tuttlingen, Germany)

23.6.2 Instrumentation

- Midline marking
  The midline of the vertebral body in the sagittal plane is usually determined from the following anatomic landmarks: position of the longus colli muscles, axis of symmetry of the anterior vertebral surface, and midline between the processi uncinati (see Fig. 23.4). The midline is most reliably determined in AP X-rays from the position of the spinous processes and the midline between the uncinate processes. The midline must be permanently marked with a bone chisel or high-speed drill or by inserting midline pins/Caspar. After verification of the midline position, the pins can be removed and replaced with the Caspar screws, using the same bone hole screws (see Fig. 23.5a, b). *Note*: A final check of the midline should be made after placing the trial implant in the disc space.
- Preparation of the disc space
  Discectomy is performed using standard procedures. The cartilaginous end plate has to be removed completely, but care should be taken to avoid any damage to the integrity of the bony end plates. Decompression of neural elements has to be precise and complete (microsurgical technique). In lateral soft disc prolapse, the posterior longitudinal ligament can be preserved as a tension band on the asymptomatic side and in the midline. Burrs, cutters, reamers, or drills can be used for foraminal decompression or cutting off the posterior osteophytes. Bone preparation should be kept

a
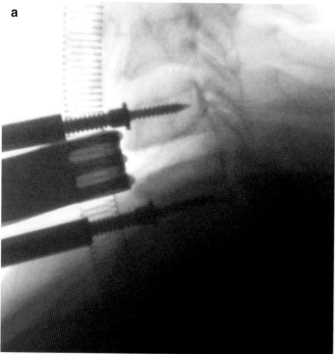

b
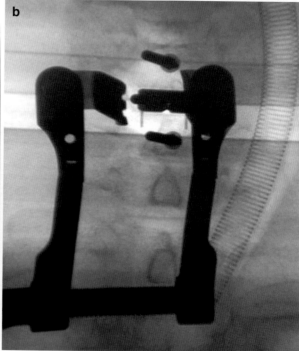

Fig. 23.5 Position of the midline marking pins or Caspar screws (**a** – lateral; **b** – AP view)

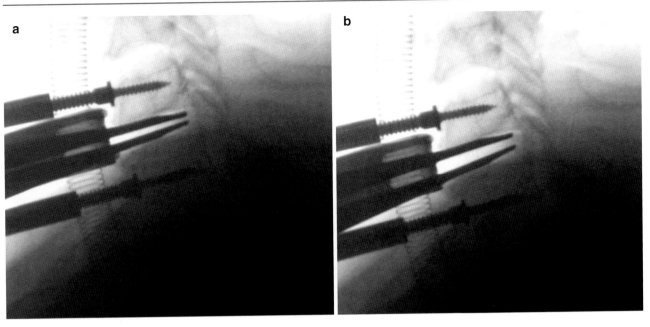

Fig. 23.6 Distraction forceps are used for distracting the treated segment. (**a**) without and. (**b**) with distraction

minimal in order to avoid creating too much bone powder as this can serve as a focal point for later ossification. Preparation of the posterior uncus should be limited to one-third of the total structure to avoid instability of the segment.

- Distraction with Caspar retractor or distraction forceps
  Once the midline has been determined and the disc compartment prepared (partial discectomy), the Caspar screws for the distractor are inserted.
  Note: For fusion procedures, the Caspar screws are usually applied centrally in lateral alignment, and the distraction force is transmitted via their shafts. In activ C implantation, however, the Caspar distractor serves as a distraction holding device. The self-locking mechanism assures its stability and keeps the vertebral end plates parallel. Maximal distraction force is created by means of distraction forceps, and the interbody distance enlargement is passively followed by moving the distractor longitudinally.
  Distraction forceps are used for distracting the treated segment. The forceps are applied to the posterior part of the intervertebral space under fluoroscopic control. Distraction is increased gradually in parallel fashion. Step-by-step distraction allows relaxation of the ligaments (see Fig. 23.6a, b). The height of the space in the treated segment should be compared with adjacent segments to avoid over-distraction. Careful observation of joint fissure enlargement can be helpful. The forceps are equipped with a locking mechanism to hold the distance.
- Trial implant (see Fig. 23.7a, b)
  Inserting the trial implant – verifying the size of the required disc implant.

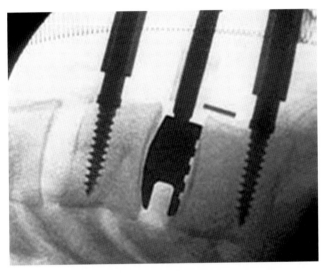

Fig. 23.7 Under X-ray control, tap the trial implant into the disc compartment until the safety stop touches the anterior side of the vertebral body

The safety stop position is adjusted in the AP direction with the adjusting wheel. The safety stop is moved forwards by turning the adjusting wheel counterclockwise and backwards by turning the adjusting wheel clockwise. Initially, the safety stop is moved forwards as far as possible. The trial implant is then tapped into the disc compartment until the safety stop touches the vertebral body from anterior. The size (depth and height) of the trial implant is inspected under X-ray control. If necessary, adjusting wheel is turned clockwise to move the safety

Fig. 23.8 (**a**, **b**) Preparation of the keel groove. The figures show burr holes (No. 1 and 2) in lateral X-ray view. The latter runs immediately next to the trial implant. Both burr holes end 1.5 mm in front of the posterior edge of the trial implant

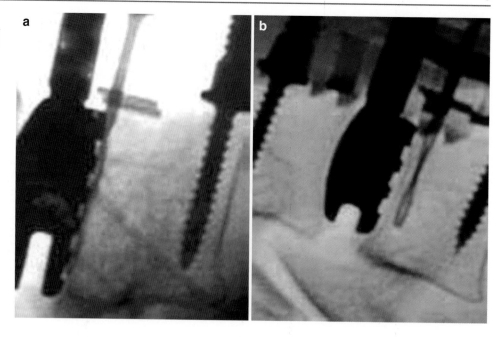

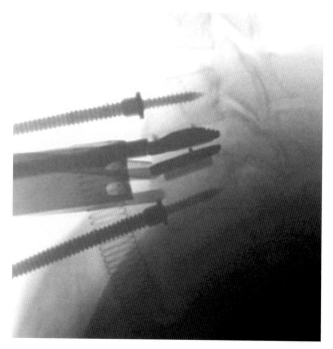

Fig. 23.9 Implantation of the prosthesis. The prosthesis is carefully inserted in the disc compartment by guiding the keel into the prepared keel groove

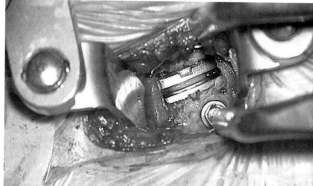

Fig. 23.10 Prosthesis in situ

trial implant is introduced in the distracted position. Over-distraction must be avoided. The trial implant should not be introduced too far posterior. *The midline and sagittal midplane must be respected.* Once the keel groove has been reamed, the position of the prosthesis is fixed and can no longer be changed.

- Preparation of the keel bed, keel groove, and reaming (see Fig. 23.8a, b)
- Implantation of the artificial disc (see Figs. 23.9 and 23.10)
  – Corresponding to the trial implant used
  – Apply slight distraction with the Caspar distractor
  – Attach the appropriate prosthesis to the insertion instrument
  – Introduce the artificial disc under lateral fluoroscopic control

stop back and push the trial implant in a posterior direction. Once the final position has been reached, the distraction is released to see the actual angulation of the segment. The distractor can be removed completely for a better view. The trial holder is unlocked and removed. *Note*: The

– Detach the insertion instrument
– Check the final position in AP and lateral view
– Correct the position if necessary
– Release distraction
– Check the position of the artificial disc

23.7   Tips and Tricks

• The surgeon naturally has a duty to explain the potential complications of disc prosthesis.
The operation can lead to infection, occasionally even sepsis and meningitis; secondary bleeding with or without respiratory problems; injury of the oesophagus, trachea, carotid artery, and jugular vein; injury of the recurrent nerve, spinal cord, and nerve roots; and cerebrospinal fluid fistula. Dislocation and migration of the implant must also be considered. With regard to the cervical spine itself, the possible complications are a loss of lordosis and increase in kyphosis, narrowing of the disc space, fracture of the end plates and heterotopic ossification (HO).

• When explaining the operation, it is important to describe alternative methods such as fusion techniques, dorsal decompression, and conservative treatment (physiotherapy, manual therapy osteopathy, and pain treatment).

• The dorsal edges of the bones should be sealed with bone wax.

• Choosing the appropriate prosthesis size and insertion position should prevent subsidence or extrusion of the prosthesis.

References

1. Anderson PA, Rouleau JP (2004) Intervertebral disc arthroplasty. Spine 29:2779–2786
2. Anderson PA, Sasso RC, Rouleau JP et al (2004) The Bryan cervical disc: wear properties and early clinical results. Spine J 4:303S–309S
3. Boden SD, Balderston RA, Heller JG et al (2004) An AOA critical issue. Disc replacements: this time will we really cure low-back and neck pain? J Bone Joint Surg Am 86:411–422
4. Chang UK, Kim DH, Lee MC et al (2007) Changes in adjacent level disc pressure and facet joint force after cervical arthroplasty compared with cervical discectomy and fusion. J Neurosurg Spine 7:33–39
5. DiAngelo DJ, Puttlitz CM (2006) Biomechanical aspects associated with cervical disk arthroplasty. In: Kim DH, Cammisa FP, Fessler RG (eds) Dynamic reconstruction of the spine. Thieme, New York/Stuttgart
6. Jaramllo-de La Torre J, Grauer JN, Yue JJ (2008) Update on cervical disc arthroplasty: where are we and where are we going? Curr Rev Musculoskelet Med 1:124–130
7. Kim SW, Shin JH, Arbatin JJ et al (2008) Effects of a cervical disc prosthesis on maintaining sagittal alignment of the functional spinal unit and overall sagittal balance of the cervical spine. Spine 17:20–29
8. Lafuente J, Casey AT, Perzold A et al (2005) The Bryan cervical disc prosthesis as an alternative to arthrodesis in the treatment of cervical spondylosis. J Bone Joint Surg Br 87:508–512
9. Leung C, Casey AT, Goffin J et al (2005) Clinical significance of heterotopic ossification in cervical disc replacement: a prospective multicenter clinical trial. Neurosurgery 57:759–763
10. Lin EL, Wang JC (2006) Total disk arthroplasty. J Am Acad Orthop Surg 14:704–714
11. Mummaneni PV, Haid RW (2004) The future in the care of the cervical spine: interbody fusion and arthroplasty. J Neurosurg Spine 1:155–159
12. Nabhan A, Ahlhelm F, Shariat K et al (2007) The Pro-Disc C prosthesis: clinical and radiological experience 1 year after surgery. Spine 32:1935–1941
13. Sekhon LH (2004) Cervical arthroplasty in the management of spondylotic myelopathy: 18-month results. Neurosurg Focus 15:E8

Overview of Surgical Techniques and Implants

24

Stefan Schären

24.1 Introduction and Core Messages

A posterior approach to the cervical spine is indicated in posteriorly situated lesions or as a supplement to anterior surgery. Great advancements in posterior instrumentation have been made over the last decades. Today, modern versatile rod-screw systems allow easy and stable fixation from the occiput to the upper thoracic spine. If surgery is indicated, the choice of the approach depends on etiology and location of the pathology and the functional spinal stability considering the options for appropriate decompression and stabilization. Posterior decompressive approaches are suited for cases of posteriorly situated lesions compressing the spinal cord and/or the exiting nerve roots. As an advantage, the posterior approach is relatively simple not being compromised by neural or vascular structures and can easily be extended if necessary. Also, the posterior bony elements are usually very strong, providing excellent purchase for implants even in the osteoporotic spine. Nevertheless, intact anterior column is an important prerequisite for a stable long-term result. In cases of anterior column defect or kyphotic deformity, anterior or combined approaches are indicated. Thanks to the continuous evolution of spinal instrumentation technology over the last decades, versatile and powerful implants are available that meet the specific demands of the cervical spine, adding immediate stability and increasing the fusion rate. The strength of the constructs allows minimal, if any, external bracing. In addition, the latest generation of implants is designed to be compatible with MRI and allows to rapidly asses adequate decompression of neural structures or progression of pathological lesions being treated. Due to the specific

characteristics the techniques of stabilization for the craniocervical junction, the atlantoaxial articulations, and the subaxial cervical spine will be discussed separately. In reality, pathologies rarely respect artificial boundaries but cross the various regions. Frequently, techniques must be combined. The modern modular implants which have been developed in the past decade are adapted to meet these specific anatomical characteristics.

24.2 Approach and Positioning

The patient is placed in prone position with cushion under his chest. Alternatively, a vacuum mattress or a spine frame may be used. The head is fixed in slightly flexed position on a padded U-shaped headrest. Alternatively, a Mayfield clamp can be used. A laterally placed image intensifier should be installed in fixed position. As with occipitocervical fusion, the neutral position of the head must be verified under image intensifier and compared to preoperative standard lateral radiograph. Reduction and traction (always under image intensifier) are possible if necessary (fracture dislocation, rheumatoid arthritis). The shoulders are pulled down with adhesive straps. Shaving of the back of the head and of the neck is required (patient must be informed prior to surgery!). A standard midline approach is performed, and the posterior elements of the spine of the levels to be addressed are exposed.

24.3 Occipitocervical Fusion

The craniocervical junction comprising occiput, atlas, and axis represents a complex transition zone from the cranium to the cervical spine. Its characteristic anatomy differs fundamentally from the subaxial spine. More than 50% of the flexion/extension and rotation of the head and neck occur in

S. Schären, M.D.
Department of Orthopaedic Surgery/Spine, University Hospital, Spitalstrasse 21, 4031 Basel, Switzerland
e-mail: sschaeren@uhbs.ch

U. Vieweg, F. Grochulla (eds.), *Manual of Spine Surgery*,
DOI 10.1007/978-3-642-22682-3_24, © Springer-Verlag Berlin Heidelberg 2012

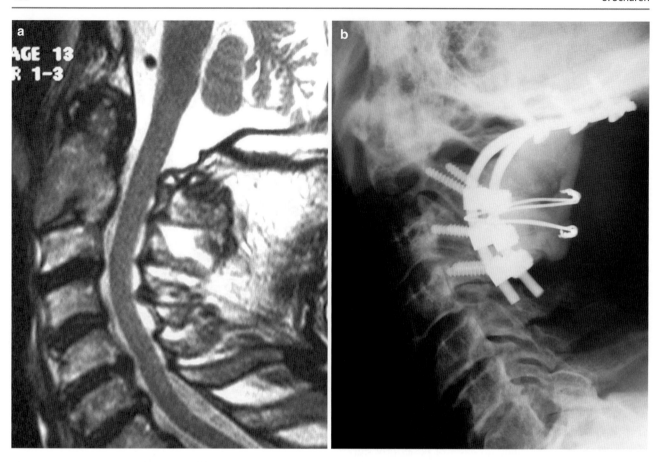

Fig. 24.1 (**a, b**) T2-weighted sagittal MRI of an 81-year-old patient with invalidating neck pain shows infiltration of corpus and dens axis by plasmocytoma (1A). Occipitocervical (C0–C4) stabilization with Cervifix® (Synthes, Oberdorf, Switzerland) was performed. In view of the malignant underlying disease of the lesion, the construct was augmented with PMMA (1B)

this area. As a result, high biomechanical forces and strong lever arms are acting and challenging the attempt of surgical stabilization. In order to neutralize these biomechanical forces, instrumentation constructs must therefore have adequate dimensions and sufficient rigidity. At the same time, the systems must offer great flexibility to be easily adapted to the multiple anatomical variations and leave enough room for grafting, allowing for bony fusion to take place. The first occipitocervical fusion was reported in 1927 by Foerster [7], who inserted a fibular graft between the occiput and C7 to stabilize a progressive atlantoaxial dislocation after an odontoid fracture. Since then, multiple methods of fusion in this area have been developed: simple onlay bone grafts with halo immobilization; wire, pin, or hook constructs; rigid metallic loops or rectangles fixed to the bone with wires or screws. Today, modular rod-screw systems have become the standard for occipitocervical stabilization in adults [1, 12, 17]. The systems can be fixed either by lateral mass screws or transpedicular screws to the subaxial spine and be attached to the suboccipital bone by plates. They are easy to contour and provide rigid internal fixation allowing immediate mobilization with no or minimal external support, while the fusion is taking place. High fusion rates are reported [1, 22]. In several biomechanical studies, superior stability of the rod-screw systems could be demonstrated [15, 17]. Most stable are constructs including C2 reducing the number of segments to be included in the fusion [6]. For good and safe anchoring to the suboccipital bone, it is essential to study preoperatively the thickness of the bone and the position of the dural sinuses on CT scans. In an anatomical study, the thickness was found to be 8 mm and more extending from the occipital protuberance bilaterally for 23 mm [5]. In pediatric patients, internal fixation techniques have been applied more hesitantly partly because fusion without internal fixation is achieved more easily and partly because the implants did not suit the smaller anatomy. Today, smaller implants are available, and there is a tendency toward internal fixation also in children [3]. Only anatomic constraints in children less than 1 year old usually still require fusion with onlay techniques (Fig. 24.1).

24.4 Atlantoaxial Fusion

Techniques for isolated C1–2 fusion have gradually evolved over the last several decades since Gallie described the placement of a notched bone graft between the posterior arch of the atlas and the spinous process of C2 secured by sublaminar

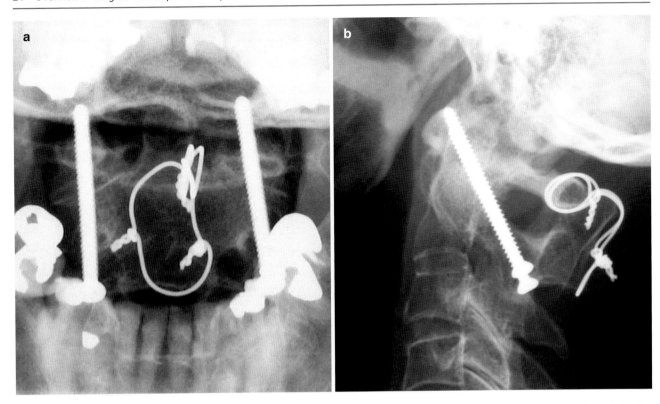

Fig. 24.2 (**a, b**) A 73-year-old female patient with painful atlantoaxial osteoarthritis. Transarticular screw fixation C1–C2 was performed showing solid fusion and stable implants at 24 months postoperatively

wires in 1939 [8]. The single midline fixation point provided only limited rotational stability requiring rigid postoperative immobilization, preferably a halo. Modifications by Brooks and Sonntag aimed to increase the rotational stability [4, 23]. The introduction of transarticular screws fixing the lateral masses of C1 and C2 by Magerl presented a major breakthrough in posterior atlantoaxial fixation [14]. The transarticular screws provide immediate stabilization. Mostly, a Gallie-type interspinous bone graft with or without wires is added providing a very stable three-point fixation. In case of incomplete or fractured posterior arch of the atlas, the atlantoaxial joints can be opened and packed with bone graft. Preoperatively, the diameter of the isthmus of C2 must be determined on CT reconstructions for safe passage of the screws without injury to the vertebral artery. If no safe screw can be inserted, unilateral C1–2 facet screw fixation with interspinous bone graft wiring was reported to still provide excellent stability leading to high fusion rates [10]. Drilling and insertion of the screws are performed under lateral fluoroscopic control. A specific aiming device and computer assistance can further increase safety of the technically demanding procedure [9, 18]. Olerud modified the Magerl technique in 2001, adding a clamp for C1 posterior arch fixation obviating the need for posterior wiring [16].

The only true contraindication for transarticular screws remains fixed/irreducible subluxation of C1–2. Trying to

overcome this shortcoming, Harms and Melcher described a novel technique of atlantoaxial stabilization in 2001 using polyaxial head screws inserted in the lateral mass of C1 and the pedicle of C2 [11]. The screws are bilaterally connected by rods. Fluoroscopically guided reduction of the atlantoaxial articulation can be performed if necessary, and a cancellous onlay bone graft can be used for fusion. In contrast to the transarticular screws, the lateral atlantoaxial joints are not affected, allowing removing the implants if only temporary fixation is required. Biomechanically, several studies demonstrated superior almost identical rigid internal fixation for the Magerl and the Harms technique [20]. Regarding safety, C2 pedicle screw placement was reported to have nearly the same anatomic risk of vertebral artery injury as transarticular screw placement (Fig. 24.2) [24].

24.5 The Subaxial Cervical Spine

Originally, various wiring techniques and laminar clamps systems have been used to stabilize the subaxial spine. Both methods provided only limited stability especially in rotation and translation, necessitating prolonged external fixation. Nevertheless, the incidence of nonunion and loss of correction was high. Sublaminar wires and laminar hooks also carried the risk of neurovascular injury. Lateral mass

Fig. 24.3 (**a–c**) Transdiscal fracture C5/6 in a 61-year-old patient with ankylosing spondylitis (3A). Considering the highly unstable injury in ankylosing spondylitis, posterior stabilization of C3/T2 using a polyaxial screw and rod system (Synapse, Synthes, Oberdorf, Switzerland) and fusion of C5/6 using iliac crest autograft were performed

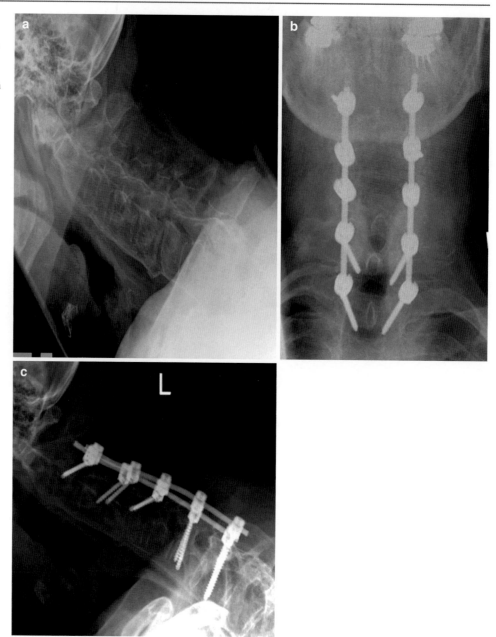

plate systems first described by Roy-Camille were biomechanically superior to laminar wire or clamp fixation [21]. In addition, unlike posterior laminar wiring or clamping, lateral mass plates did not require the presence of the posterior elements, which are often removed to facilitate decompression. However, the plates still were associated with a number of disadvantages like the given position of the screw holes, the limited insertion angle, and the insufficient angular stability between screw and plate. Subsequently, various versatile screw-rod systems have been developed which have become the standard for posterior stabilization [13, 19]. Its modular design allows easy contouring and offers almost unlimited flexibility regarding orientation and location of the screws. If necessary, the stabilization can easily be extended to the occiput and/or the thoracic spine. The screw-rod systems are anchored with lateral mass screws inserted according to the technique of Magerl or An [2, 13]. In recent years, pedicle screws for the cervical spine have been established as an alternative [1, 19]. Safety and accuracy of the technically demanding pedicle screws could be improved using computer navigation [18]. Biomechanically, the modern angle-stable screw-rod systems particularly with transpedicular fixation provide the most rigid stability reducing the risk of implant failure and until fusion takes place and allowing instrumentation of fewer segments (Fig. 24.3).

References

1. Abumi K, Takada T, Shono Y et al (1999) Posterior occipitocervical reconstruction using cervical pedicle screws and plate-rod systems. Spine 24:1425–1434

2. An HS, Gordin R, Renner K (1991) Anatomic considerations for plate-screw fixation of the cervical spine. Spine 16:S548–S551

3. Anderson RC, Ragel BT, Mocco J et al (2007) Selection of a rigid internal fixation construct for stabilization at the craniovertebral junction in pediatric patients. J Neurosurg 107(1 Suppl): 36–42

4. Brooks AL, Jenkins EB (1978) Atlanto-axial arthrodesis by the wedge compression method. J Bone Joint Surg Am 60:279–284

5. Ebraheim NA, Lu J, Biyani A et al (1996) An anatomic study of the thickness of the occipital bone. Implications for occipitocervical instrumentation. Spine 21:1725–1730

6. Finn MA, Fassett DR, Mccall TD, Clark R et al (2008) The cervical end of an occipitocervical fusion: a biomechanical evaluation of 3 constructs. Laboratory investigation. J Neurosurg Spine 9: 296–300

7. Foerster O (1927) Die Leitungsbahnen des Schmerzgefühls und die chirurgische Behandlung der Schmerzzustände. Urban & Schwarzenburg, Berlin

8. Gallie WE (1939) Fractures and dislocations of the cervical spine. Am J Surg 46:495–499

9. Gebhard JS, Schimmer RC, Jeanneret B (1998) Safety and accuracy of transarticular screw fixation C1-C2 using an aiming device. An anatomic study. Spine 23:2185–2189

10. Grob D, Bremerich FH, Dvorak J et al (2006) Transarticular screw fixation for osteoarthritis of the atlanto axial segment. Eur Spine J 15:283–291

11. Harms J, Melcher RP (2001) Posterior C1-C2 fusion with polyaxial screw and rod fixation. Spine 26:2467–2471

12. Jeanneret B (1996) Posterior rod system of the cervical spine: a new implant allowing optimal screw insertion. Eur Spine J 5:350–356

13. Jeanneret B, Schaeren S (2004) Posterior stabilization of the cervical and upper thoracic spine with the CerviFix®. Oper Orthop Traumatol 16:89–116

14. Magerl F, Seemann PS (1987) Stable posterior fusion of the atlas and axis by transarticular screw fixation. In: Kehr P, Weidner A (eds) Cervical spine, vol 1. Springer, Vienna

15. Oda I, Abumi K, Sell LC et al (1999) Biomechanical evaluation of five different occipito-atlanto-axial fixation techniques. Spine 24:2377–2382

16. Olerud S, Olerud C (2001) The C1 claw device: a new instrument for C1-C2 fusion. Eur Spine J 10:345–347

17. Richter M, Wilke HJ, Kluger P et al (2000) Biomechanical evaluation of a new modular rod-screw implant system for posterior instrumentation of the occipito-cervical spine: in-vitro comparison with two established implant systems. Eur Spine J 9:417–425

18. Richter M, Mattes T, Cakir B (2004) Computer-assisted posterior instrumentation of the cervical and cervico-thoracic spine. Eur Spine J 13:50–59

19. Richter M (2005) Posterior instrumentation of the cervical spine using the neon occipito-cervical system part 2: cervical and cervicothoracic instrumentation. Oper Orthop Traumatol 17:579–600

20. Richter M, Schmidt R, Claes L et al (2002) Posterior atlantoaxial fixation: biomechanical in vitro comparison of six different techniques. Spine 27:1724–1732

21. Roy-Camille R, Saillant G, Judet T et al (1983) Traumatismes Recents Des Cinq Dernieres Vertebres Cervicales Chez L'Adulte (Avec et sans complication neurologique). Sem Hop 59:1479–1488

22. Schaeren S, Jeanneret B (2002) Occipitocervical instrumentation. Tech Orthop 18:87–95

23. Sonntag VKH, Dickman CA (1993) Craniocervical stabilization. Clin Neurosurg 40:243–272

24. Yoshida M, Neo M, Fujibayashi S, Nakamura T (2006) Comparison of the anatomical risk for vertebral artery injury associated with the C2-pedicle screw and atlantoaxial transarticular screw. Spine 31:E513–E517

Foraminotomy

25

Frank Grochulla

25.1 Introduction and Core Messages

Posterior foraminotomy at the cervical spine is a minimal invasive microsurgical technique for the posterior decompression of nerve roots affected by lateral soft disc herniations or spondylotic formations in the foramen. The nerve root should be decompressed without affecting the stability of the cervical spine. Furthermore, this procedure is a motion – preservation technique.

25.2 Indications

- Lateral/foraminal soft disc herniation with nerve root compression and associated radicular symptoms
- Osteophytic foraminal nerve root compression with radicular symptoms

25.3 Contraindications

- Pathology near the midline, myeloradiculopathy
- Instability of the motion segment

25.4 Technical Prerequisites

High-speed burr, microscope, fluoroscopy, microsurgical instruments, Mayfield frame.

F. Grochulla, M.D.
Department for Spinal Surgery, Hospital for Orthopaedics, Trauma Surgery and Spinal Surgery, Euromed Clinic, Europa-Allee 1, 90763 Fürth, Germany
e-mail: frank.grochulla@euromed.de

25.5 Positioning

- Patient is placed in a prone position (Fig. 25.1).
- Three-point pin fixation device such as Mayfield tongs to secure the head (Fig. 25.2).
- *Note*: The neck should be slightly flexed and keep in a horizontal plane. Extreme flexion should be avoided as it may produce spinal cord ischemia.
- The table is placed in a head-up position (20–30°).
- Cushions or rolled blankets are applied under the chest and the pelvis to avoid abdominal compression (with secondary elevation of venous pressure of the epidural venous plexus).
- The patient is positioned in a prone position with rigid pin fixation to the skull.
- The cervical spine and head are in a neutral position or slightly flexed.
- X-ray is performed to determine the target level and to plan exactly the minimal invasive approach.

25.6 Surgical Technique [1–6]

- "Classic" median 2.5–3 cm skin incision across the target level and incision of the fascia.
- Subperiosteal dissection of the muscular and ligamentous tissues along the laminae of interest.
- The facet joint is exposed with the lateral mass above and below the target level.
- A tubular retractor system with black-coated surfaces (to avoid glare under microscopical view) is applied (Fig. 25.3).
- An alternative to the classic approach is the minimally invasive paramedian approach with 1.5-cm skin incision (under microscope or endoscope assistance).
- X-ray at this time is essential to confirm the correct level.
- Using a high-speed burr under the microscope, the foraminotomy is started at the junction between the lateral aspect

U. Vieweg, F. Grochulla (eds.), *Manual of Spine Surgery*,
DOI 10.1007/978-3-642-22682-3_25, © Springer-Verlag Berlin Heidelberg 2012

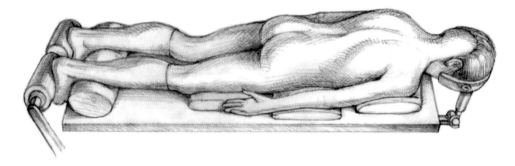

Fig. 25.1 Positioning in the prone position

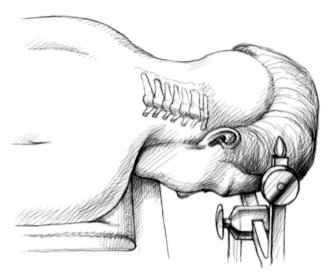

Fig. 25.2 Optional pin fixation of the head

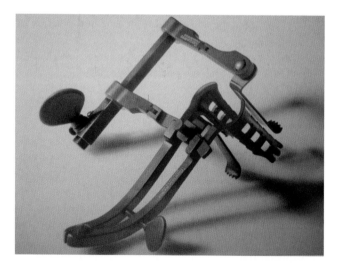

Fig. 25.3 Caspar tubular retractor system

- The size of the keyhole foraminotomy is approximately 8–10 mm in diameter.
- Careful blunt dissection and resection of the ligamentum flavum will expose at first the lateral portion of the dura as an anatomical landmark. Epidural venous bleeding from the perineural plexus or from the epidural plexus in the lateral spinal canal is a frequent problem at this time. A series of careful coagulations of the epidural tissues followed by cuttings with microscissors will avoid major epidural venous bleedings. If persistent venous bleeding occurs after coagulation, the use of hemostatic agents (e.g., Floseal, Fa. Baxter) is helpful to achieve absolute hemostasis.
- The nerve root, the axilla of the nerve root, and the lateral part of the dura is exposed.
- Soft disc sequestrations are often located in the axilla of the nerve root. When the compressed root has been exposed, a short blunt nerve hook is placed in the axilla, and the nerve root is retracted superiorly. It is important to be certain that the entire nerve root is retracted (separate dural sleeves of the motor and sensory roots may occur!). In the case of separated dural sleeves, the smaller motor nerve root is located anterior and caudal to the larger sensory root.
- After retraction, a blade is used to open the posterior longitudinal ligament, and disc herniation is then removed with small forceps. An adequate decompression is achieved, when the nerve root expands with CSF pulsations (Fig. 25.5).
- After removal of disc fragments, there is often additional space so that the foramen can be better explored and enlarged.
- Hemostasis and thorough irrigation of the wound.
- Wound closure: the paravertebral muscles, nuchal ligament, subcutaneous tissues, and skin are sutured.

of the interlaminar space and the medial border of the facet joint (Fig. 25.4a, b). One-third of the upper and lower laminae are drilled away, and laterally one-third but never more than one half of the facet joint is removed. The bone where the superior articular facet of the inferior vertebra meets the pedicle is also removed to gain access to the nerve root axilla.

25.7   Postoperative Care

- Soft collar for 2–4 weeks
- Anti-inflammatory medication and muscle relaxant
- Progressive neck exercise program

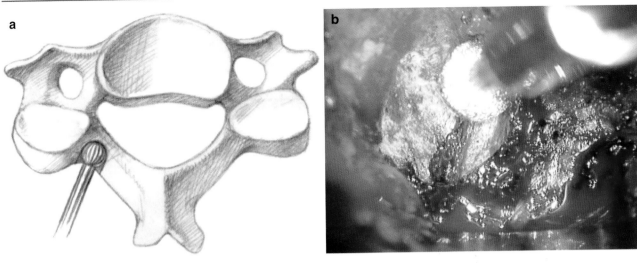

Fig. 25.4 (**a**) The foraminotomy is started at the junction between the lateral aspect of the interlaminar space and the medial border of the facet joint. (**b**) High-speed burr under microsurgical view

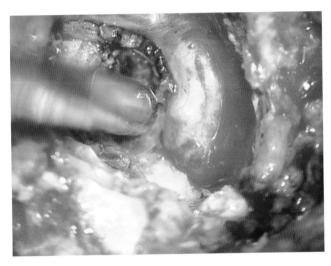

Fig. 25.5 Nerve root C8 after decompression

25.8 Complications and Pitfalls

Spinal cord and/or nerve root injury, CSF leakage, postoperative compressive hematoma, laceration of the vertebral artery, inadequate removal of the disc herniation or spondylotic bars with persistent radicular symptoms, deep paraspinous, or epidural wound infection.

25.9 Tips and Tricks

- Correct and careful positioning is important to reduce bleeding.
- The lateral facet capsule should be spared.

- When bleeding from the epidural venous plexus is encountered, it can be managed by the use of hemostatic agents such as Floseal (Baxter).

References

1. Burke TG, Caputy A (2000) Microendoscopic posterior cervical foraminotomy: a cadaveric model and clinical application for cervical radiculopathy. J Neurosurg 93:126–129
2. Chen BH, Natarajan RN, An HS, Andersson GB (2001) Comparison of biomechanical response to surgical procedures used for cervical radiculopathy: posterior keyhole foraminotomy versus anterior foraminotomy and discectomy versus anterior discectomy with fusion. J Spinal Disord 14:17–20
3. Clark CR (2005) The cervical spine, 4th edn. Lippincott Williams & Wilkins, Philadelphia, pp 1031–1042
4. Collias JC, Roberts MP (2000) Posterior surgical approaches for cervical disk herniation and spondylotic myelopathy. In: Schmidek HH, Sweet WH (eds) Operative neurosurgical techniques: indications, methods and results, 4th edn. WB Saunders, Philadelphia, pp 2016–2027
5. Fessler RG, Khoo LT (2002) Minimally invasive cervical microendoscopic foraminotomy: an initial clinical experience. Neurosurgery 51:S37–S45
6. Gala VC, O'Toole JE, Voyadzis JM et al (2007) Posterior minimally invasive approaches for the cervical spine. Orthop Clin North Am 38:339–349

Laminoplasty

26

Frank Grochulla

26.1 Introduction and Core Messages

The aims of the laminoplasty are to expand the spinal canal, to secure spinal stability, and to preserve the protective function of the spine. Preservation of mobility is also a goal of this procedure for multiple-level involvement. Cervical laminoplasty was developed in the early 1970s for the treatment of cervical myelopathy due to multilevel spondylosis or multilevel ossification of the posterior longitudinal ligament. Since then, a variety of laminoplasty techniques have been described (Fig. 26.1–26.3). In this chapter, the laminoplasty with the hardware-augmented open-door technique is described.

26.2 Indications

- Patients with cervical spinal canal stenosis (AP spinal canal diameter <13 mm) due to developmental multilevel spondylotic and ossification of the posterior longitudinal ligament origin, with straight or lordotic cervical alignment.

26.3 Contraindications

- Cervical spine instability
- Severe cervical kyphosis

26.4 Technical Prerequisites

High-speed burr, microscope, X-ray, microsurgical instruments, Mayfield frame, special laminoplasty systems (e.g., New Bridge Laminoplasty System (Blackstone Medical)).

26.5 Planning, Preparation, and Positioning

- Patient is placed in a prone position (Fig. 26.4).
- Three-point pin fixation device such as Mayfield tongs to secure the head.
- The neck should be slightly flexed and kept in a horizontal plane. Extreme flexion should be avoided as it may produce spinal cord ischemia.
- The table is placed in a head-up position (20–30°).
- Cushions or rolled blankets are applied under the chest and the pelvis to avoid abdominal compression (with secondary elevation of venous pressure of the epidural venous plexus).

F. Grochulla, M.D.
Department for Spinal Surgery, Euromed Clinic,
Europa-Allee 1, 90763 Fürth, Germany
e-mail: frank.grochulla@euromed.de

U. Vieweg, F. Grochulla (eds.), *Manual of Spine Surgery*,
DOI 10.1007/978-3-642-22682-3_26, © Springer-Verlag Berlin Heidelberg 2012

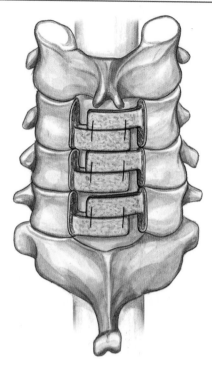

Fig. 26.1 Z-laminoplasty

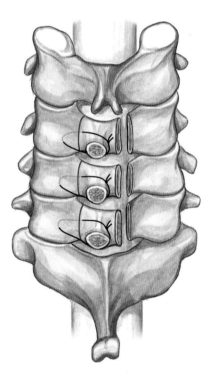

Fig. 26.2 Open-door laminoplasty

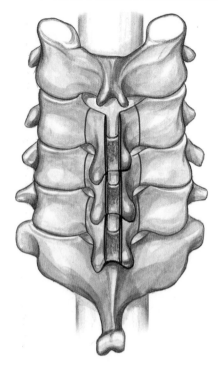

Fig. 26.3 Kurokawa laminoplasty

26.6   Surgical Technique

- Midline skin incision across the target region. For a C3–C7 laminoplasty, a 10–12-cm incision from the spinous processes C2 to C7/T1 may be adequate.
- Midline fascia incision to the level of the ligamentum nuchae.
- Dissection along the margin of this deep fascia to avoid bleeding. In the conventional posterior median approach, major blood vessels are not encountered.
- Careful dissection of the paraspinous muscles in a subperiosteal plane with Cobb, curved periosteal elevator, and cautery. Exposure until the lateral portion of the facet joint capsules is identified.
- Care should be taken not to violate the attachment of the semispinalis cervicis muscles at the inferior tip of the C2 spinous process (important for the maintenance of cervical lordosis).
- The open-side gutter is made first with a steel burr at the junction of the laminae and the facet joints. Perforation and resection of the ventral cortex with a diamond burr and/or a thin-bladed Kerrison rongeur.

Fig. 26.4 (**a–c**) Positioning of the patient

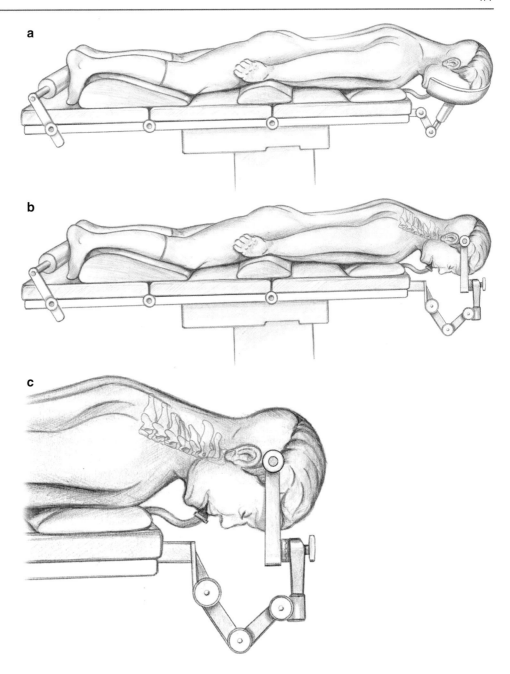

- Resection of the ligamentum flavum at the upper and lower end of the laminar door, usually at C2/3 and C7/Th1 with a thin-bladed Kerrison rongeur.
- The hinge-side gutter is made with a high-speed steel burr (Fig. 26.5 and 26.6). A thin rim of bone – a part of the ventral cortex – is left.
- Opening procedure (Fig. 26.7): The tip of one side of the laminar elevator is placed under the ventral surface of the lamina at the open side, and the lamina is lifted slightly to expand the gap. The spinous process can be held in the expanded position by an assistant. Then the next lamina is lifted in the same manner. During the opening procedure, the remaining soft tissues and adhesions in the open side should be excised with microdissectors and scissors to avoid tension.
- With the lamina in expanded position, the appropriate miniplate size can be determined by inserting the trial implants into the laminar gap (Fig. 26.8).
- A single- or double-bend miniplate is selected by placing the plates on the laminar expansion (Fig. 26.9).
- A variety of screws (self-tapping and self-drilling) are available to secure the miniplate.

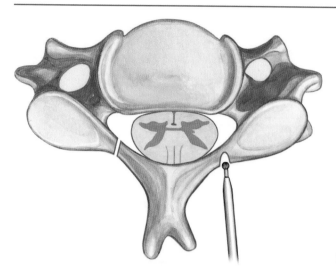

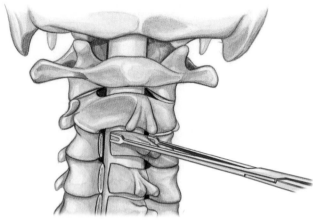

Fig. 26.7 Posterolateral view showing the elevation of the lamina

Fig. 26.5 With a thin cut the lamina is separated on the side with predominant symptoms. On the opposite side, a hinge is created in the lamina (Springer)

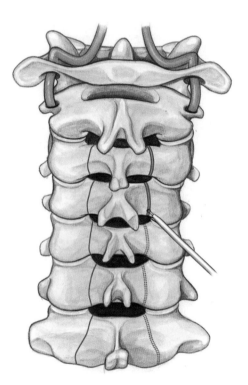

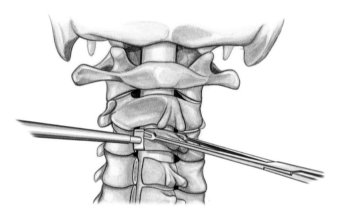

Fig. 26.8 Determination of the appropriate size and shape of the allograft with a trail spacer

Fig. 26.6 Posterior view of the vertebral levels showing the laminar cuts and the hinges

- The first screw of proper size should be placed immediately lateral to the gap. Self-tapping screws require drilling prior to insertion.
- Two screws on each side of the gap should be placed (Fig. 26.10).
- Insertion of the remaining miniplates (Fig. 26.11).
- A drainage tube is placed subfascial/epidural.
- The paravertebral muscles, nuchal ligament, subcutaneous tissues, and skin are sutured.

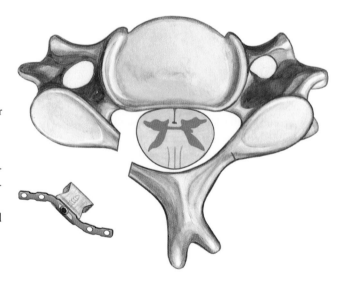

Fig. 26.9 Introducing of the construct with the miniplate and a bone piece or spacer

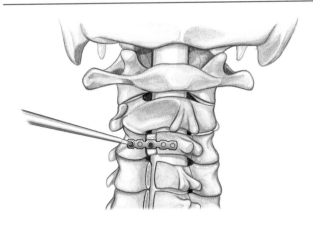

Fig. 26.10 Fixation of the miniplate with self-tapping screws on the right side

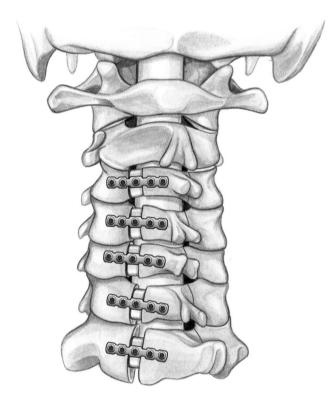

Fig. 26.11 Illustration after open-door laminoplasty of the cervical spine using a spacer plate system

26.7 Postoperative Care

- The patients are allowed to mobilize 4–6 h postoperatively.
- Soft cervical collar for 3–4 weeks.
- Instructions for general neck movement after 3–4 weeks, mild progressive neck exercise program.

26.8 Tips and Tricks

- Correct and careful positioning is important to reduce bleeding.
- When bleeding from the epidural venous plexus is encountered, it can be managed by the use of hemostatic agents such as Floseal (Baxter).
- Care should be taken during repair of the nuchal ligament for maintained good alignment postoperatively.

References

1. Nakamura K, Seichi A (2003) History of laminoplasty. In: Nakamura K, Toyama Y, Hoshino Y (eds) Cervical laminoplasty. Springer, New York, pp 3–11
2. Kawai S, Sunago K, Doi M et al (1988) Cervical laminoplasty (Hattori's method). Procedure and follow-up results. Spine 13:1245–1250
3. Hirabayashi K, Watanabe K, Wakano K et al (1983) Expansive open-door laminoplasty for cervical spinal stenotic myelopathy. Spine 8:693–699
4. Kurokawa T, Tsuyama N, Tanaka H et al (1982) Enlargement of the spinal canal by the sagittal splitting of the spinous processes (in Japanese). Bessatu Seikeigeka 2:234–240
5. Chiba K, Ogawa Y, Ishii K et al (2006) Long term results of expansive open-door laminoplasty for cervical myelopathy – average 14 year follow up study. Spine 31:2998–3005
6. Ratliff JK, Cooper PR (2003) Cervical laminoplasty: a critical review. J Neurosurg 98(Spine 3):230–238

Occipital Cervical Stabilization with Rod-Screw Systems

27

Michael A. Finn and Meic H. Schmidt

27.1 Introduction and Core Messages

Modern screw-based occipitocervical constructs enable immediate stabilization of the craniocervical junction [1, 2, 4]. Various screw trajectories allow for concomitant decompression and the creation of biomechanically stable constructs in a broad array of conditions. Bony fusion is successful in >95% of cases without requiring the use of rigid external immobilization. The goals of segmental instrumented occipitocervical fusion are stabilization of the craniocervical junction, reduction of deformity, minimization of segments immobilized, and bony fusion of instrumented segments.

27.2 Indications

- Traumatic instability
- Rheumatoid disease/inflammatory arthropathies
- Degenerative disease
- Infection
- Congenital malformations
- Neoplasia

M.A. Finn, M.D.
Department of Neurosurgery,
School of Medicine, University of Colorado,
12631, East 17th Avenue, C307, Aurora, CO 80045, USA
e-mail: michaelfinn76@gmail.com

M.H. Schmidt, M.D., FACS (✉)
Division of Spine Surgery, Department of Neurosurgery,
Clinical Neurosciences Center, University of Utah,
175 N. Medical Drive East, Bldg 550,
Salt Lake City, UT 84132-2303, USA
e-mail: meic.schmidt@hsc.utah.edu

27.3 Contraindications

- Aberrant vertebral artery anatomy may preclude the use of some screw contructs

27.4 Technical Prerequisites

Fluoroscopy, positioning device (e.g., padded rolls), rigid head holder (e.g., Mayfield), and adequate implants and instruments are mandatory for the procedure.

In addition, neural monitoring consisting of somatosensory evoked potentials and motor evoked potentials is used in cases of significant instability or cervicomedullary compression. We additionally plan our screw trajectories on a three-dimensional workstation (StealthStation, Medtronic, Inc., Minneapolis, MN) preoperatively. More recently, we have begun using the O-arm (Medtronic, Inc.) in lieu of fluoroscopy for intraoperative navigation and confirmation of the adequacy of hardware placement. This system, however, makes the immediate confirmation of alignment upon positioning in the highly unstable spine difficult, and fluoroscopy is still used in these circumstances.

27.5 Planning, Preparation, and Positioning

Prior to surgery, a plan is created that is specific for the patient's anatomy and the goals of the procedure. Particular attention is given to the anatomy of the vertebral arteries as they course through the pars of the atlas. Three-dimensional multiplanar reconstructed images are helpful in planning screw trajectories across this area (Fig. 27.1). Anatomy permitting, transarticular screws are the preferred option as they provide excellent fixation and are the lowest cost construct. If another construct variant, including C1 lateral mass screws, C2 pars or pedicle screws, or C2 laminar screws, is planned, the placement is also planned in advance. The use of laminar screws is reserved as an option of last

U. Vieweg, F. Grochulla (eds.), *Manual of Spine Surgery*,
DOI 10.1007/978-3-642-22682-3_27, © Springer-Verlag Berlin Heidelberg 2012

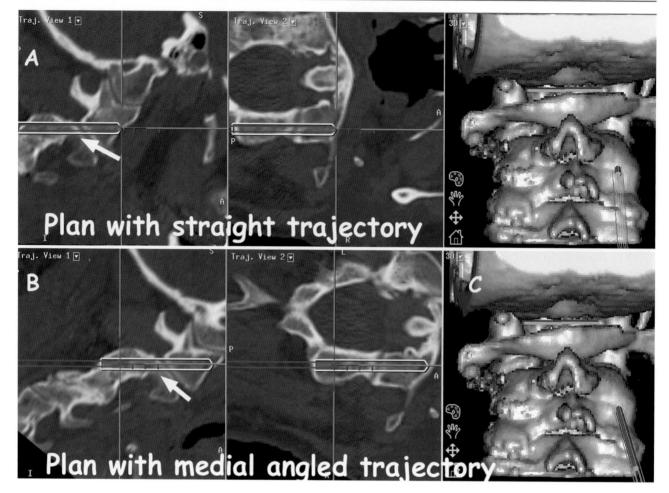

Fig. 27.1 Multiplanar three-dimensional reconstructions on the Stealth Workstation. (**a**) A straight screw trajectory results in violation of the vertebral canal. (**b**) A slight medial trajectory enables placement of transarticular screw entirely within bone. (**c**) Three-dimensional surface anatomy shows trajectory and allows for easy identification of starting position relative to bony landmarks. (With permission of Finn and Apfelbaum [2])

resort as laminar screws reduce the area over C2 for graft placement and bony fusion and have been shown to be biomechanically inferior to other options in occipitocervical constructs. In cases of significant instability, awake fiberoptic intubation is performed. Baseline evoked potentials are obtained, the patient's head is fixed in a cranial fixator, and the patient is rolled into the supine position onto padded rolls. The patient's head is kept in a neutral position and locked into place. Immediate postpositioning lateral fluoroscopic imaging is performed to ensure adequacy of alignment, and postpositioning evoked potentials are obtained. Loss of potentials mandates a return to supine position and the performance of a wake-up test. It is critical that the patient be placed in a gaze-neutral or slight downward position as fusion of the craniocervical junction in an upward position can lead to gait problems. The patient is prepped and draped from just above the inion to the upper thoracic spine to allow for the placement of guide tubes if transarticular screws are used.

27.6 Surgical Technique

27.6.1 Approach

- A midline incision is created from the level of the inion to the spinous process of C3.
- The avascular midline raphe is developed to expose the dorsal bony elements, which are dissected in a subperiosteal fashion. The occiput is exposed from the inion to the foramen magnum and laterally to the medial edge of the mastoids.
- The atlas is exposed laterally to its articulation with the axis if placement of lateral mass screws is planned. Bleeding from the epidural venous plexus may be encountered at this time and is controlled with bipolar electrocautery and powder Gelfoam (Pfizer, New York, NY) and thrombin. If Songer cables are to be used to secure the bone graft, the soft tissues are circumferentially dissected off the arch of atlas with curettes.

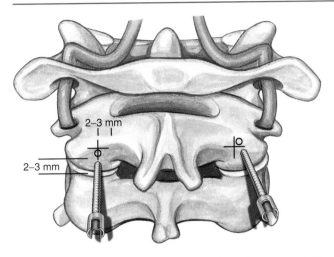

Fig. 27.2 The typical entry points for transarticular/pars screws (*left*) and pedicle screw (*right*) in C2 are illustrated with crosshairs indicating the midline. Transarticular/pars screws enter 2–3 mm cephalad to C2–3 lateral mass articulation and 2–3 mm medial to the canal. They are typically angulated at 40° in the sagittal plane and 0–10° medially in the axial plane. C2 pedicle screws enter in the upper outer quadrant of the C2 pars and are angulated approximately 20° medially and superiorly

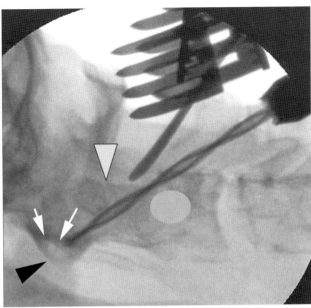

Fig. 27.3 The drill trajectory for TAS placement is demonstrated. The drill is aimed toward the upper part of the anterior arch of C1 (*black arrowhead*) to its final exit site through the anterior cortex of the lateral mass of C1 (*white arrows*). Resistance is felt as the drill passes through the C1–2 joint (*white arrowhead*) and again as the drill passes through C1 anteriorly. The Penfield dissector is placed on the pars and used as a marker to correlated intraoperative observations with fluoroscopic imaging. The *shaded circle* represents the area of the vertebral canal. (With permission of Gluf et al. [4])

- The axis is exposed laterally to the pars and the facet articulation of C2–3, with care taken not to disrupt the joint.
- Exposure of the subaxial spine is undertaken if an extended construct is planned. The interspinous ligaments between C2 and C3 are preserved.

27.6.2 Instrumentation

- Atlantoaxial screw fixation is undertaken first. The use of C3 screws may preclude placement of transarticular and C2 pars screws.

27.6.2.1 Transarticular Screw Fixation
- The entry point is identified (Fig. 27.2), and the medial edge of the pars is developed with curettes to identify the lateral boundary of the spinal canal. The typical entry point is 2–3 mm medial to this edge and 2–3 mm superior to the C2–3 joint. The entry site can vary depending on patient-specific anatomy.
- The entry site for the percutaneous drill guide is identified using fluoroscopy and a radiopaque marker (e.g., drill bit) placed alongside the patient in the trajectory of the screw. The typical entry site is at the level of the high thoracic spine. Here, a small (~1.5 cm) incision is created, and a subcutaneous/intramuscular tunnel is created to the screw entry site.

- Once the percutaneous drill guide has been placed, the inner drill guide is removed, and a starting awl is placed through the drill guide to create a starter hole at the entry site. The screw tract is then created by using a power drill with fluoroscopic guidance (Fig. 27.3). An instrument (e.g., a Penfield 4 dissector) can be placed on the dorsum of the pars as a radiographic marker for the dorsum of the pars. The drill should be aimed to exit on the upper half of the C1 lateral mass.
- The tract is tapped, and a 4.0-mm polyaxial screw is placed.

27.6.2.2 C1 Lateral Mass Screws
- The C2 nerve root is retracted caudally, and the entry point on the C1 lateral mass is identified. The typical entry point is on the middle prominence of the lateral mass. The posterior arch may need to be drilled to access this point.
- The tract is started with a high-speed burr. A high-speed drill with a protective drill guide is then used to create the pilot hole. The trajectory is slightly medial in the axial plane and parallel to the arch of C1 in the sagittal

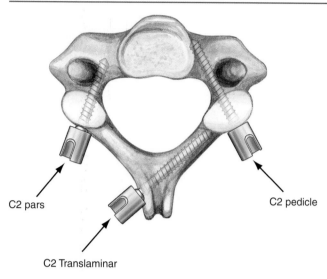

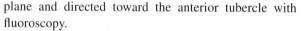

Fig. 27.4 Varying trajectories for C2 pars, pedicle, and laminar screws

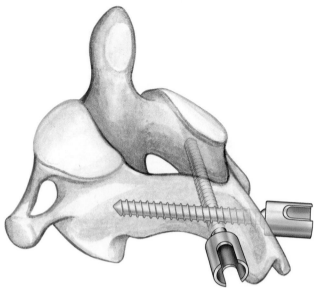

Fig. 27.5 Illustration demonstrating trajectories of crossed laminar screws

plane and directed toward the anterior tubercle with fluoroscopy.

- The tract is tapped, and a partially threaded polyaxial screw is placed, which may reduce the incidence of occipital neuralgia.

27.6.2.3 C2 Pars Screws

- The entry point, trajectory, and setup are identical to those used in transarticular screw fixation (Fig. 27.4). The length of the screw is determined on preoperative image reconstructions.

27.6.2.4 C2 Pedicle Screws

- The typical entry point is identified in the upper outer quadrant of the C2 lateral mass and marked with a high-speed drill (Fig. 27.2). Preoperative image reconstructions help determine the exact entry point, trajectory, and screw length.
- The screw tract is created with a high-speed drill at a typical trajectory of approximately 20° medial and 20° cephalad.

27.6.2.5 C2 Laminar Screws

- The typical entry point is identified and marked at the junction of the spinous process and lamina, with a cephalad entry on one side and a caudal entry on the opposing side (Fig. 27.5). The entry point should be in line with the slope of the contralateral lamina.

- The screw tract is drilled and tapped, and the screw is placed. Up-going curettes can be used to confirm absence of anterior screw breakout.
- The contralateral screw is placed just caudal to the first screw.

27.6.2.6 Occipital Plate

- Many occipital plate variants are commercially available [1] (Fig. 27.6). Key attributes to consider include ease of use, bulk, and location of screw placement. The bone is the thickest in the midline and thins out rapidly laterally (Fig. 27.7). Screws placed in the midline therefore provide the greatest resistance to pullout.
- Bony ridges on the subocciput are smoothed out with the high-speed burr to provide for a flush plate fit. The upper screw in the plate is placed first. For midline screws, a pilot hole is created with a power drill to a depth of 6 mm. The drill stop is increased in 2-mm increments until the deep cortex is penetrated. For lateral screws, bony thickness is measured on preoperative computed tomography scan, and prospective tracts are created in the same manner.
- The entire depth of the pilot tract is tapped, and 4.5-mm blunt-tipped screws are placed. The first screw is completely tightened after placement of the second screw.
- 3.5-mm rods are shaped to fit the screw heads and the plate. Hinged rods and right-angle connectors can be used to aid in connecting elements. Adequacy of head position is confirmed prior to final tightening of the construct.

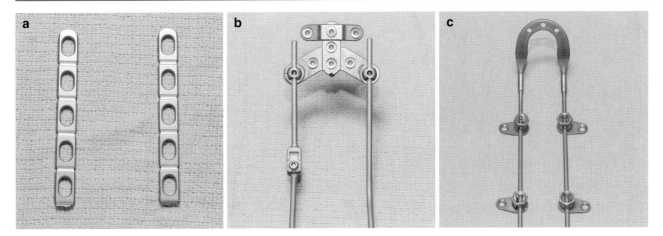

Fig. 27.6 Variations of screw-based occipitocervical instrumentation constructs. Those shown in (**b** and **c**) allow for the placement of a midline screw. (With permission of Finn et al. [3])

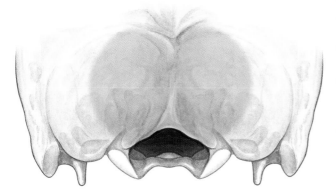

Fig. 27.7 Illustration demonstrating the optimal locations for placement of occipital screws, with *whiter areas* representing areas of thicker bone

- Tricortical iliac crest allograft is preferred in most patients and has been shown to have good fusion results. The graft is shaped to fit flush against the posterior bony elements. A V-shaped notch is cut into the bottom to accommodate the spinous process of C2. The fusion bed is decorticated, and Songer cables are used to secure the graft. A screw is placed in the cephalad end of the graft to secure it to the occiput.
- Postoperative orthoses are typically not used in nontrauma patients with good bone quality and good screw purchase.

27.7   Tips and Tricks

- Careful examination of patient-specific anatomy is critical to planning screw combinations and trajectory.
- Preoperative planning on a three-dimensional workstation can be invaluable in planning screw trajectories in difficult cases.
- Occasionally, patients are placed in a halo vest preoperatively and allowed to walk to ensure adequacy of head position. If adequate, the patient is positioned in the halo vest, which is removed only after the halo ring is secured to the operative bed. This technique ensures the patient's final head position will be adequate for ambulation and deglutition.

References

1. Dickman CA, Sonntag VK, Papadopoulos SM et al (1991) The interspinous method of posterior atlantoaxial arthrodesis. J Neurosurg 74:190–198
2. Finn MA, Apfelbaum RI (2010) Atlantoaxial transarticular screw fixation: update on technique and outcomes in 269 patients. Neurosurgery 66(3 Suppl):184–192
3. Finn MA, Bishop FS, Dailey AT (2008) Surgical treatment of occipitocervical instability. Neurosurgery 63(5):961–968
4. Gluf WM, Schmidt MH, Apfelbaum RI (2005) Atlantoaxial transarticular screw fixation: a review of surgical indications, fusion rate, complications, and lessons learned in 191 adult patients. J Neurosurg Spine 2:155–163

Posterior Transarticular C1/C2 Screw Technique

28

Michael Winking

28.1 Introduction and Core Messages

Several techniques are known for treatment of an atlanto-axial instability. Posterior transarticular screw fixation first published by Grob and Magerl (1987) is the most rigid way to achieve this aim [4-6]. The C1–C2 joint functions primarily in rotation and secondarily in flexion and extension. Therefore, in stabilization of this segment, it is mandatory that flexion-extension, lateral bending, and axial rotation are restricted. The direction of the screws in the transarticular screw technique reduces motion in all degrees of freedom, which results directly in high segmental stability. Additionally, this technique prevents a slippage of the segment. However, only the interlaminar bone graft between C1 and C2 will achieve the final stability through bony fusion [1-11].

28.2 Indications

Instability of C1–2 due to:
- Rheumatoid arthritis
- Odontoid fractures
- Os odontoideum
- Arthrosis of C1–2

28.3 Contraindications

- Aberrant course of the vertebral artery between C1 and C2.
- Physical size of the C2 isthmus is too small.

M. Winking, M.D., Ph.D.
Department of Spine Surgery,
ZW-O Spine Center, Zentrum für Wirbelsäulenchirurgie am
Klinikum Osnabrück, Am Finkenhügel 3, 49076 Osnabrück, Germany
e-mail: info@zw-o.de

- Irreducible deformity of the C1–2 junction.
- Prominent kyphosis of the cervico-thoracic junction.
- Destruction of the lateral mass of C1.

28.4 Technical Prerequisites

Preoperative 3D-CT for planning of the virtual screw pathway, navigation system (optional), fluoroscopy, Mayfield clamp, cannulated screws (optional), and titanium wiring cable.

28.5 Planning, Preparation, and Positioning

To avoid any intraoperative surprise, detailed preoperative planning using CT is mandatory. Several questions have to be answered before starting the surgery:
- What is the distance between the estimated pathway of the screws and the vertebral artery?
- Does the vertebral artery have an aberrant course?
- Is the diameter of the C2 interarticular portion big enough for a 3.5-mm screw?
- Is there a risk of drill deviation due to osteochondrosis of the joints?
- The best way to answer these questions is via a preoperative 3D-CT scan for virtual assessment of the navigation of the screws (Fig. 28.1).

Additionally, flexion/extension X-rays will identify the amount of mobility in the C1–2 segment and the chance of reducing a dislocation of the joints (Fig. 28.2). The correct drilling direction can be limited by a prominent kyphosis in the cervico-thoracic junction. Preoperatively, the estimated drilling trajectory should be checked. The MRI is more a supplemental imaging to identify the pathology as well as the spinal cord and the course of the vertebral arteries (Fig. 28.3). For surgical plannings, its information is not sufficiently enough. When the patient is still lying in supine position, the Mayfield clamp is fixed. Take care the patient has not had previous cranial

U. Vieweg, F. Grochulla (eds.), *Manual of Spine Surgery*,
DOI 10.1007/978-3-642-22682-3_28, © Springer-Verlag Berlin Heidelberg 2012

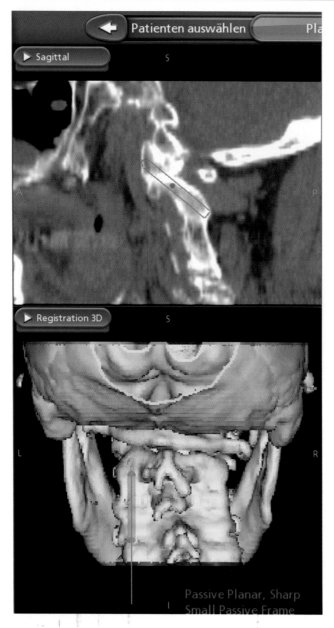

Fig. 28.1 Sagittal CT scan (3D reconstruction) with trajectory for the screws

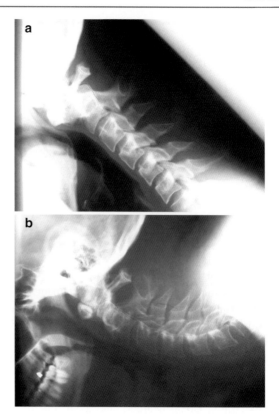

Fig. 28.2 Preoperative flexion and extension X-ray in a patient with atlanto-axial instability due to rheumatoid arthritis

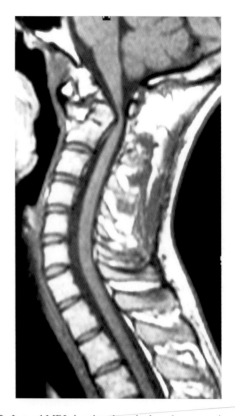

Fig. 28.3 Lateral MRI showing the spinal cord compression

surgery (an X-ray of the cranium before surgery is necessary). Now the patient is turned over on the operating table into prone position.

Definitive fixation of the Mayfield clamp to the operating table is done after AP and lateral fluoroscopy. The upper cervical spine should be positioned in exact derotation and a slight extension. A potential atlanto-axial deviation should be adjusted. Check the estimated drilling trajectory. A prominent kyphosis of the cervico-thoracic junction can limit the access. Pull back the cervical spine slightly to adjust the trajectory. The shoulders should be positioned alongside the body fixed with a slight pull in caudal direction (Fig. 28.4). This will reduce intraoperative bleeding because the intramuscular veins are compressed. Make sure that the intravenous catheters work

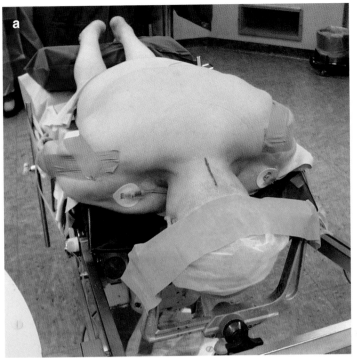

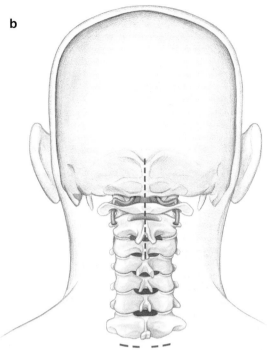

Fig. 28.4 (**a**) The patient is positioned while monitoring vertebral position under lateral fluoroscopy. (**b**) Illustration of the midline skin incision and the additional skin incisions lateral to C7

well. During surgery, the treatment of any anesthesiological emergency can be complicated by the prone position of the patient and the sharp fixation of the head.

28.6 Surgical Technique

28.6.1 Approach

- A midline incision from the occiput to C7 is performed (Fig. 28.4a,b).
- Cut the subcutaneous tissue until you identify the nuchal ligament.
- Stay accurately in the midline to reduce venous bleeding.
- Identify the spinous processes from C2 to C4.
- By electrocautery, remove the splenius and semispinalis muscle from the spinous processes (Fig. 28.5).
- Remove the muscles bilaterally from C3 and C4 by blunt preparation.
- Leave the capsules from C2/3 and C3/4 protected. Identify the C2/3 facet.
- Dissect bilaterally the lower part of the obliquus capitis inferior muscle to identify the arch of C2.
- Remove the rectus capitis minor muscle insertions from the dorsal arch of C1. With blunt preparation, the lamina of C1 is dissected, stopping short of the sulcus of the vertebral artery (Fig. 28.5).
- Remove the atlanto-axial membrane. The preparation should be done with a sharp dissector subperiosteally.

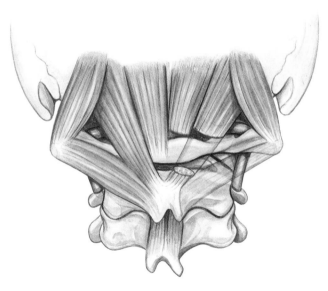

Fig. 28.5 Anatomical situation after resection of M. rectus capitis posterior and M. obliquus capitis inferior

Now the lamina of C1 can be identified for later wiring. Identify the joint of C1. During this step, the periradicular venous plexus can be damaged. The bleeding can be controlled by bipolar coagulation, better by compression with hemostatic substances.

- Identify the inner cortical border of the isthmus of C2 with a nerve hook, which will guide the later drilling direction.

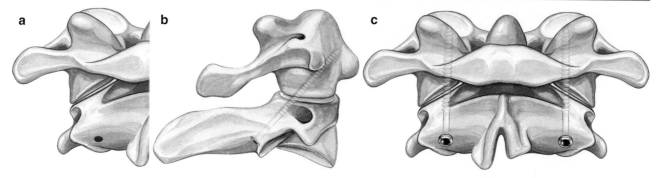

Fig. 28.6 (**a–c**) Drill placement, starting point, and drilling direction for transarticular screwing

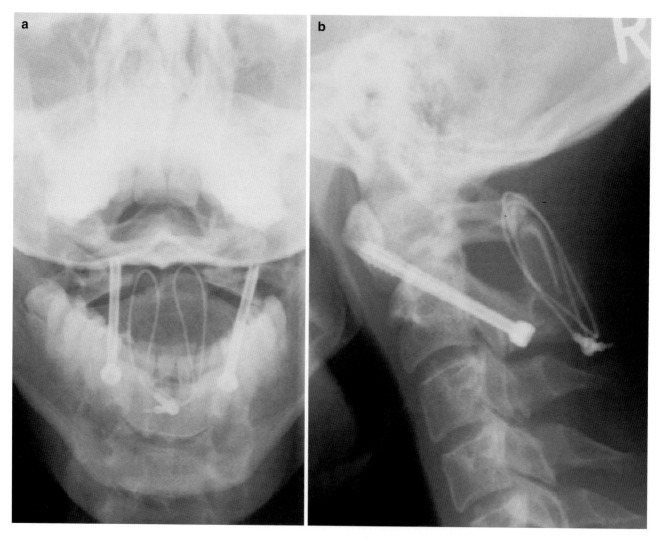

Fig. 28.7 (**a** and **b**) Postoperative X-ray after C1–C2 transarticular screwing in a patient with os odontoideum

28.6.2 Instrumentation

- The starting point for screw placement is typically 2–3 mm cephalad to the lower border of the C2 facet and 2–3 mm lateral to the medial cortical border of the C2 isthmus (Fig. 28.6a).

- The entry point is opened with an awl (Fig. 28.8).
- Using lateral fluoroscopy, a guide wire is drilled toward the superior aspect of the anterior C1 ring (Fig. 28.6b).
- Sometimes percutaneous skin incisions (beneath C7) are necessary to ensure the right angulation toward C1 (Figs. 28.13). The drilling direction is orientated slightly

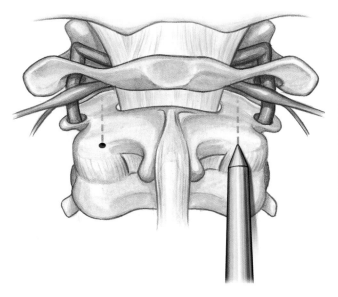

Fig. 28.8 Details of the surgical anatomy. The desired screw placement is just lateral to the edge of the spinal canal. It will traverse the isthmus of C2 and the C1–C2 articulation

medially, parallel to the inner wall of the isthmus of C2. During drilling, the direction is controlled with a nerve hook attached to the isthmus.

- In cases of an osteochondrotic C1 joint, the guide wire may drift from its planned direction as it passes the joint space. Drilling with reduced pressure under continuous fluoroscopy will help keep the right trajectory. After positioning, a guide wire is used as a track for the cannulated 3.5-mm drill. Use fluoroscopic guidance to ensure that the guide wire is not moved forward during drilling.
- After threading, screws with a length between 38 and 50 mm are inserted.
- AP and lateral fluoroscopy will assess the screw direction.
- In case of a persistent dislocation between C1–2 joint, C1 can be pulled back using a towel clamp which is fixed at the C1 lamina. Alternatively, you can push C2 spinous process. Under lateral view fluoroscopy, you see the adjustment. Using a guide wire for first drilling the cannulated instruments and screws gives the advantage that the drilling channel can be recovered at the temporarily fixed C1–2 joint. After having inserted both screws, the spinous process of C2 should be gripped with a towel clamp and pulled back to check the C1–2 stability (Figs. 28.10, 28.11, 28.12, and 28.13).

28.6.3 Bone Graft

- For fusion and long-term stability, an additional bone graft is necessary.
- Best stability will be achieved by a tricortical bone graft from the iliac crest.

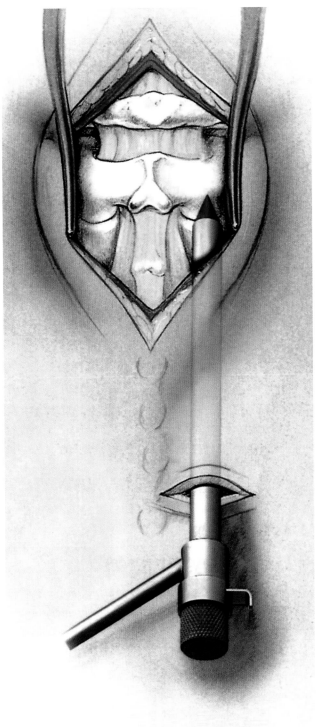

Fig. 28.9 Placement of the guide tube (with obturator) through a stab wound into the field

- To prepare the implantation bed, the surface of the C1 and C2 lamina is decorticated. Proceed with caution with the thin C1 lamina, which may be fractured by a brisk debridement.
- The cable loop passes beneath the dorsal arch of the atlas in midline from caudally to cranially. A notch, which is

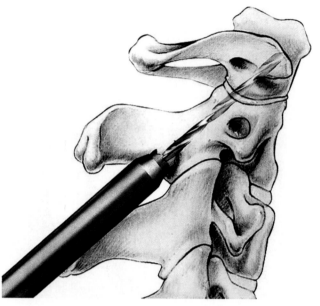

Fig. 28.10 Drilling (With permission of Aesculap AG, Tuttlingen, Germany)

cut into the lamina near the spinous process of C2, will hold the loop. The bone graft is clamped between both laminae. The two free ends of the cable are pulled slightly and crimped over the bone block. Additional spongious bone chips can be used to cover the remaining decorticated areas (Fig. 28.14).

- For closure, the detached deep cervical muscles are fixed to the spinous process of C2. The wound is closed in multilayer fashion.

28.7 Postoperative Treatment

A cervical (Philadelphia) collar is applied for 6 weeks. For follow-up, radiographs are taken immediately after surgery, after 6 days and 6–8 weeks, respectively (Fig. 28.7a,b). Especially in rheumatoid arthritis, a long-term follow-up is necessary to detect a later subaxial instability. Isometric exercises are started once it has been established that there is no screw loosening.

28.8 Tips and Tricks

The complication feared most of all is an injury of the vertebral artery. The symptom is severe bleeding (pulse synchronous) out of the borehole. In these cases, transarticular screwing should be avoided on this side. Bleeding can be

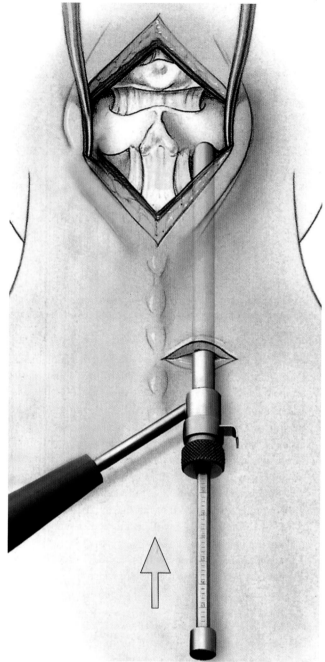

Fig. 28.11 Measurement of the screw length (With permission of Aesculap AG, Tuttlingen, Germany)

stopped only by closing the hole with hemostatic agents. Unilateral screwing with bone graft apposition will give sufficient stability in these cases. A postoperative angiography is recommended. In rare cases of split atlas, bone apposition is limited. In those cases, bone graft must be attached to the C1–2 facet.

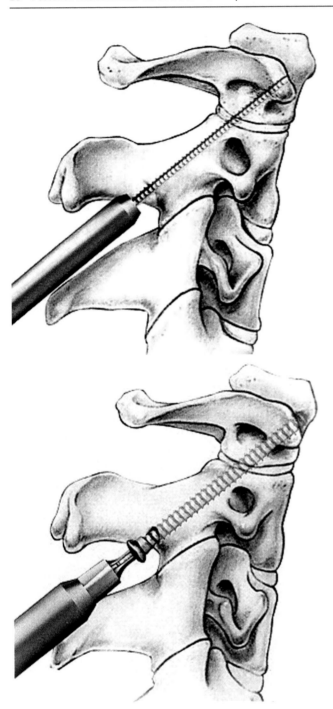

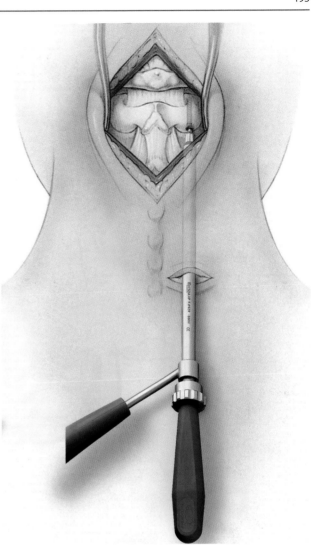

Fig. 28.13 Introducing of the transarticular screw in the AP view (With permission of Aesculap AG, Tuttlingen, Germany)

Fig. 28.12 Taping and introducing of the transarticular screw in the lateral view (With permission of Aesculap AG, Tuttlingen, Germany)

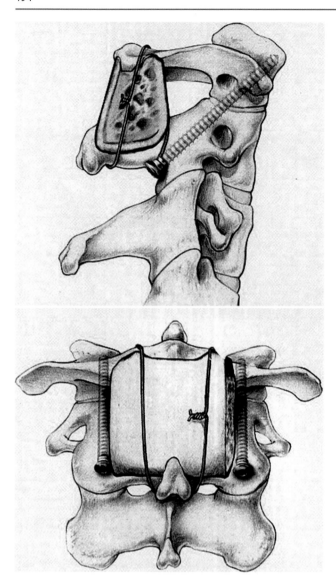

Fig. 28.14 Illustration after transarticular fixation and wiring C1/C2 with an additional bone graft between the arch of C1 and C2 (With permission of Aesculap AG, Tuttlingen, Germany)

References

1. Brooks AL, Jenkins EB (1978) Atlanto-axial arthrodesis by the wedge compression method. J Bone Joint Surg Am 60:279–283
2. Dickman CA, Sonntag VKH, Papadopoulos S et al (1991) The interspinous method of posterior atlantoaxial arthrodesis. J Neurosurg 74:190–198
3. Gallie WE (1939) Fractures and dislocations of the cervical spine. Am J Surg 46:495–499
4. Grob D, Crisco JJ, Panjabi MM et al (1992) Biomechanical evaluation of four different posterior atlantoaxial fixation techniques. Spine 17:480–490
5. Grob D, Jeanneret B, Aebi M, Markwalder T (1991) Atlanto-axial fusion with transarticular screw fixation. J Bone Joint Surg Br 73B:972–976
6. Grob D, Magerl F (1987) Operative Stabilisierung bei Frakturen von C1 und C2. Orthopäde 16:46–54
7. Jeanneret B, Magerl F (1992) Primary posterior fusion C1 in odontoid fractures: indications, technique, and results of transarticular screw fixation. J Spinal Disord 5:464–475
8. Magerl F, Seeman PS (1987) Stable posterior fusion of the atlas and axis by transarticular screw fixation. In: Kehr P, Weidner A (eds) Cervical spine. Springer, Berlin
9. Mandel IM, Kambach BJ, Petersilge CA et al (2000) Morphologic considerations of C2 isthmus dimensions for the placement of transarticular screws. Spine 25:1542–1547
10. Marcotte P, Dickman CA, Sonntag VKH et al (1993) Posterior atlantoaxial facet screw fixation. J Neurosurg 79:234–237
11. Weidner A, Wähler M, Chiu ST et al (2000) Modification of C1-C2 transarticular screw fixation by image-guided surgery. Spine 25:409–414

C1–C2 (Harms) Technique

29

Christian Schultz

29.1 Introduction and Core Messages

There is a broad range of options for stabilization of the atlantoaxial complex. To achieve stability, often fusion was used between the laminar arches C1/C2. The persisting motion was the reason for the high failure rates for this kind of single posterior fusion. To increase the fusion rate, Magerl introduced the transarticular screw fixation C1/C2 in 1987 [1]. The Harms technique of stabilizing C1–C2 using fixation of the C1 lateral mass and the C2 pedicle with polyaxial screws and rods is a further option when utilizing the posterior approach. Advantages are reduction of C1/C2, protection of the C1/C2 joint, and possibility of screw removal after healing to regain C1/C2 range of motion. Moreover, the Harms technique reduces the risk of vertebral artery lesion in comparison to the transarticular screw fixation because the screw angulation is easier in patients with kyphotic spine compared to the transarticular screw fixation according to Magerl.

29.2 Indications

- C1/C2 instability caused by trauma, tumor, and inflammatory conditions
- Nonfusion of odontoid fractures
- Revision after failed odontoid screw fixation
- Unstable Jefferson fractures

- Disruption or laxity of the transverse ligament caused by trauma, local disease processes, or local effects of systemic diseases
- Nonfusion, instability after alternative fixation techniques

29.3 Contraindications

- Anatomical variation of the vertebral artery

29.4 Technical Prerequisites

Utilization of C-arm for intraoperatively lateral and AP fluoroscopy control, the use of navigation could be useful. Endotracheal anesthesia, positioning device (e.g., Mayfield head clamp), and adequate implants and instruments (the distal part of the screw should not be threaded to preserve the C2 nerve). The S4 Cervical System (Aesculap) is one suitable implant for the C1/C2 Harms technique. Other suitable implants are, e.g., the Oasys System (Stryker) or the Axon System (Synthes).

29.5 Planning, Preparation, and Positioning

Preoperative CT scan is performed to estimate the pathology, the run of the vertebral artery, and to examine anatomical variation. Furthermore, information about the pedicle anatomy is obtained to choose suitable implant sizes. The patient is placed in the prone position, head and neck are secured with the desired sagittal alignment, and positioning is done while monitoring vertebral position under lateral fluoroscopy. Preoperative closed reduction may be done by positioning if possible. After final supporting of the head in a pin head holder, again preoperative alignment is confirmed by using a lateral fluoroscopy.

C. Schultz, M.D., M.B.A.
APEX SPINE Center,
Helene-Weber-Allee 19, 80637 Munich, Germany
e-mail: schultz.christian@gmx.de

U. Vieweg, F. Grochulla (eds.), *Manual of Spine Surgery*,
DOI 10.1007/978-3-642-22682-3_29, © Springer-Verlag Berlin Heidelberg 2012

29.6 Surgical Technique

29.6.1 Approach

- Surgical approach with a midline incision from the occiput to the spinal process C3 and further preparation similar to the C1/C2 transarticular screw fixation.
- Preparation in lateral direction and exposure of the posterior elements of C1/C2. Dissection of the lamina of C2 and the C2 pars interarticularis to remove soft tissue and to identify the landmarks for the C2 pedicle screw insertion.
- To dissect the entry point in the C1 lateral mass, the greater occipital nerve (dorsal ramus of C2) has to be retracted in a caudal direction.

29.6.2 Instrumentation (Using the S4 Cervical System)

Insertion of the C1 Lateral Mass Screw
- The landmarks for the C1 lateral mass screw are below the posterior lamina of C1, above the C1/C2 joint in the center of the posterior lateral mass (see Fig. 29.1) [3].
- The use of a guiding tube is recommended to ensure a safe procedure without endangering the greater occipital nerve as well as the vertebral artery which both lie very close to the screw entry point.
- The cortical bone is opened by using a bone awl through the guiding tube (see Fig. 29.2).
- The hole is drilled with the 2.9-mm-diameter drill for 4.0-mm-diameter screws under fluoroscopy control. The appropriate trajectory is 10–20° ascending direction, parallel to the plane of the C1 posterior arch in the lateral view and 10° toward the midline in the axial plane. Drilling must be bicortical; the drill has a scale for length measurement and the possibility of a safety stop (see Fig. 29.3).
- Although the screws are self-tapping, cortical tapping is recommended (see Fig. 29.4) [2].
- Bicortical screw insertion under fluoroscopy control (see Fig. 29.5), to preserve the C2 nerve and the dorsal ramus, the distal part of the screw is not threaded (smooth shank screw) (see Fig. 29.6).

Insertion of the C2 Pedicle Screw
- The landmarks for the C2 pedicle screws are the medial and cranial part of the pars interarticularis in the middle between the upper and lower articular surfaces of C2. This technique was first described by Judet in 1962 [2].
- After opening, the cortical bone drilling is performed with the 2.4-mm-diameter drill for 3.5-mm-diameter screws (if favored angle screw is preferred, 2.9-mm drill is used

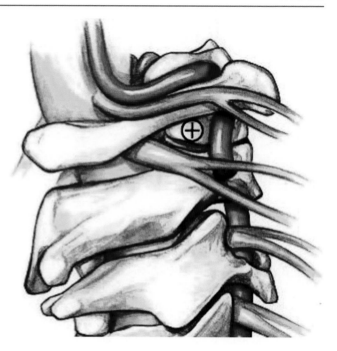

Fig. 29.1 Landmarks for the C1 screw insertion (With permission of Aesculap AG, Tuttlingen, Germany)

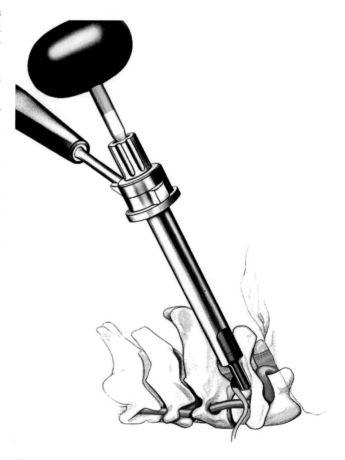

Fig. 29.2 Opening the cortical bone by using a bone awl through the guiding tube (With permission of Aesculap AG, Tuttlingen, Germany)

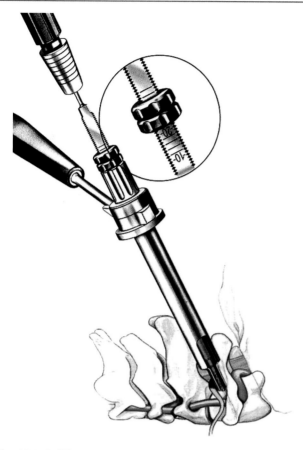

Fig. 29.3 Drilling the bicortical hole (With permission of Aesculap AG, Tuttlingen, Germany)

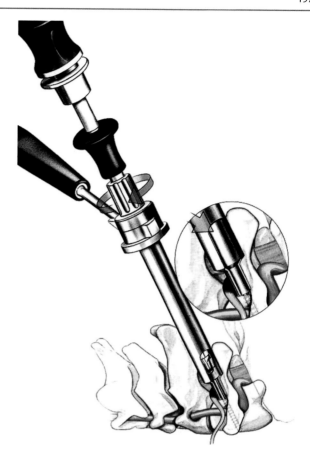

Fig. 29.5 Screw insertion (With permission of Aesculap AG, Tuttlingen, Germany)

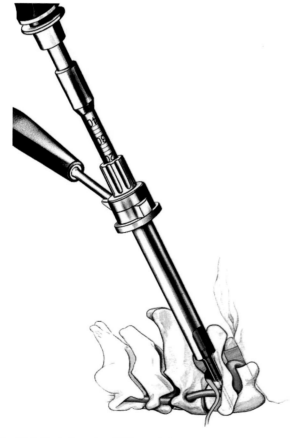

Fig. 29.4 Cortical tapping (With permission of Aesculap AG, Tuttlingen, Germany)

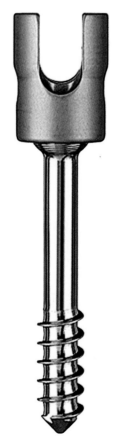

Fig. 29.6 Smooth shank screw (With permission of Aesculap AG, Tuttlingen, Germany)

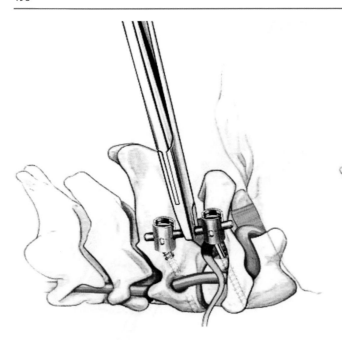

Fig. 29.7 Rod insertion (With permission of Aesculap AG, Tuttlingen, Germany)

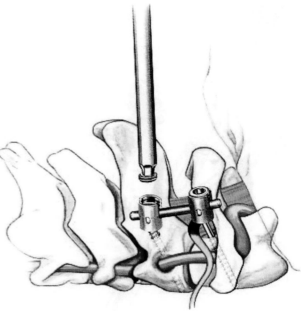

Fig. 29.8 Set screw insertion (With permission of Aesculap AG, Tuttlingen, Germany)

for 4.0-mm-diameter screw) under fluoroscopy control. The drill trajectory is 20–30° cranially under lateral fluoroscopy control and 20–25° in a convergent direction in the axial plane.

- Bicortical insertion of a polyaxial screw with suitable length.
- If necessary reduction C1/C2 in the desired position by adjusting the screws or by manipulation the head.

Rod Insertion

- Insertion of the rod and with the rod in place the set screws can be inserted to tighten the construct and fix the rod with the polyaxial screws (see Figs. 29.7, 29.8, and 29.9).
- To achieve fusion between the laminar arches, bone grafting can be considered.

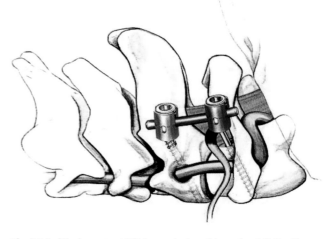

Fig. 29.9 Final construct (With permission of Aesculap AG, Tuttlingen, Germany)

29.7 Postoperative Care

Soft collar for a period of 6–8 weeks.

29.8 Tips and Tricks

Opening the cortical bone and drilling frequently causes bleeding of the venous plexus; bleeding control by bipolar electrocautery may risk a nerve injury, as an alternative quick insertion of the screw and compression with the screw head controls bleeding.

References

1. Harms J, Melcher RP (2001) Posterior C1-C2 fusion with polyaxial screw and rod fixation. Spine 26:2467–2471
2. Magerl F, Seeman PS (1987) Stable posterior fusion of the atlas and axis by transarticular screw fixation. In: Kehr P, Weidner A (eds) Cervical spine. Springer, Wien, pp 322–327
3. Stulik J, Vyskocil T, Sebesta P et al (2005) Harms technique of C1-C2 fixation with polyaxial screws and rods. Acta Chir Orthop Traumatol Cech 72:22–27

Rod-Screw Stabilization of the Posterior Cervical Spine

30

Uwe Vieweg

30.1 Introduction and Core Messages

Posterior rod-screw systems have a history of successful clinical use. The posterior rod-screw technique, with the screw positioned in the lateral mass or transpedicularly, provides a stable tension band system. For fixation to the occiput, an occiput plate has been designed. The complete system includes top-loading screws, rods, offset connectors, cross connectors, clamps, laminar hooks, and occiput screws and plates.

30.2 Indications

- Upper and lower cervical spine instabilities (rheumatoid arthritis, anomalies, traumatic instabilities, infections, tumours, deformities)
- Anterior fusions requiring additional posterior stabilization
- Instability associated with deficiency of the posterior elements from laminectomy or fractures

30.3 Contraindications

- Significant damage to the vertebral bodies

U. Vieweg, M.D., Ph.D.
Clinic for Spinal Surgery, Sana Hospital Rummelsberg,
90593 Schwarzenbruck, Germany
e-mail: uwe.vieweg@yahoo.de

30.4 Technical Prerequisites

Fluoroscopy, positioning device (e.g. padded rolls), rigid head holder (e.g. Mayfield), and adequate implants (polyaxial rod-screw systems) and instruments are essential for the procedure.

30.5 Planning, Preparation, and Positioning

A CT for preoperative planning is recommended (anatomical variation, confirm pedicle orientation, planning of implant size, etc.). The patient is placed on the operating table in the prone position and secured with the desired sagittal alignment. Accurate positioning is especially important when fixing the occiput to the cervical and thoracic spine. Confirm proper alignment using an image intensifier or radiograph prior to draping. The neck and shoulder are prepped and draped in the usual manner. The sitting position is an alternative.

30.6 Surgical Technique

30.6.1 Approach

- A posterior midline incision is performed.
- The incision is taken down through the subcutaneous tissue and facia with electrocautery.
- If fusion is to include the occiput, exposure should be extended to the external occipital protuberance.
- All soft tissue is removed from the posterior bone structures, and the lateral mass is identified. The medial border of the lateral mass is the valley at the junction of the lamina and lateral mass. The lateral boundary is the far edge of the lateral mass. The superior and inferior borders are the respective cranial and caudal facet joints.

U. Vieweg, F. Grochulla (eds.), *Manual of Spine Surgery*,
DOI 10.1007/978-3-642-22682-3_30, © Springer-Verlag Berlin Heidelberg 2012

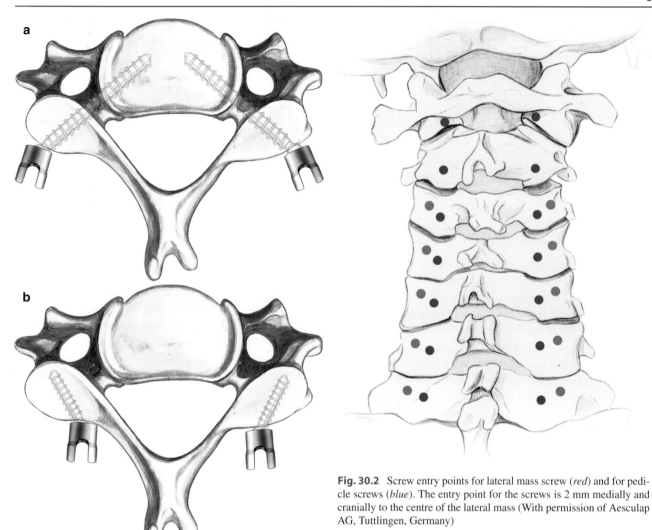

Fig. 30.1 Pedicle screw (**a**) and lateral mass screw (**b**) (With permission of Aesculap AG, Tuttlingen, Germany)

Fig. 30.2 Screw entry points for lateral mass screw (*red*) and for pedicle screws (*blue*). The entry point for the screws is 2 mm medially and cranially to the centre of the lateral mass (With permission of Aesculap AG, Tuttlingen, Germany)

30.6.2 Instrumentation [1–3]

Rod-Screw Stabilization Without Occiput

- In general, the screws can be placed in two different ways – either (a) transpedicular, with pedicle screws inserted from lateral to medial through the pedicle or (b) lateral mass, with lateral mass screws inserted from medial to upper lateral (see Fig. 30.1a, b). Though there are dangers associated with the insertion of cervical pedicle screws, their use is advantageous in some clinical conditions when increased load bearing is necessary [4].

- Depending on the anatomy, different entry points for the screws may have to be chosen. The entry point for the lateral mass screws is more medial than the entry point for the pedicle screws. The entry point for the lateral mass screws lies 2 mm medially and cranially to the centre of the lateral mass (see Fig. 30.2).

- The lateral mass screws are placed as described by Magerl [5] (see Fig. 30.3). Note: in order to achieve the correct drilling direction, partial resection of the spinous process, which is in the way, may be helpful.

- The screw trajectory is about 20–25° outwards (lateral to the spinous process) and 30–40° cranially. The cranial angulation attempts to parallel the facet joint. *Note*: the inclination of the surface can be determined by inserting a fine dissector into the joint.

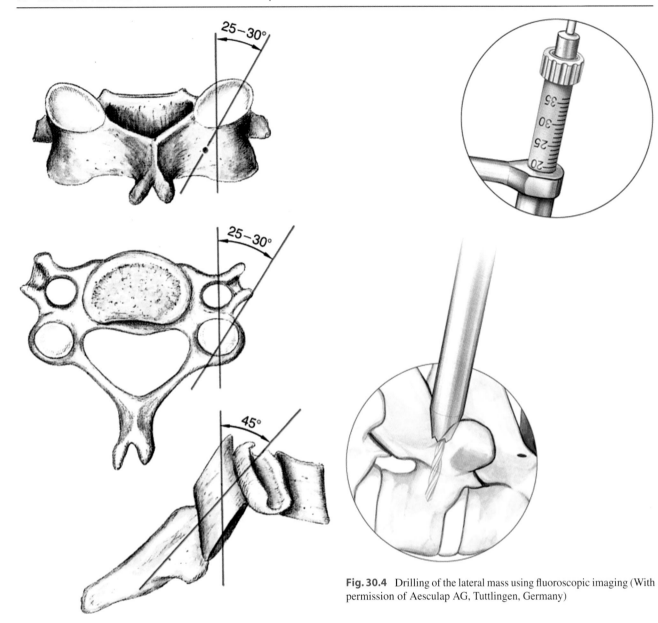

Fig. 30.3 Positioning of the lateral mass screws as described by Magerl. The screw orientation is about 20–25° outwards (lateral to the spinous process) and 30–40° cranially. The cranial angulation attempts to parallel the facet joint (With permission of Aesculap AG, Tuttlingen, Germany)

Fig. 30.4 Drilling of the lateral mass using fluoroscopic imaging (With permission of Aesculap AG, Tuttlingen, Germany)

- An awl may be used to open the cortex. Alternatively, a 1–2-mm drill hole can be made using a small decortication burr.
- The lateral mass is drilled with an adjustable drill guide using fluoroscopic imaging. Note: the drill guide is initially set at 12 mm. The depth of the hole is checked with a depth sounder (see Fig. 30.4 and 30.5). The

length of the adjustable drill guide is increased in 1- to 2-mm increments until the drill penetrates the far cortex.
- With the pedicles or lateral mass prepared and the proper screw length determined, the appropriate screws are inserted into the predrilled holes bilaterally, using the self-holding polyaxial screwdriver (see Figs. 30.6 and 30.7).
- Once the screw is inserted, the position of the polyaxial head is optimized for rod insertion using a screw body manipulator.

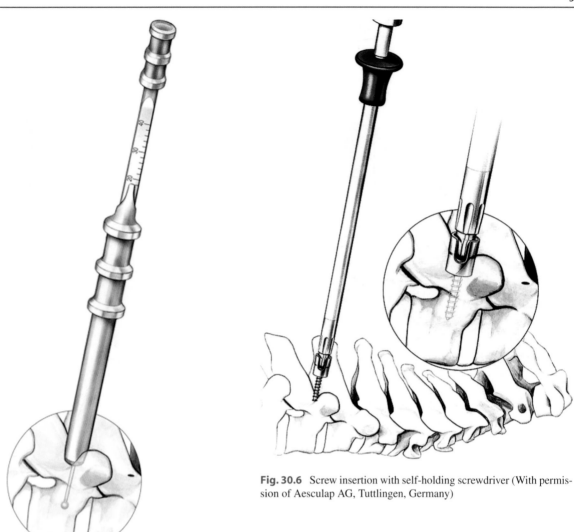

Fig. 30.6 Screw insertion with self-holding screwdriver (With permission of Aesculap AG, Tuttlingen, Germany)

Fig. 30.5 The hole is checked for penetration with a depth gauge (With permission of Aesculap AG, Tuttlingen, Germany)

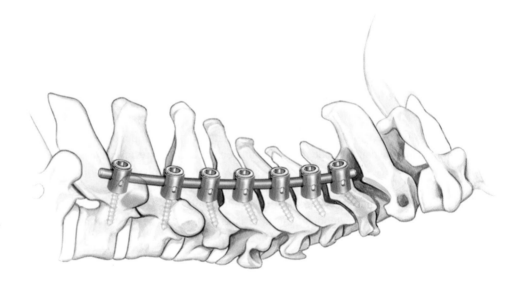

Fig. 30.7 Complete rod-screw construct C3-Th2 (With permission of Aesculap AG, Tuttlingen, Germany)

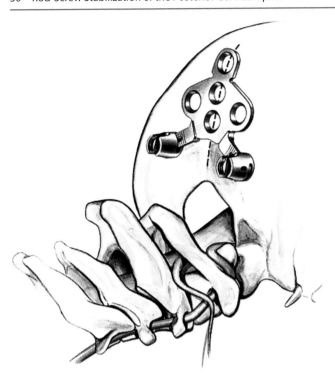

Fig. 30.8 Positioning of the occipital plate (With permission of Aesculap AG, Tuttlingen, Germany)

- After the insertion of the screws, and prior to insertion of the rods, the lordotic alignment of the cervical spine should be verified via intraoperative lateral fluoroscopy. A trial rod template can be used to aid in rod contouring or trimming to the required length.
- Insertion of the set screw in the polyaxial body is started by turning the instrument counterclockwise until a click is heard or felt. The set screws are hand tightened with the set screw starter and then finally tightened to the predefined optimum torque with a torque-limiting screwdriver and the countertorque handle.
- Cancellous bone graft is applied over the decorticated laminae and articular masses.

Rod-Screw Stabilization with Occiput

- The occiput plate should be placed medial to the external occipital protuberance and the foramen magnum. The greatest stability of the plate is achieved by midline fixation at the inion where the bone thickness is highest (see Fig. 30.8).
- A drill guide can be used to hold the plate onto the occiput. Note: even if the drill depth was measured before surgery,

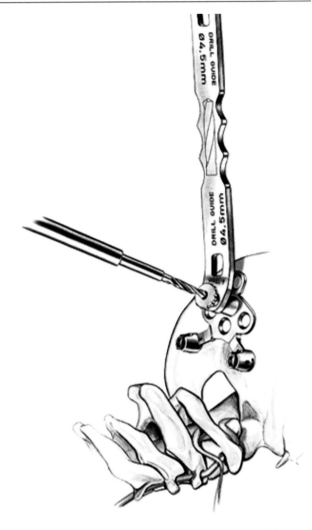

Fig. 30.9 Drilling of the occipital bone (With permission of Aesculap AG, Tuttlingen, Germany)

proceed with care to prevent damage to the dura (see Fig. 30.9).
- By using the tap guide and the tap, the drilled hole is further prepared for insertion of the occipital screws.
- The occipital screws are inserted, and the plate is fixed on the occipital bone. The occipital screws can be inserted in the appropriate holes using a screwdriver (see Fig. 30.10).
- To connect the occipital plate to the cervical spine, a prebent rod is inserted into the rod receptacles and fixed with set screws.
- Finally, the set screws have to be locked using a torque wrench and countertorque handle (see Fig. 30.11).

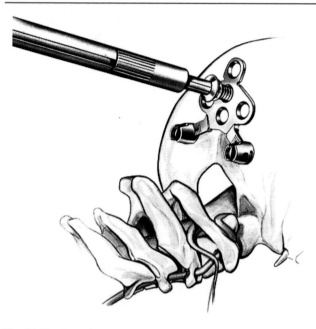

Fig. 30.10 Screw insertion in the occipital bone (With permission of Aesculap AG, Tuttlingen, Germany)

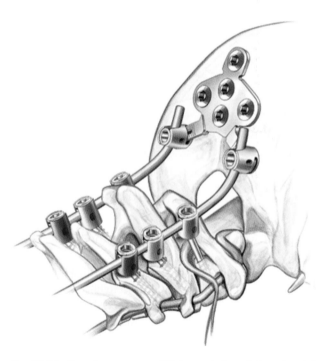

Fig. 30.11 Complete construct (With permission of Aesculap AG, Tuttlingen, Germany)

References

1. Aebi M, Thalgott JS, Webb JK (1998) Chapter 6: Posterior techniques lower cervical spine. In: AO ASIF Principles in spine surgery. Springer, Berlin/Heidelberg, pp 54–76
2. Dickman CA, Sonntag VKH, Marcotte P (1992) Techniques of screw fixation for the upper cervical spine. BNI Q 8:9–26
3. Dickman CA, Douglas R, Sonntag VKH (1990) Occipitocervical fusion: posterior stabilization of the craniovertebral junction and upper cervical spine. BNI Q 6:2–14
4. Dunlap BJ, Karaikovic EE, Park HS et al (2010) Load sharing properties of cervical pedicle screw-rod constructs versus lateral mass screw-rod constructs. Eur Spine J 19(5):803–808, Epub 2010 Feb 2
5. Magerl F, Grob D (1987) Dorsal fusion of the cervical spine with the hook plate. In: Kehr P, Weidner A (eds) Cervical spine, 2nd edn. Springer, Berlin

Part V

Anterior Thoracic Spine

Overview of Surgical Techniques and Implants

31

Christian Schultz

31.1 Introduction and Core Message

The chapter gives an overview to the different approaches (extended anterior cervical approach, periscapular approach and cervical thoracic approach with osteotomy of the manubrium to the upper thoracic spine; posterolateral transthoracic approaches to the mid-level and lower thoracic spine), different approach techniques (open/mini-open approach, microendoscopic approach) and different implants (plate-screw systems, rod-screw systems, vertebral body replacements) for the anterior thoracic spine.

31.2 Approaches

31.2.1 Open/Mini-Open Anterior Approach to the Cervicothoracic Junction (T1 to T2)

- Caudally extension of the standard anterior lower cervical approach to dissect between the trachea and the esophagus medially and the innominate vessels inferolaterally
- Exposure of the anterior wall of the vertebral bodies and the intervening discs (Fig. 31.1)
- Identification of internal jugular vein, common carotid artery, the recurrent laryngeal nerve and the thoracic duct
  With this approach, it is usually possible to attain the vertebral bodies T1 and T2; in some individual cases, one can reach the T3/T4 level. For more caudal access, there is a need for median sternal bone resection [1].

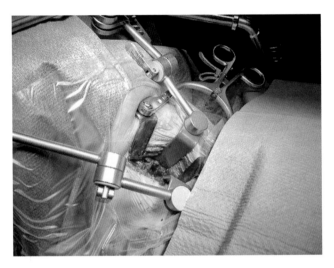

Fig. 31.1 Anterior approach to the cervicothoracic junction

31.2.2 Open/Mini-Open Anterior Approach to the Upper Thoracic Spine (Level T3–T4)

- Common cervicosternal approach with an osteotomy of the clavicle and an individual-sized sternotomy depending on the extend of the pathology.
- In case of sternotomy, the brachiocephalic vein has to be ligated.
  Because of the ligation and section of the left brachiocephalic vein, the risk of injury of the thoracic duct increases. The superior intercostal vessels should be preserved.
  Alternative to decrease the morbidity:
- Exposure of the level T1 to T4 between the right brachiocephalic vein and the brachiocephalic artery.
  The level T4 to T5 can be exposed between the superior vena cava and the ascending aorta using a transmanubrium approach without ligation and section of the left brachiocephalic vein.

C. Schultz, M.D., M.B.A.
APEX SPINE Center,
Helene-Weber-Allee 19, 80637 Munich, Germany
e-mail: schultz.christian@gmx.de

U. Vieweg, F. Grochulla (eds.), *Manual of Spine Surgery*,
DOI 10.1007/978-3-642-22682-3_31, © Springer-Verlag Berlin Heidelberg 2012

31.2.3 Lateral Approach to the Upper Thoracic Spine

- Skin incision at the inferior scapula
- Dissection of the latissimus dorsi and the serratus muscle to fold away the scapula
- Intercostal opening or resection of the ribs depending on the extend of pathology

This approach can lead to significant morbidity because of the extensile muscle dissection [2].

31.2.4 Open/Mini-Open Approaches to the Mid-level Anterior Thoracic Spine (Level T5 to T9)

Standard anterior approach until the level T9 is by a right posterolateral thoracotomy:
- Positioning on the left side (vacuum bed), abduction of the right arm 120°
- Skin incision depending on the level and extend of pathology
- Dissection of the latissimus dorsi muscle if necessary and as distal as possible
- Dissection of the serratus muscle also as distal as possible to avoid lesions of the long thoracic nerve and the lateral thoracic artery
- Intercostal approach to the spine, in rare cases rib resection

On the T4 level, the azygos arch ends in the superior vena cava. The azygos arch crosses the vagus nerve running on the surface of the esophagus. The anterior intercostal veins from the higher vertebral bodies end in the vertex of the azygos arch crossing the vertebral bodies perpendicularly (Fig. 31.2). The sympathetic trunk and ganglia continue to be nearby the rib heads [3].

31.2.5 Open/Mini-Open Approaches to the Lower Anterior Thoracic Spine (Level T10 to T12)

Standard anterior approach to the lower levels is the left lateral thoracotomy:
- Skin incision on the tenth rib
- Dissection of the latissimus dorsi muscle and intercostal thoracotomy (Fig. 31.3).

This approach leads into the costodiaphragmatic recess, and with an additional diaphragm, split it is possible to reach the level L2 [4].

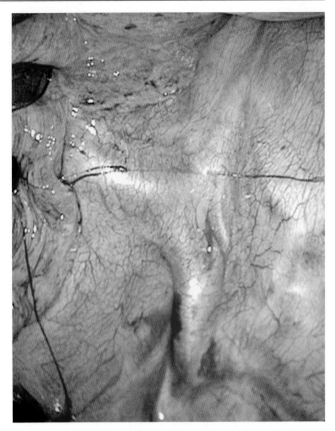

Fig. 31.2 View at the azygos vein at the level T5

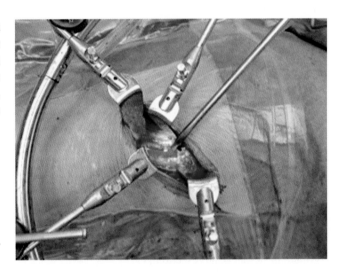

Fig. 31.3 Open approach to the lower anterior thoracic spine with the SynFrame Retractor System (Synthes)

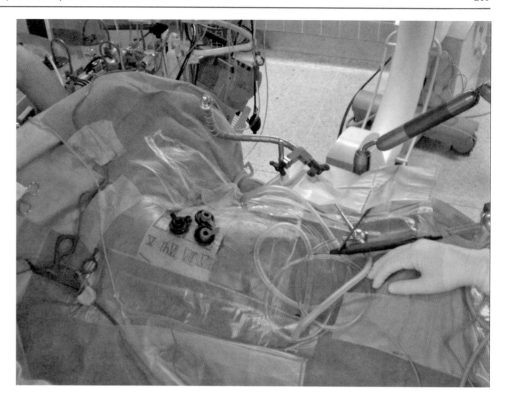
Fig. 31.4 Trocar positioning for the endoscopic approach to the level T6 from the *right side*

31.2.6 Endoscopic Approaches Upper Anterior Thoracic Spine (Level T2 to T4)

Demanding nearly transaxillary approach for experienced surgeons:
- Positioning on the left side, arm lifted upwards
- Four portals with the working portal above the pathology, the camera portal caudal in the same line, suction and irrigation portal anterocranial and the retractor portal caudal

The thoracodorsal and axillary vessels, the long thoracic nerve and the brachial plexus could be compromised. For these thoracic levels, the open approach still is the standard approach [5].

31.2.7 Endoscopic Approaches Mid-Level Anterior Thoracic Spine (Level T5 to T8)

Because of the position of the great vessels and the heart approach from the right side:
- Lateral position on the left side
- Portal position as stated above (Fig. 31.4)

The side of approach depends on the position of the aorta; therefore, a preoperatively CT or MRI is desirable.

31.2.8 Endoscopic Approaches Lower Level Anterior Thoracic Spine (Level T9 to T12)

Because of the liver, the lower levels have to be approached from the left side:
- The working portal is also located above the pathology, the camera portal is located two intercostal spaces cranial to the working portal and suction and retractor portal are each located anterior.

31.3 Implants

31.3.1 Rod-Screw and Plate-Screw Systems

These implants for stabilisation of the anterior spine are usually used combined with bone graft or additional implants like vertebral body replacements (VBR). The new implants provide an angle-stable constrained construct with four-point stability like the Telefix System (Synthes, Umkirch) or the MACS TL System (Aesculap, Tuttlingen) (Fig. 31.5) with:
- Low profile, smoothed edges and a safe screw insertion due to monocortical screw design
- A design for open and endoscopic procedures with
- Cannulated instruments and implants to simplify the endoscopic application with k-wire-guided instrumentation

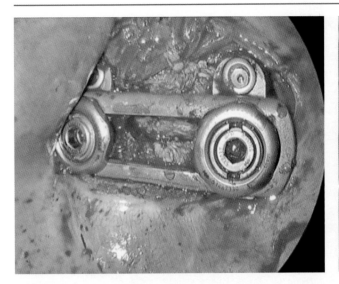

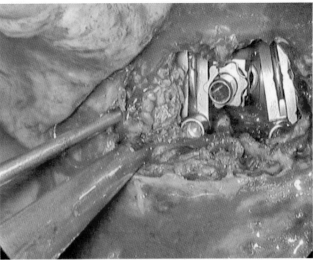

Fig. 31.5 MACS TL Implant (Aesculap, Tuttlingen, Germany) with iliac crest bone graft T12

Fig. 31.6 Hydrolift VBR (Aesculap AG, Tuttlingen, Germany) T10

31.3.2 Vertebral Body Replacement (VBR)

For special indications like multilevel corporectomy in tumour cases, there are still non-expandable cages like the titanium mesh cylinder, so-called Harms Cage (DePuy) or the SynMesh (Synthes). They are designed to fill with bone to achieve a healing in and resulting stability. Alternatives are the tantalum cages (Zimmer Spine). Among other things, the endoscopic approaches and the request for primary stability have the use of expandable titanium cages for vertebral body replacement well established. Commonly, today's devices are mechanically expandable like the Obelisc (Ulrich), the Synex II Cage (Synthes), VLift (Stryker) and Xtenz (Königsee). Advantages of these devices:

- Small size of the compressed VBR
- Adjustment of the height of the VBR to the length of the cavity
- High primary stability

Because of the manually application until the VBR fits tight into the resection area, there is no reliable feedback of the applied forces. An overextension could lead to an impression of the end plates. The new Hydrolift (Aesculap) is a new generation of VBR (Fig. 31.6) with special features to avoid these complications:

- Hydraulic manometer-controlled distraction
- Continuously adjustable endcaps to improve force transmission at the bone-cage interface

References

1. Xiao ZM, Zhan Xin Li, Gong De Feng et al (2007) Surgical management for upper thoracic spine tumors by a transmanubrium approach and a new space. Eur Spine J 16:439–444
2. Anderson TMMK, Jl M (1993) Approaches to anterior spinal operations: anterior thoracic approaches. Ann Thorac Surg 55:1447–1452
3. Cauchoix J, Binet JP (1957) Anterior surgical approaches to the spine. Ann R Coll Surg Engl 21(4):234–243
4. Ikard Robert W (2006) Methods and complications of anterior exposure of the thoracic and lumbar spine. Arch Surg 141:1025–1034
5. Cheung KMC, Al Ghazi S (2008) Approach-related complications of open versus thoracoscopic anterior exposures of the thoracic spine. J Orthop Surg 16:343–347

Anterolateral Endoscopic Stabilization

Oliver Gonschorek

32.1 Introduction and Core Messages

The use of minimally invasive techniques in thoracoscopically assisted procedures allows the reconstruction of the anterior column after vertebral fractures of the thoracolumbar region with reduced approach morbidity. Further indications are secondary reconstruction after malalignment and nonunion and resection of tumour and metastasis. After resection of the destroyed discs and vertebra, vertebral body replacement together with an angle-stable double-rod instrumentation results in a biomechanical stable anterior column. The aims of this procedure are: reconstruction and stabilization of the anterior column, decompression of the spinal canal, resection of destroyed discs, restoration of the sagittal alignment, early functional treatment and reduced comorbidity by using the minimally invasive approach.

32.2 Indications [1, 2]

32.2.1 General

- Unstable fractures between T3 and L3
- Fractures A1.2, A1.3 and A2 with kyphosis >15° [5]
- Burst fractures A3 (main indication) [5]
- Tumour and metastasis
- Secondary operations, i.e., after malalignment and nonunion

32.2.2 Monosegmental Anterior Spondylodesis

- Incomplete burst fracture A3.1 and A1.2 fractures
- Good bone quality (young patient, no osteoporosis)
- One destroyed disc

32.2.3 Bisegmental Anterior Spondylodesis

- Burst (split) fractures A3.2/A3.3, Pincer fracture A2.3 [5]
- Two destroyed discs

32.3 Contraindications

- Limited general condition
- Restricted cardiopulmonary function
- Severe thoracic trauma
- Acute posttraumatic lung failure

32.4 Technical Prerequisites

Fluoroscopy, carbon table, vacuum mattress, thoracoscopy unit (see Fig. 32.1), special thoracoscopical instruments (Fig. 32.2), monosegmental cages (i.e., Tantalum, Zimmer Spine, monosegmental procedure), expandable cages (i.e., Hydrolift, Aesculap, bisegmental procedure), angle-stable double rod system (MACS, Aesculap). For monosegmental spondylodesis, bone grafts may be used. Due to the harvest morbidity, we prefer to use a nonexpandable cage, i.e., Tantalum (Fig. 32.3). Small expandable cages may be used as well. However, in most cases they are too big. For bisegmental spondylodesis, expandable cages are advantageous (Fig. 32.4). Beside the mentioned Hydrolift (Aesculap), there are many other products (VLift, Stryker; Obelisk, Ulrich; Xtenz, Königsee). For lateral stabilization, an angle-stable

O. Gonschorek, M.D.
Department of Spine Surgery, Trauma Center,
Berufsgenossenschaftliche Unfallklinik Murnau,
Prof. Küntscher Strasse 8, 82418 Murnau, Germany
e-mail: oliver.gonschorek@bgu-murnau.de

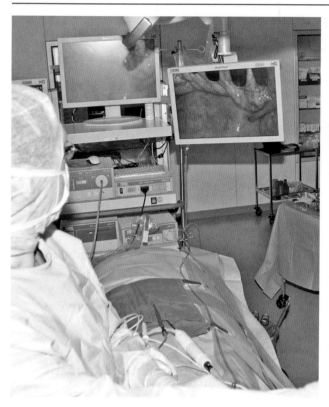

Fig. 32.1 The thoracoscopy unit with three HD screens allows all participants an excellent view

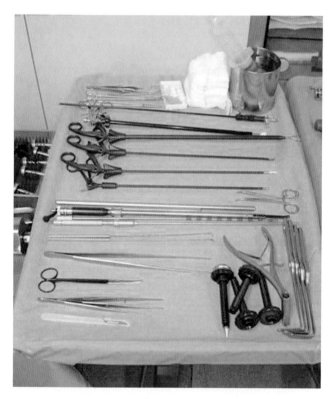

Fig. 32.2 Special instruments are necessary to operate under endoscopical control

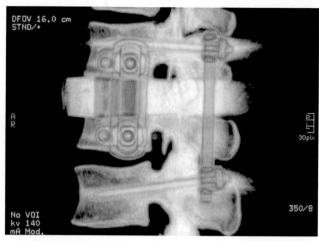

Fig. 32.3 Monosegmental spondylodesis with Tantalum cage and MACS shown as 3D-CT scan

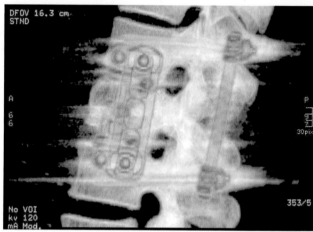

Fig. 32.4 Bisegmental spondylodesis with Hydrolift and MACS shown as 3D-CT scan

system should be used. Alternatives to the MACS system are Xia anterior (Stryker) and Telefix or Arcofix (Synthes), respectively [3, 6].

32.5 Planning, Preparation and Positioning

The CT scan is used to measure the sizes of all implants to be used during the anterior spondylodesis. During the operation, measurements are re-evaluated using intraoperative special measuring devices and fluoroscope. Navigation may be useful. Stable lateral positioning on the right side of the patient on a carbon table is performed using a vacuum mattress. Free tilt of the C-arm must be checked. Entrance points for the working and optical channels and the target area are marked on the skin using the fluoroscope (see Fig. 32.5).

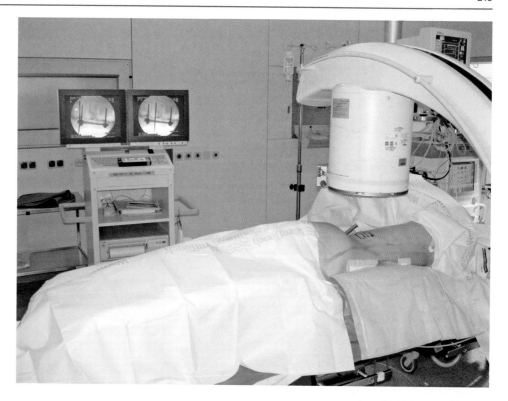

Fig. 32.5 Patient in lateral position on a vacuum mattress, approaches are marked under fluoroscopic control

32.6   Surgical Technique

32.6.1 Approach

- Four trocars are placed after the one-lung ventilation has started, the first one using a mini-open procedure to avoid lung lesions (see Fig. 32.6).
- From this point, all operative steps are under thoracoscopic control.
- Lung retractor and suction instrument are inserted using the anterior portals; the working channel is caudal posterior.
- To reach L1–3, a diaphragm split is necessary [4].

32.6.2 Instrumentation

- A K-wire is placed in the vertebra superior to the fractured one using the K-wire impactor under fluoroscopic control. The correct position is close to the ground plate ~1 cm from the posterior border (see Fig. 32.7).
- The entry hole is prepared using a cannulated punch (see Fig. 32.8).
- The posterior polyaxial screw, the polyaxial plate and the centralizer have to be preassembled and then placed over the K-wire (see Fig. 32.9).
- To avoid the risks by pushing forward the K-wire, it has to be removed after the initial turns.
- The polyaxial plate is then screwed down but not tightened. The precise alignment may be controlled by fluoroscope.

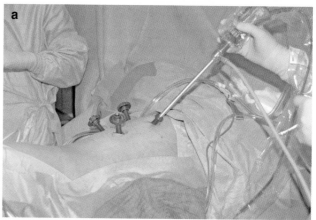

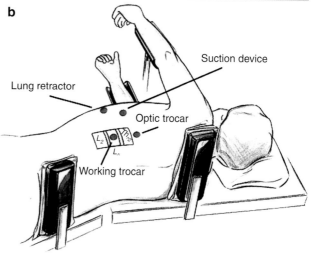

Fig. 32.6 (**a**) Situs with the portals for endoscopic operation technique. (**b**) Illustration of the portal placements (With permission of Aesculap AG, Tuttlingen, Germany)

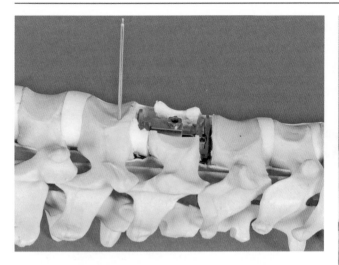

Fig. 32.7 K-wire placed close to the end plate of the vertebra

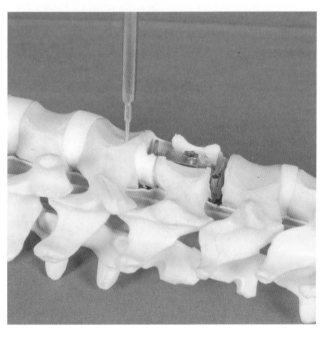

Fig. 32.8 Entry hole prepared by punch

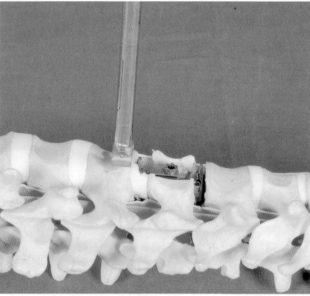

Fig. 32.9 The polyaxial screw together with the polyaxial plate is placed over the K-wire

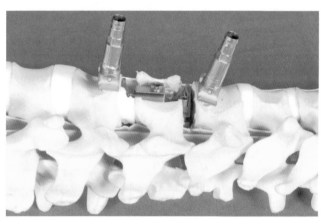

Fig. 32.10 Both polyaxial plates and screws together with the centralizer in place

- Same procedure has to be performed with the second screw (see Fig. 32.10).

32.6.3 Monosegmental Procedures

- The second screw has to be placed close to the ground plate of the fractured vertebra.
- The ruptured intervertebral disc and the fractured parts of the vertebra are resected.
- The cancellous bone of the remaining vertebra is compressed by using the probes of the cage.
- The Tantalum cage is then inserted in a "press-fit technique".

32.6.4 Bisegmental Procedures

- The second screw has to be placed close to the end plate of the adjacent vertebra.
- Both discs are resected and partial corpectomy is performed.
- The expandable cage is inserted and expanded.
  - Cancellous bone graft (from the resected vertebra) is attached laterally.
  - The double rod system configured as a frame plate is laid onto the clamping elements (see Fig. 32.11) and fixed by nuts, using a torque of 15 Nm (see Fig. 32.12).
  - The posterior screws are tightened down to press the plate firmly to the vertebra (see Fig. 32.13).

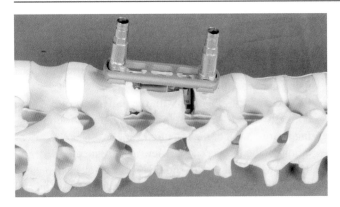

Fig. 32.11 Insertion of the frame plate

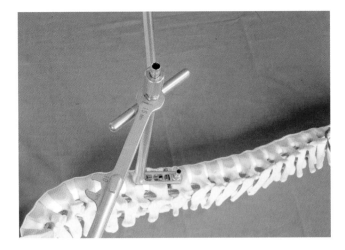

Fig. 32.12 The frame plate is fixed to the clamping elements firmly using a torque wrench

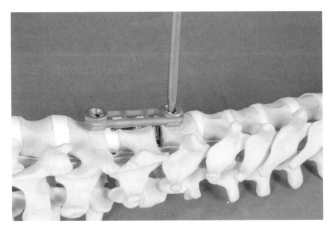

Fig. 32.13 The frame plate is tightened to the vertebra

- A guide sleeve is inserted to place the anterior screw after opening the cortex using a punch (see Fig. 32.14).
- The anterior screws are inserted through the guide sleeve (see Fig. 32.15).

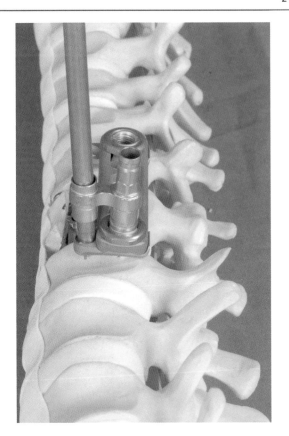

Fig. 32.14 Entry hole for the anterior screw is prepared by punch

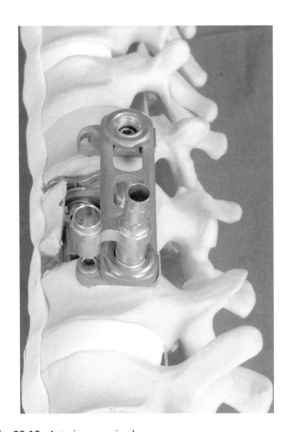

Fig. 32.15 Anterior screw in place

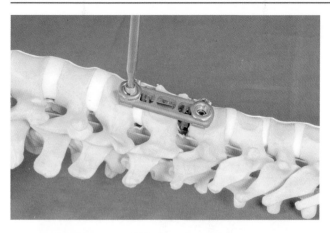

Fig. 32.16 Locking of the polyaxial mechanism

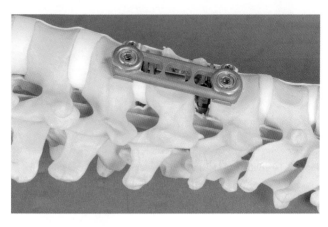

Fig. 32.17 Final construction of the MACS in a bisegmental anterior spondylodesis (with Hydrolift as expandable cage)

- The guiding sleeve is then removed and the polyaxial mechanism is locked by inserting a locking screw (see Figs. 32.16, 32.17).
- If a diaphragma split has been performed, the gap in the diaphragma is closed using adaptive sutures.
- A chest tube is placed with its end in the costodiaphragmatic recess, and all instruments and trocars are removed, the portals closed.

32.7 Tips and Tricks

- Screwdrivers should be inserted perpendicular to the screws. This is facilitated by "switching over the rib" using one working portal.
- Posterior screws together with the polyaxial plate – once correctly placed – may serve as a "navigation frame" during the resection of the fractured vertebra. Thereby, orientation on the thoracoscopic view is facilitated.
- The K-wires and screws should be placed close to the end plates. So it is very unlikely to set lesions to the segmental vessels.

References

1. Beisse R, Potulski M, Beger J et al (2002) Entwicklung und klinischer Einsatz einer thorakoskopisch implantierbaren Rahmenplatte zur Behandlung thorakolumbaler Frakturen und Instabilitäten. Orthopade 31:413–422
2. Gonschorek O, Bühren V (2006) Verletzungen der thorakolumbalen Wirbelsäule. Orthop Unfall Up2date 1:195–222
3. Josten C, Katscher S, Gonschorek O (2005) Therapiekonzepte bei Frakturen des thorakolumbalen Überganges und der Lendenwirbelsäule. Orthopade 34:1021–1032
4. Kim DH, Jahng TA, Balabhadra RS et al (2004) Thoracoscopic transdiaphragmatic approach to thoracolumbar junction fractures. Spine 4:317–328
5. Magerl F, Harms J, Gertzbein SD et al (1990) A comprehensive classification of thoracic and lumbar injuries. Eur Spine J 3:184–201
6. Raju S, Balabhadra V, Kim DH (2005) Thoracoscopic decompression and fixation (MACS-TL). In: Kim DH, Fessler RG, Regan JJ (eds) Endoscopic spine surgery and instrumentation. Thieme, New York

Vertebral Body Replacement

33

Jürgen Nothwang

33.1 Introduction and Core Messages

The anterior support in thoracolumbar spine fractures and in some special cases of tumour diseases is one of the most important steps for reconstructing the shape of the vertebral column to preserve satisfying long-term results. A lot of biomechanical and clinical investigations confirm the necessity of anterior reconstruction in bisegmental posterior stabilizations to avoid posterior implant failure. Potential of healing of a bisegmental corticocancellous graft is limited. With vertebral body replacements (VBR), the loss of correction after removal of the posterior stabilization device is small. VBRs with expandable components (see Fig. 33.1) allow an adapted anterior defect bridging and open the possibility of anterior reduction.

33.2 Indications

Indication of vertebral body replacement is depending on the entity of the lesion, bone quality and general condition of the patient. We have to remind that even in endoscopic techniques, the perioperative risk [1, 6] is respectable:

- Fractures of thoracolumbar spine: (a) Type A2.3, A3.2. and A3.3. (b) Type B and C1 fractures in combination of bisegmental fractures of the vertebral body. (c) Type C2.2 and C3 fractures with severe destruction of the vertebral body.
- Total corporectomy/vertebrectomy in primary tumour treatment.
- Metastases of vertebral body in epithelial tumours with mild prognosis: corporal destruction >40% (lumbar spine) and 60% (thoracic spiy[12].
- Persistent instability after total vertebral collapse due to osteoporosis.
- Postinfectious deformities.

33.3 Contraindications

- Reduced general conditions of the patient: pulmonary and cardiac risk factors (ASA risk score ≥IV, NYHA score IV).
- Pre-existing lung diseases with major reduction of vital capacity, pleural diseases as pleural rind, adhesions of the lung, and residuals after lung contusion may disable a thoracic transpleural approach and one-lung ventilation in endoscopic approach.
- Disturbance of haemostasis.
- Extensive osteoporosis with severe pre-existing deformities.
- Bad prognosis in tumour diseases and reduced general conditions of the patient.
- Malformation of the thorax and its cavity.

J. Nothwang, M.D.
Department of Traumatology and Orthopedics,
Rems-Murr-Kliniken gGmbH,
Schlichener Strasse 105, 73614 Schondorf, Germany
e-mail: jnothwang@khrmk.de

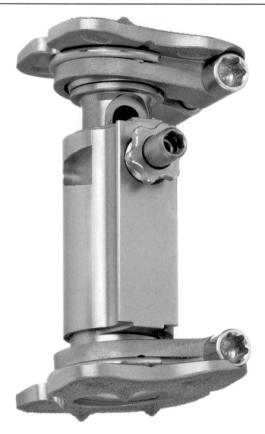

Fig. 33.1 Expandable vertebral body replacement system Hydrolift (Aesculap) (With permission Aesculap AG, Tuttlingen, Germany)

33.4 Technical Prerequisites

Fluoroscopy, radiolucent operating table, retraction device, rib raspatory, rib resector, light source, long instruments, thoracotomy set, lung retractor, electric scissor and hook for preparation of the pleura parietalis, osteotomes, hook probes, sharp and blunt rongeurs, Kerrison rongeur, curettes, clip applicator and, if disposable, shaver for disc preparation. *Not only for endoscopic preparation ultrasound dissector is helpful and enables an operation technique with reduced blood loss.*

For endoscopic techniques, there is further need of: three chip camera, 30°-angled rigid scope, light source, monitors, video recorder and printer, irrigation/suction unit and fan retractor

In endoscopic technique, double-tube tubage for one-lung ventilation intraoperatively is mandatory

33.4.1 Basic Clinical and Biomechanical Messages

- Reduced load bearing capacity of the anterior column (i.e., burst fractures, extended vertebral body defects) is

the major risk for loss of correction and implant failure [7, 10, 12].
- Several biomechanical investigations have demonstrated the breakage of the posterior implant under cyclic load [2, 3].
- In vitro biomechanical investigations showed that the maximum load was lower in the strut-grafted spines when compared with those with pedicle fixation only [5]. It is also of concern that the potential of healing of a bisegmental corticocancellous graft is limited. Pseudarthrosis and even fractures of the grafts are described [4].
- To minimize principle loss of correction, a metallic titanium expandable vertebral body replacement can offer higher guarantee [8].
- Collapse of the VBR implant into the vertebral body remains a point of concern [10, 11].
- Currently, little is known about the amount of loads which is created by VBRs and which stresses the end plates under daily life movements [9]. Additional axial loads in upright position in interaction with individual factors due to bone mineral density further modify the resistance capabilities.

33.5 Planning, Preparation and Positioning

- Analysis of the preoperative X-rays and CT scans to evaluate the region of lesion and special conditions of the vessels (King-King phenomenon, atypical veins). In some special cases, angio-MRI may provide further information of blood supply and FSU.
  Attention is demanded to the number of lumbar vertebrae and stump ribs to identify the correct segment level.
- Measurement of FSU height is recommendable, especially cranial T9. In small patients, the predetermined space is smaller than the smallest expandable VBR, and strategy of treatment has to be modified. (*In endoscopic approaches, the patient should be informed of switching to open procedure techniques if endoscopic approach has to be quit by technical reasons or complications.*)
- Preparation of the patient should include shaving of the operative field and catheter of urinary bladder. (In our experience in transthoracic operations, further preparations as intestinal preparation by laxatives are dispensable, even if a split of diaphragma is necessary.)
- Right side positioning is chosen in all lesions of T9 and lower, left side positioning above T9. (This decision is due to the course of the vessels which by trend prefer a dexter course lower than T9 and a sinistral one in the upper regions.)
- A straight lateral position should be favoured. With fluoroscopy, the posterior wall has to form a singular line, and the end plates should be hit perpendicular to the radiologic beam.

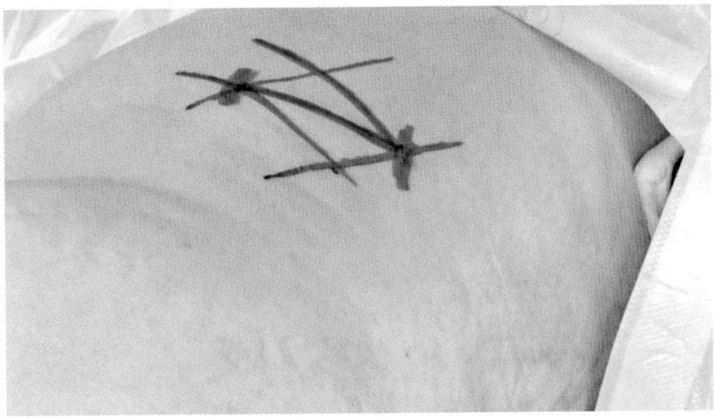

Fig. 33.2 *Incision line – exactly in projection to the target area*

- The patient has to be fixed in pillars with anterior and posterior support. To avoid decubital problems to the legs, we use a special bedding pillow, so-called tunnel.
- Before starting the operation under fluoroscopic control, the incisions are marked. Especially in endoscopic approach, the definition of the portals is one of the most important steps.
- In minimal, open and endoscopic approaches, the incision of the working channel should be exactly in projection to the target area. The length of the skin incision depends on the presumed size of the vertebral body replacement (see Fig. 33.2).
- In endoscopic technique, which we prefer in thoracic spine surgery, the portal for the endoscope should be marked two segments above the working channel; the incisions of the fan retractor and the suction form a trapezoid.

33.6 Surgical Technique

33.6.1 Approach

- We always start the operation with the working channel. (It has the largest size, and the success of one-lung ventilation can be controlled without danger of lung damage even in case of adhesions.)
- *In thoracolumbar junction, attention should be given to the course of the diaphragmal line, especially in cases of raised dome position.*
- If elasticity of the chest is obviously limited, we recommend a limited resection of the rib in projection to the target segment to reduce stress and risk of rib fracture. If required, the bone of the rib can be saved for grafting.

- *Usually in the upper thoracic spine, the resection of the rib is necessary due to the horizontal and narrow course of the ribs.*
- In terms of the further steps in endoscopic approach, see the specific chapter.
- If diaphragma's split is necessary, we expose the line of insertion with the fan retractor and then incise it with the help of an electric hook or scissor. After having opened the diaphragma in the line of insertion, a split of the diaphragma follows, and the fan retractor can be placed into the diaphragma's gap. With the same instruments, the parietal pleura is incised in a T-shape and mobilized anteriorly and posteriorly.
- The segmental vessels of the target vertebral body are mobilized, closed with clips and dissected.
- The adjacent discs are identified and cut in by a long-armed scalpel.
- With a raspatory, the disc is separated from the end plates and finally removed with Kerrison rongeurs.
- If decompression of the spinal canal is necessary, the lower border of the pedicle is identified, and the base of the pedicle is then resected in a cranial direction with the help of a Kerrison rongeur and punches.
- Having finished the resection, the clearance of the spinal canal can be performed.
- The bed for the vertebral body replacement has to be prepared and modelized by chisels. Angulated chisels are available to shape the corners precisely (see Fig. 33.3).
- The end plate and the suitable length of the vertebral replacement can be appreciated by test implants (see Figs. 33.4 and 33.5).
- Choose a size close to the measured length to create high stiffness of the spacer and avoid weakening of the implant by long expansion's distance.
- Ex situ, the angle of the end plate can be gently fixed as well as the safety screw for distraction.
- With a holding device, the VBR is inserted (see Fig. 33.6).
- Under fluoroscopic control, the VBR is placed in a midline position in both planes (see Fig. 33.7).
- The safety screw is opened, and the spacer can be expanded hydraulically controlled (see Fig. 33.8).
- The compression forces should not pass 30 atm.
- The screws for end plate fixation are opened to allow optimal adaption to the end plates of the next segments.
- If ideal positioning is achieved, all screws have to be tightened by torque wrench.
- With the preparation of the spacer's bed, usually plenty enough cancellous bone graft can be harvested, used for lateral spondylodesis and covering of the VBR.

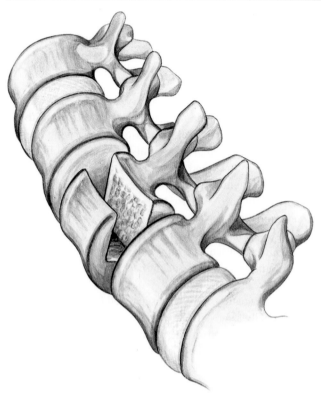

Fig. 33.3 Preparation of the implant bed (With permission Aesculap AG, Tuttlingen, Germany)

- In osteoporosis, vertebroplasty of the adjacent vertebral bodies is recommendable to avoid subsidence of the implant. The cement augmentation should be applied close to the end plates.
- In tumorous diseases, cement augmentation should be considered to enlarge local stability (so-called compound spondylodesis).

33.7   Tips and Tricks

- A strict lateral positioning of the patient is extremely important to avoid malposition of the VBR. *Respecting the correct position means eliminating any risk of spinal canal compromising.*
- If the collapse of the lung has not been succeeded totally, it is possible to push the lung back by an abdominal cloth.
- To reduce the frequency of fluoroscopic control, we mark the midline of the adjacent vertebral bodies in the lateral view by K-wires before starting the vertebral body resection. In our experience, further fluoroscopy is not required until the definite implantation of the VBR.

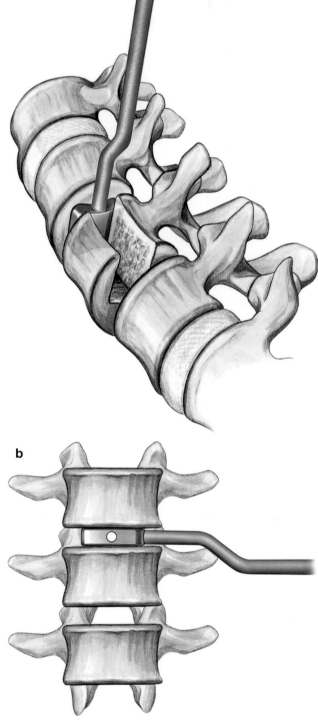

Fig. 33.4 Test implant for the suitable size of the end plates (**a**, **b**) (With permission Aesculap AG, Tuttlingen, Germany)

- Use the largest implant which can be inserted in the prepared cavity without additional forces.
- If reduction is desired, the angle of the VBR end plates must be definitely fixed in the favoured position before

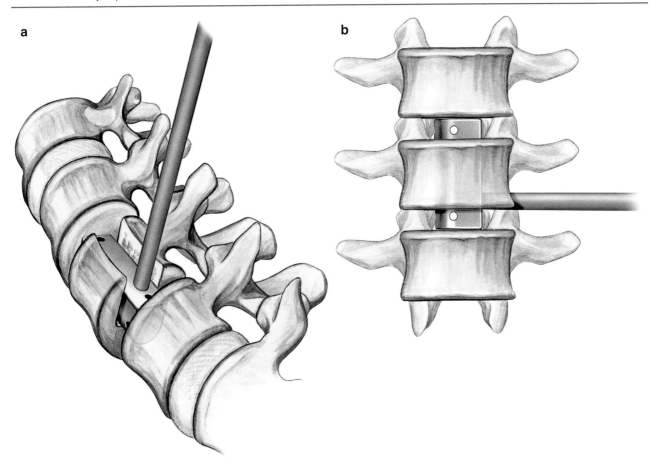

Fig. 33.5 Measurement device for the ident length of the implant (**a**, **b**) (With permission Aesculap AG, Tuttlingen, Germany)

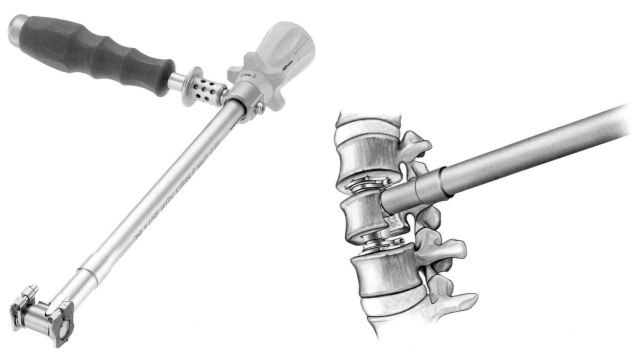

Fig. 33.6 Holding instrument for the vertebral body replacement (VBR) device (With permission Aesculap AG, Tuttlingen, Germany)

Fig. 33.7 Positioning of the VBR under pressure control (With permission Aesculap AG, Tuttlingen, Germany)

Fig. 33.8 Intraoperative situation with positioning of the VBR under pressure control

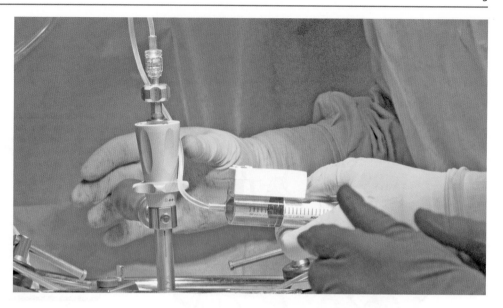

introduction of the spacer. For this procedure, special templates are provided by the companies.

- The aim of the vertebral replacement is to achieve high contact zones between the VBR end plates and the end plates of the adjacent vertebral bodies. The larger the contact zone, the lesser the risk of implant penetration.

- Infiltration of intercostal space where the thoracic drainage is inserted reduces postoperative pain. If harvesting bone graft from the anterior or posterior iliac crest is required, we recommend periosteal denerving by electric knife and finally infiltration with Naropin®.

References

1. Beisse R (2005) Complications of endoscopic surgery of the spine. Trauma Berufskrankh 7(Suppl 2):321–326
2. Cripton PA, Jain GM, Wittenberg RH et al (2000) Load sharing characteristics of stabilized lumbar spine segment. Spine 25:170–179
3. Cunningham BW, Sefter JC, Shono Y (1993) Static and cyclic biomechanical analysis of pedicle screw spinal constructs. Spine 18:1677–1688
4. Knop C, Blauth M, Bühren V et al (2001) Operative treatment of thoracolumbar fractures – results of a prospective multicenter study by the working group "spine" of the German Society of Trauma Surgery Part 3 Follow-up. Unfallchirurg 104:583–600
5. Maiman DJ, Pintar F, Yoganandan N et al (1993) Effects of anterior vertebral grafting on the traumatized lumbar spine after pedicle screw-plate fixation. Spine 18:2423–2430
6. Matschke S, Wagner C, Davids D et al (2006) Complications in endoscopic anterior thoracolumbar spinal reconstructive surgery. Eur J Trauma 23:215–226
7. McLain RF, Sparling D, Benson DR (1993) Early failure of short segment pedicle instrumentation for thoraco-lumbar fractures. A preliminary report. J Bone Joint Surg Am 75:162–167
8. Nothwang J, Ulrich C (2000) The reconstruction of the anterior column of thoracolumbar spine fractures. Osteosynthese Int 8:1–6
9. Rohlmann A, Graichen F, Bender A et al (2008) Loads on a telemeterized vertebral body replacement measured in three patients within the first postoperative month. Clin Biomech 23:147–158
10. Sasso RC, Cottler HB (1993) Posterior instrumentation and fusion for unstable fractures and fracture dislocations of the thoracic and lumbar spine. Spine 18:450–560
11. Reinhold M, Schmölz W, Canto F et al (2007) An improved vertebral body replacement for the thoracolumbar spine. A biomechanical in vitro test on human lumbar vertebral bodies. Unfallchirurg 110(4):327–333
12. Taneichi H, Kaneda K, Takeda N et al (1997) Risk factors and probability of vertebral body collapse in metastases of the thoracic and lumbar spine. Spine 22:239–245

Part VI

Posterior Thoracic Spine

Paulo Tadeu Maia Cavali

34.1 Introduction and Core Messages

Currently, the instrumentation of thoracic spine is a rigid construction. There is no dynamic instrumentation system for the thoracic spine, except for early onset scoliosis, where growing systems can be applied. This means that achieving an arthrodesis is the goal of an ideal spine stabilization, and the use of implants does not substitute the procedure of bone grafting. Many factors are involved in selecting the type of system (screws, hooks, wires, plates, rods, etc.), and which function (tension band, bridge fixation, buttressing, derotation, compression, etc.) must be employed. The surgeon has to always understand the following factors: surgeon familiarity with techniques, host bone quality, mechanism of injury, direction of instability, degree of instability, expected level of patient loading, graft bone quality, availability of implants, necessity of postoperative immobilization, and time of tissue healing. Harrington in the 1960s developed the first generation of spinal instrumentation using a hook-based distraction, Luque in the 1970s and 1980s developed the second generation of instrumentation, using a segment fixation technique with sublaminar wires, and Cotrel and Dubousset, in the 1980s, first brought up rigid segmental hook-based fixation which gave rise to all kinds of new types of implants using screws and hooks with enormous biomechanical versatility [7]. The objectives of this chapter are to discuss the different implants and different techniques for the treatment of scoliosis, kyphosis, and fracture.

34.2 Implants

The implants employed in the posterior thoracic spine constructs are wires, hooks, and pedicle screw systems from different companies (see Figs. 34.1a and 34.1b).

34.2.1 Wiring Systems

Although the sublaminar wiring techniques are no longer common in the thoracic spine, a number of wire-rod techniques continue to be routinely employed. The Luque technique is the most common and employs sublaminar wires in each vertebra as additional anchors. These wires are then wrapped around rods of nonrigid segmental spine constructs. Indications commonly include the neuromuscular scoliosis (see Figs. 34.2a and 34.2b), scoliosis including a thoracic lordosis and some cases of osteoporotic spine, where they are used as a hybrid construct with pedicle screw. Wiring techniques do not provide axial stability, and they are a poor choice for stabilization of pathologic processes including anterior column insufficiency such as tumors and fractures. Another limitation of these techniques is the lacking rotation correction of scoliosis. In addition, these methods have a high risk of iatrogenic neurologic injury with the sublaminar wires passage being in the spinal canal and moving there during the fixation and reduction maneuvers. The contraindications to wiring system are patients with kyphosis or canal stenosis and those related to biomechanic insufficiencies.

34.2.2 Hooks

There are a variety of hooks with different characteristics. Basically, three types of hooks can be used: pedicle hooks, laminar hooks, and transverse process hooks (see Fig. 34.3). Pedicle hooks, resting on the lamina of the instrumented vertebrae and the superior articular process

P.T.M. Cavali, M.D.
Department of Scoliosis, Hospital AACD,
Rua. Diogo Jacome n. 954, compl. 2711,
Sao Paulo 04512-001, Brazil
e-mail: paulo.escolioseaacd@uol.com.br

U. Vieweg, F. Grochulla (eds.), *Manual of Spine Surgery*,
DOI 10.1007/978-3-642-22682-3_34, © Springer-Verlag Berlin Heidelberg 2012

Fig. 34.1 (**a**) Sublaminar Wires. The Luque instrumentation. (**b**) Types of pedicles screws and hooks. Implants of S4 System by Aesculap

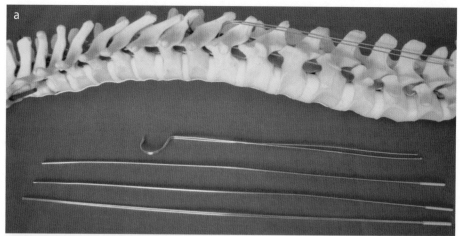

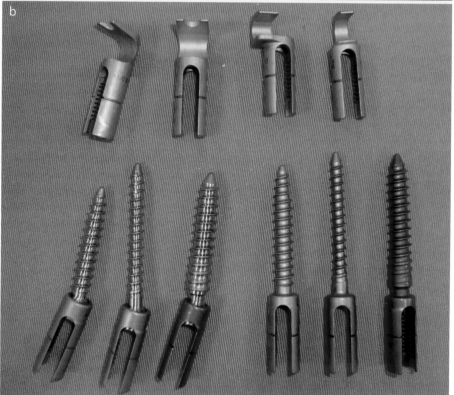

of next distal vertebrae, are the strongest hooks. They are always directed cephalad so that their "u" shaped tip embraces the pedicle and provides maximal stability concerning rotation and translation maneuvers. These implants can be placed from T1 to T10. Some of these hooks have additional features such as the possibility of being locked to the pedicle. Laminar hooks are available in a variety of designs. Variations in the blade width and style allow for an optimized hook-bone interface. These hooks may be placed in supralaminar or infralaminar positions dependent upon the required distraction or compression forces. Transverse process hooks have less risk of iatrogenic cord injury because they are out of the spinal canal. Usually, these implants are combined with a pedicle hook or a pedicle screw. This claw is the strongest hook construct, and it is very helpful in hyperkyphosis correction and can be added to transpedicular constructs to protect the screws from pullout.

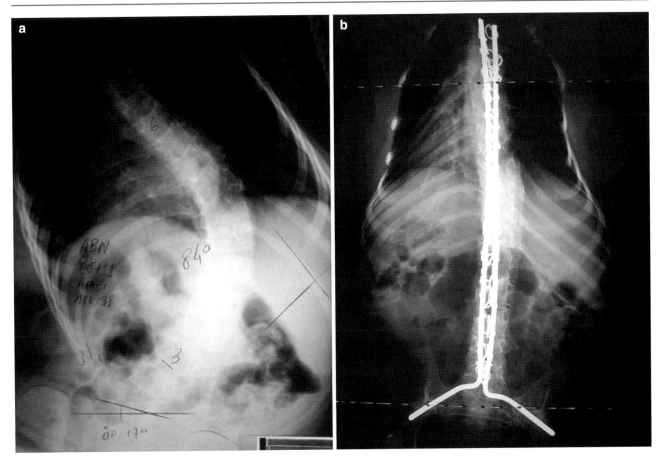

Fig. 34.2 (**a**) Preoperative image of neuromuscular scoliosis. (**b**) Surgical treatment of neuromuscular scoliosis with sublaminar wires technique

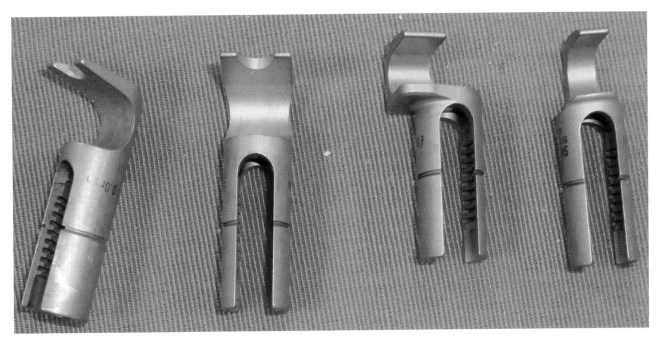

Fig. 34.3 Three types of hooks – pedicle, transverse process and laminar hooks. Implants of S4 System by Aesculap

34.2.3 Pedicle Screw

The pedicle screw is the strongest implant because it is inserted into the vertebral body.

34.3 Special Surgical Techniques

34.3.1 Correction of Kyphosis [2–6]

The operative surgery for kyphosis is based on cantilever maneuvers and compression forces. Compression causes shortening of posterior column of the thoracic spine. Distraction is not allowed because of the high neurological risk. The standard construction for the treatment of a flexible thoracic kyphosis includes instrumentation reaching from T2 to L1. For the rigid kyphosis, prior to the posterior instrumentation, any kind of osteotomy (pedicle subtraction or Smith-Petersen) or anterior disc and ligaments release should be performed when necessary. Cranial implants are inserted using a claw on each side. The claw can be combined with a pedicle screw in T3 and a transverse process hook in T2 or a pedicle hook in T3 and transverse process hook in T2. In either construction, the superior laminar hook can be substituted by a transverse process hook. The important feature of the claw mechanism is the compression between the two superior vertebrae on either side to avoid a pullout of the cranial implants. The claw can also be used by leaving one vertebra in between (for example T2 and T4). If necessary, more than one claw construct per side can be done on the superior part of instrumentation. Pedicle screws or hooks are inserted as preoperatively planed. The preference at the caudal end is the use of pedicle screws. These can be supplemented with laminar hooks to resist the pullout force. Depending upon the curve rigidity, it may be necessary to insert pedicle screws in all vertebrae. Using the rod benders, the 6-mm rods are precontoured to the desired sagittal plane kyphosis. The rods are then inserted into the upper pedicle screws or specialized pedicle hooks. With the rods applied in the correct sagittal plane, the claw constructs are locked. The rods are then reduced to the next caudal implants by applying uniform force on each rod with a rod pusher or rod holder. Compression is then applied to the implant in direction of the proximal claw construct. The nut can then be tightened to maintain the achieved correction before moving on to the next distal implants and repeating the procedure. At the end of the construct, two rod holders are applied to the rods, which are gently pushed down together onto the pedicle screws at T12 and L1. Once the rods are reduced onto these distal implants, the connectors and nuts are screwed on, and compression is applied against the proximally adjacent fixed implant or a rod holder placed in between. Then the nuts are tightened.

Finally, two cross-links are applied close to the ends of the instrumentation.

34.3.2 Correction of Scoliosis [1, 6, 7]

The most common pattern of idiopathic scoliosis is the right thoracic curve, and it will be the example to illustrate the principles of correction. The surgical treatment of scoliosis is based on many factors: age of patient, curve flexibility, Lenke classification (or other), frontal and sagittal balance, quality of bone, bone graft, patient clinical condition, structure of hospital, and availability of implants, as well as the surgeon's familiarity with the techniques among others. There are many ways to surgically reduce a scoliosis. It is utmost important to correctly apply the principles of correction. The follow technique using USS by Synthes is one option. The proximal and distal end vertebrae are identified on AP standing and lateral bending, fulcrum bending, or traction and lateral standing X-rays. The classic instrumentation of the right thoracic curve extends from T4 to L1. After posterior approach and intraoperative imaging to confirm the appropriate levels, the implants can be inserted, starting from the concave side and going to the convex side. The amount of implants (pedicle screws or hooks) depends upon the preoperative plan. The more implants are used and the more vertebrae are instrumented, the greater the potential of correction is. The foundation of the construct is established with pedicle screws placed in T12 and L1 caudally and in T4 and T5 cranially, on the concave side. On the convex side cranially, the implants are inserted as a claw construct, and it is applied between T4 and T5. Caudally, pedicle screws are inserted also at T12 and L1. The apical vertebra is usually T8 or T9 and is instrumented with pedicle screws, if possible on both sides. Additional instrumentation can usually be placed at alternating levels; however, additional implants must be used in larger and stiffer curves. A 6-mm rod template is placed in the desired sagittal plane on the concave side between the T4 and L1 screws. This template is used for the calculation of the final rod length while keeping in mind that the spine will automatically and passively elongate during the correction maneuvers. The rod template is then removed, and the appropriate size rod is contoured to the desired sagittal plane and cut to length. The rod can then be inserted into the T4 and L1 implants on the concave side, and collars and nuts are applied on both levels, but the nut is only tightened at L1 while maintaining the sagittal orientation of the rod. Using the complex reduction forceps (persuader), the intervening implants are brought to the rod using translation force. It is important not to apply force beyond that which the bone can withstand. In flexible curves, the apical implants are brought to the rod with the persuader. If the curve is stiff, do not primarily proceed to the reduction of apical implants and direct your attention to the convex side. The convex-contoured rod is now applied as a kind of lateral cantilever maneuver. The rod is inserted into the proximal claw inserted at T4 and T5. The claw is then compressed, and the nuts are tightened (T4 and T5) to ensure stability of the implants while the rod is maintained in a strict sagittal position. The convex rod is then pushed toward the midline using the rod holder to laterally engage the pedicle screws at T6, repeating the procedure at T8, T10, T12, and finally at L1. It is important not to tighten these nuts at this stage because this would prevent further correction on the concave side. At this moment, only the pedicle screw at L1 on concave side and the screws of the claw on the convex side have the nuts tightened to the rod, all the other implants connected to the rods have the nuts loose. The apical screws on the concave side will now have to be translated toward the concave rod using persuader forceps. After completing the coupling of implants to the rod on both sides of the spine in this way, the spine will have passively found its own length. The individually instrumented vertebrae are then sequentially derotated as they are secured to the rod starting from each end. This is achieved by placing a derotation force through the sticks attached to each of the implants, using the L handle and 6-mm socket wrench to tighten the nuts. It is important to hold the end vertebrae in their normal, neutral position prior to commencing this process in order to avoid transference of the torque force from instrumented to the uninstrumented spine. Cross-links are applied at the extremities of the instrumentation. Decortication of the posterior elements and osteotomy of the facet joints are important steps before the bone grafting procedure.

34.3.3 Stabilization of Fractures

The principles of treatment of fractures of the thoracic spine are to correct the deficient part of the injured spine using appropriate forces, support, and stabilization methods. The use of any type of fracture classification will be helpful to choose the principles and proper implant system.

A good example for using these principles is the Universal Spine System – fracture module by Synthes. This system can be used in the middle and low thoracic spine. It is not recommended in the upper thoracic spine because the pedicles are too small and the instrumentation may be too prominent at these levels. In this system, the implants act as a tension band, a buttress, and a neutralization system. USS allows a lordosation, distraction, compression, as well as fixation, in a neutral position. Another important point is that the fulcrum of corrective forces can be adjusted by applying half rings. The important features of this system are: Schanz screws, clamps with separate fixation for rods,

and Schanz screws and the half-ring clamps. The use of Schanz screw allows easy reduction of the vertebral body in the sagittal plane. The USS fracture clamps have separate fixations for rods and Schanz screws; it allows a range motion of + or $-18°$ in the sagittal plane of the Schanz screws. Also, it is possible to do compression or distraction independently of the Schanz screw angle. The half-ring clamps can move the fulcrum of the corrective forces away from the posterior wall of the vertebral body. When all four Schanz screws have been inserted, the rods of the fracture module are applied to the Schanz screws using fracture clamps with the rods lying medially to the Schanz screws. The clamps are left loose.

34.3.3.1 Reduction and Fixation of Fractures with Intact Posterior Wall

The posterior ends of the Schanz screws are manually approximated until the desired correction of the kyphosis has been attained. The set screws on the clamps must remain loose so that the clamps can slide freely toward each other during the reduction maneuver. The center of rotation then lies at the posterior edge of the vertebral body. By creating the lordosis, the vertebral body will be distracted anteriorly, and the disc space and disc height can be restored by ligamentotaxis. Place the cannulated socket wrenches over the caudal Schanz screws and tilt them cranially to create lordosis in the spine. The posterior nuts are then locked. The same procedure is performed on the cranial Schanz screw in order to reestablish the correct sagittal plane. The appropriate posterior nuts are tightened to fix the angle between the Schanz screws and the rods. At this stage, it is necessary to distract the Schanz screws to reestablish the normal height of the injured disc and vertebra. A half-ring clamp is placed and locked in the center of each rod between the clamps. Distract the spreader forceps and check the procedure with the image intensifier. When the desired distraction is obtained, tighten the set screws and remove the rings.

34.3.3.2 Reduction and Fixation of Fractures with Fractured Posterior Wall

In this type of fractures, there is a danger that the posterior wall fragments might displace posterior into the spinal canal during the correction of the kyphosis by compressing the posterior ends of the Schanz screws. It is important to protect the posterior wall against compression. Distraction is used to reconstitute the height of the vertebral body and disc space.

Two half rings are placed on each of the 6-mm rods prior to reduction with the Schanz screws. A distance of 5 mm between the half rings and the clamp is allowed for every 10° of attempted kyphosis correction. When approximating the ends of the Schanz screws, the clamps will soon touch the half rings, and the center of rotation is transferred posterior to the level of the rods instead of the posterior wall. The lordosis is checked with a lateral image intensifier view. The posterior-opening nuts are tightened to secure the correction, and the set screws on the clamps are fixed. This procedure is repeated for the other Schanz screws. The half rings are then removed. Distraction is performed between the Schanz screws to obtain the height of the vertebral body.

After fracture reduction and stabilization, anterior surgery may be required for biomechanical purposes in case of significant vertebral body comminution, osteoporosis, or incomplete clearance of the spinal canal with persistent neurological deficit.

34.4　Tips and Tricks

- The pedicle screw is the most powerful implant because of its three-column insertion. An appropriate utilization of these implants, therefore, requires an understanding of their mechanical properties as well as the properties of alternative devices and models of constructions.
- If the placement of a pedicle screw is difficult, it is possible to open the spinal canal and, through direct visualization of pedicle, introduce the pedicle screw. If in doubt, instrumentation should be avoided, especially when optimal purchase and placement are in doubt.
- The principle of ligamentotaxis for posterior fragments reduction of fracture is valid only if the posterior longitudinal ligament is intact. When the posterior longitudinal ligament is disrupted, then indirect decompression of the spinal canal should not be done using this procedure. Images from a CT scan or an MRI can demonstrate the disruption of the posterior longitudinal ligament with the sign of a reverse cortical sign of the posterior wall fragment.
- The use of half rings can be avoided by using rod holders.
- The use of sticks or Schanz screw can be substituted by any kind of elongated screw to allow for cantilever force or other systems.

References

1. Aebi M, Arlet V, Webb JK (2007) AOSPINE manual. Principle and techniques, vol 1. Thieme, New York
2. Cho KJ, Bridwell KH, Lenke LG et al (2005) Comparasion of Smith-Petersen versus pedicle subtraction osteotomy for the correction of fixed sagittal imbalance. Spine 30:2030–2037
3. Gill JB, Levin A, Burd T et al (2008) Corrective osteotomies in spine surgery. J Bone Joint Surg Am 90:2509–2520
4. Heary RF, Bono CM (2006) Pedicle subtraction astronomy in the treatment of chronic, posttraumatic kyphotic deformity. J Neurosurg Spine 5:1–8
5. Macagno AE, O'Brien MF (2006) Thoracic and thoracolumbar kyphosis in adults. Spine 19(Suppl):S161–S170
6. Mohan AL, Das K (2003) History of surgery for the correction of spinal deformity. Neurosurg Focus 14(1):e1
7. Winter RB, Lonstein JE (2007) Congenital thoracic scoliosis with unilateral unsegmented bar and concave fused ribs. Spine 32: E841–E844

Stabilization of the Thoracic Spine with Internal Fixator

35

Robert Morrison and Uwe Vieweg

35.1 Introduction and Core Messages

The preparation of the pedicle within the thoracic spine requires precise preoperative planning. The anatomical structures marking the entry point, the pedicle orientation, and diameter must be known prior to the operation. Performing an adequate preoperative planning including CT scans is elemental for planning of the instrumentation and selection of the correct screw placement. In cases of very small pedicle diameters, especially within the middle thoracic spine, only a parapedicular screw placement may be possible. In cases of small pedicle diameter or poor intraoperative radiological picture quality (obese patient, etc.), navigational screw placement is recommended. Due to the lower axial load within the upper thoracic spine and the stabilization through the rib cage, an additional anterior stabilization is not as often necessary as in the lumbar spine.

35.2 Indications

- Fractures of the thoracic spine
- Degenerative disorders
- Deformities/scoliosis
- Tumors or infections of the spine

R. Morrison, M.D. (⌧)
Department of Spine Surgery,
Sana Hospital Rummelsberg,
Rummelsberg 71,
90592 Schwarzenbruck, Germany
e-mail: dr.r.morrison@googlemail.com

U. Vieweg, M.D., Ph.D.
Clinic for Spinal Surgery, Sana Hospital Rummelsberg,
90593 Schwarzenbruck, Germany
e-mail: uwe.vieweg@yahoo.de

35.3 Contraindications

- Osteopenia/osteoporosis (relative contraindication).
- Ongoing infection within the instrumented vertebra (relative contraindication).
- Poor medical condition of the patient (possibly absolute contraindication).
- Small pedicles make transpedicular stabilization impossible (relative contraindication).

35.4 Technical Prerequisites

Fluoroscopy, special cushions (e.g., Wilson Frame etc.), radiolucent operating table, possibly additional intraoperative electrophysiological monitoring (SSEP, MEP). Facultative, a spinal navigation system can be used.

35.5 Planning, Preparation, and Positioning

Preoperative measurement includes the pedicle diameter and especially the transverse diameter. Within the thoracic spine, this should be done with a CT scan. If the transverse diameter is large enough to carry the screws, the preoperative planning can take place. The correct *entry point* can be found after identifying the necessary landmarks. These include the facet joint with its borders and the transverse process. Intraoperatively, the entry point is located in the lateral half of the oval area of the pedicle in the AP fluoroscopy. This also includes measuring the transverse diameter of the pedicles (Table 35.1). The *orientation of the pedicle* can be gauged in lateral radiographs or even more precise using CT scans. Sagittal reconstructions of the planning-CT for the cranial-caudal angle and coronary scans for the lateral deviation are advised (Fig. 35.1). These two values show a great variation within the thoracic spine [1, 5]. The *pedicle length* also shows great variations. The correct screw length cannot be gauged intraoperatively in lateral fluoroscopy, as the anterior cortex has a

U. Vieweg, F. Grochulla (eds.), *Manual of Spine Surgery*,
DOI 10.1007/978-3-642-22682-3_35, © Springer-Verlag Berlin Heidelberg 2012

Table 35.1 Table showing the average pedicle diameter, transverse angle corresponding to the midline, and the inclination angle of the pedicle orientation corresponding to the superior end plate

Vertebra	Gender	Transversal pedicle diameter (mm)	Transversal angle of the pedicle (°)	Inclination angle of the pedicle (°)
Th 1	M	8.8	39	23
	F	10.4	29	20
Th 2	M	6	35	23
	F	6.7	28	20
Th 3	M	4.1	22	22
	F	5.3	22	19
Th 4	M	3.9	29	23
	F	3.8	19	17
Th 5	M	4.6	24	25
	F	4	17	19
Th 6	M	3.6	26	27
	F	4	15	24
Th 7	M	4.5	25	24
	F	4.6	11	19
Th 8	M	5	29	20
	F	4.6	9	18
Th 9	M	5.3	21	18
	F	5.5	12	18
Th 10	M	5.6	20	18
	F	6	17	17
Th 11	M	8.3	22	20
	F	8.8	15	19
Th 12	M	8	15	20
	F	9.4	11	18

Adapted from Ebraheim et al. [1]

convex shape. When deciding for a screw length, one must keep in mind that 60% of the pullout force is achieved in the pedicle and 15–20% additionally in the cancellous bone of the vertebral body [6]. So the screw should rather be chosen too short than too lang.

35.5.1 Anatomical Specifications of the Thoracic Spine

- Small pedicle diameter (smallest in the midthoracic spine T3–T8) [4]. The screw diameter should be 75–80% of the transverse pedicle diameter.
- The medial cortex of the pedicles is much stronger than the lateral wall, making the lateral perforation much more common [3].
- Very small pedicle diameters make transpedicular screw placement impossible in such cases.
- Plain radiographs in two planes are often not enough to plan the instrumentation in the thoracic spine; in such cases, a CT scan is necessary.

35.6   Surgical Technique

35.6.1 Approach

- Open access via a midline incision. The incision should be two segments longer than the intended length of fusion.

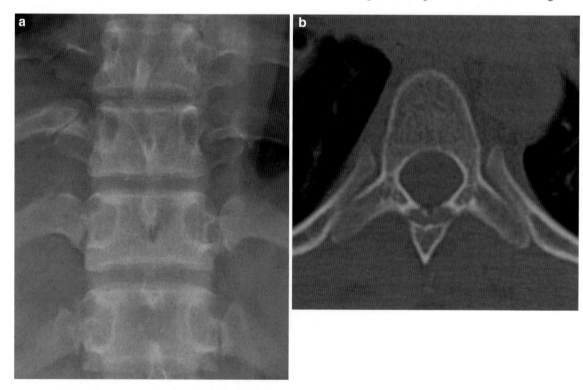

Fig. 35.1 (**a**) Plain radiograph of the thoracic spine in AP view and (**b**) corresponding CT scan in axial view showing the pedicle width and orientation

The subcutis is dissected to the fascia, and wound retractors are applied. The fascia is detached on both sides using a diathermy knife close to the bone. The paraspinal structures are retracted with a raspatory. The muscles are retracted to expose the costal processes (Fig. 35.2).

- Alternatively an additional laminotomy can be performed. This is used when a safe identification of the pedicles cannot be found during the operation. In such cases, the lamina is resected to display the medial side of the pedicles. Then the screws can be placed as described above.

35.7 Instrumentation

35.7.1 Trajectory

- Entry point can be found at the intersection of the vertical line along the middle of the superior articular process and the horizontal line through the top of the transverse process. Distances to other landmarks can be misleading in the thoracic spine due to the great anatomical variability [1] (Fig. 35.2).
- The pedicle is opened with a pedicle awl, followed by consecutive deepening with a pedicle trocar. The length of the screw can be seen on the side of the trocar. To verify the intact pedicle walls, the walls of the canal are tested with a ball-tip pedicle probe.
- Within the thoracic spine, the screws will have a decreasing convergence toward the midline (20–25° in T1 to 5° in T4–12) (Table 35.1) (Fig. 35.3).
- The screws should be placed parallel to the superior end plate if possible. Alternatively, a slanted introduction is also possible. Thereby, the tip of the screw is aimed

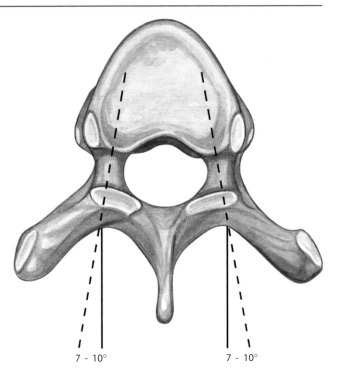

Fig. 35.3 Entry point of the transpedicular screw in the thoracic spine, with an angulation of 7–10° toward the midline

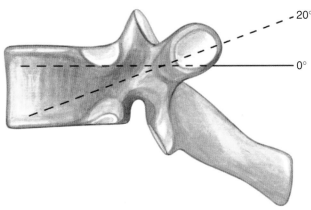

Fig. 35.4 Entry point of the transpedicular screw in the thoracic spine in a lateral view. Angulation depending upon the desired positioning

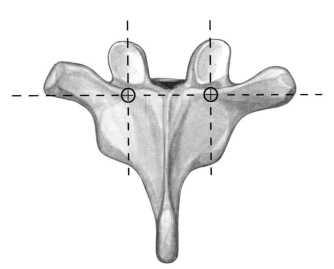

Fig. 35.2 Entry point of the transpedicular screw in the thoracic spine, when planning a screw placement parallel to the superior end plate

toward the anterior edge of the inferior end plate (Choose higher entry point!) (Fig. 35.4).
- *Parapedicular screw placement* [2]
  In cases of narrow pedicles, a transpedicular trajectory would cause a burst fracture of the pedicles. In such cases, a more lateral entry point is chosen. The trajectory starts at the tip of the transverse process and enters the vertebral body via the costotransversal joints (Figs. 35.5). This technique involves a greater risk of penetration of the pleural cavity.

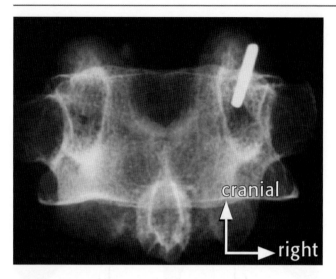

Fig. 35.5 Superior view of typical extrapedicular screw placement

35.8   Tips and Tricks

- Start out by marking the entry points with K-wires or short pins using the fluoroscopy in the AP direction.
- The correct positioning and orientation can be verified by adjusting the fluoroscopy to where the K-wire is a "point," which lies clearly within the pedicle.
- The positioning of the patient is especially important when instrumenting the mid thoracic spine (T3–6), as the scapula interferes with the lateral fluoroscopy.

References

1. Ebraheim NA, Xu R, Ahmad M et al (1997) Projection of the thoracic pedicle and its morphometric analysis. Spine 22:233–238
2. Husted DS, Yue JJ, Fairchild TA et al (2003) An extrapedicular approach to the placement of screws in the thoracic spine: an anatomic and radiographic assessment. Spine 28:2324–2330
3. Kothe R, O'Holleran JD, Liu W et al (1996) Internal architecture of the thoracic pedicle: an anatomic study. Spine 21:264–270
4. Panjabi MM, Takata K, Goel V et al (1991) Thoracic human vertebrae. Quantitative three-dimensional anatomy. Spine 16:888–901
5. Vaccaro AR, Rizzolo SJ, Allardyce TJ et al (1995) Placement of pedicle screw in the thoracic spine. Part one: morphometric analysis of the thoracic vertebrae. J Bone Joint Surg Am 77:1193–1199
6. Weinstein JN, Rydevik BL, Rauschning WJN (1992) Anatomic and technical considerations of pedicle screw fixation. Clin Orthop Relat Res 284:34–46

Transpedicular Stabilization with Freehand Technique on the Thoracic Spine

36

Paulo Tadeu Maia Cavali

36.1 Introduction and Core Messages

The use of pedicle screws has become popular during the past decade, first in applications involving the lumbar spine and subsequently in thoracic spine surgery. Pedicle screws also prevent the need to place instrumentation within the spinal canal like sublaminar wiring or hooks which create the risk of neurological injury. Transpedicular stabilization (TS) has been shown to resist flexion and extension loads as well as torsional loads better than other devices. Especially in spinal deformity surgery, the use of TS provides better correction and maintenance than system with hooks and wires. Disadvantages of pedicular screws are related to the misplacement of pedicle screws which can lead to disastrous complications such as vascular or neural injuries. Accurate and safe placement of screw within the pedicle is a crucial step during the surgery. There are many proven techniques used to insert pedicle screws, including fluoroscopic or radiographic guidance, stereotactic guidance system based on computed tomography, direct visualization of pedicle with the use of a laminotomy, and the freehand technique (without intraoperative image guidance). The freehand techniques use established surface landmarks and direct palpation of internal pedicle and vertebral structure. The objective of this chapter is to describe the freehand technique for transpedicular stabilization in the thoracic spine.

36.2 Indications

- Deformities such as scoliosis and kyphosis
- Trauma with fractures and/or dislocations
- Tumors and other pathologic fractures

36.3 Contraindications

- Intense osteoporosis
- Small pedicle with diameter smaller than 4.0 mm
- Inadequate anterior column support

36.4 Technical Prerequisites

Fluoroscopy, positioning device (e.g., Wiltse frame), intraoperative neuromonitoring with somatosensory evoked potentials (SSEP), transcranial electric motor-evoked potentials (TMEP), and electromyography (EMG). The

P.T.M. Cavali, M.D.
Department of Scoliosis, Hospital AACD,
Rua. Diogo Jacome n. 954 compl. 2711,
Sao Paulo 04512-001, Brazil
e-mail: paulo.escolioseaacd@uol.com.br

U. Vieweg, F. Grochulla (eds.), *Manual of Spine Surgery*,
DOI 10.1007/978-3-642-22682-3_36, © Springer-Verlag Berlin Heidelberg 2012

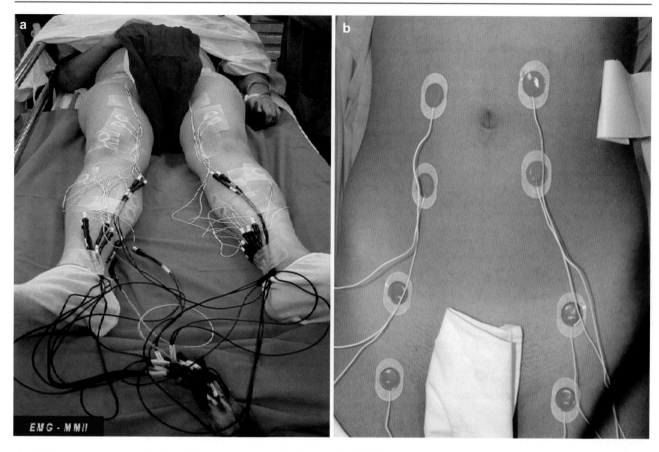

Fig. 36.1 Intraoperative monitoring with somatosensory evoked potentials (SSEP) and transcranial electric motor-evoked potentials (TMEP). The thoracic nerve roots from T6–T12 are performed with EMG from rectus abdominus muscle

SSEP and TMEP provide evaluation of cord function, and triggered EMG gives information about any contact of screw with neural structures as spinal cord or nerve roots (see Fig. 36.1). Adequate implants and instruments. There are many pedicle screw systems in the market. Most of them are able to stabilize the thoracic spine. In the thoracic spine, the area to set up the instrumentation is smaller than lumbar one; it means that the profile of head of screws, rods, and connectors must fit well for each patient to avoid prominence in the skin.

36.5   Planning, Preparation, and Positioning

Prior to surgery, the patient's X-ray is reviewed to assess pedicle diameter, length, and its orientation. Knowledge of normal pedicle morphometry is essential to proper placement of pedicle screw.

The lateral images with the patient in prone position on the operative table give orientation of screws for each vertebra

in sagittal plane (see Fig. 36.2). For deformities surgeries, the level of spine instrumentation and the number and local of screws depend on many features as: classification, stiffness, and magnitude of curve. The patient is positioned prone on a radiolucent operative table. The abdomen and thorax are permitted to hang freely.

36.6   Operative Technique

36.6.1   Approach

- The midline posterior approach is the avenue for placement of thoracic instrumentation. It is performed with wide subperiosteal exposure of the posterior bony elements to the level of the transverse processes (see Fig. 36.3). This significantly more wide exposure beyond the facet and out into the transverse process is important to identify all anatomical landmarks.
- Transverse process and the base of superior facet are used as landmarks. With a 2-mm osteotome, approximately

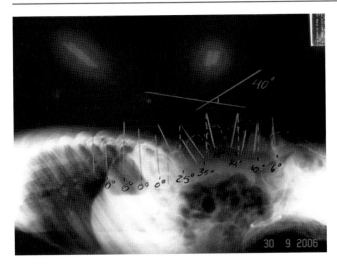

Fig. 36.2 Preoperative X-ray with the patient in prone position on the operative table. The measurement of the sagittal angle of all pedicles to be instrumented

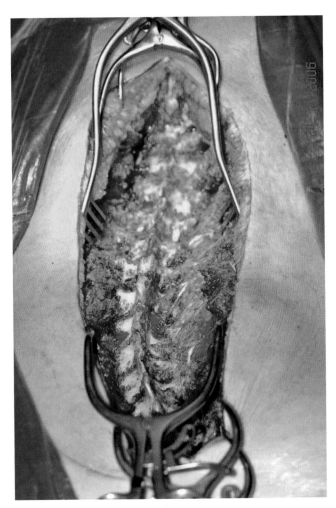

Fig. 36.3 The wide posterior exposure of the thoracic spine

5 mm of inferior articular process is removed so as to expose the base of the superior articular process.

36.6.2 Instrumentation [1–6]

- The starting point for each thoracic level is slightly variable and is based on the posterior element anatomy of the transverse process and the base of superior articular facet. The ideally entry point in the thoracic pedicle is at the junction of a horizontal line along the inferior border of facet joint and vertical line at the junction of the outer third and inner two-thirds of the facet joint. The starting point in the proximal region (T1–T3) is at the middle of transverse process; in the mid- and lower thoracic region, it is at superior third of transverse process, and in T12, the entry point is at middle and tip of transverse process (see Fig. 36.4).

- Before making the entry into the pedicle, initial neuromonitoring recordings with SSEP and TMEP are performed to establish the preinstrumentation neural status of the patient.

- The entry point is made rough with rouger or a 3.5-mm acorn-tipped burr to prevent slippage of awl, to visualize of cancellous bone, and to create space to lodge the head of pedicle screw.

- Then the further passage in the pedicle is made with appropriate amount of ventral pressure using the gearshift (2 mm blunt-tipped pedicle finder).

- The surgeon must be careful to the axial and sagittal position of vertebrae space to position the probe down the pedicle shaft appropriately. The information about the axial and sagittal angle is given by the images obtained preoperatively.

- In the thoracic spine without scoliosis and kyphosis, the pedicle finder should be angled 7–10 toward the midline and 10–20 caudally. When the spine is deformed or scoliotic, these angles are different and asymmetrical.

- The trajectory of pedicle screw is completed with the gearshift going down to the pedicle and reaching the cancellous bone near to anterior cortex of vertebra body. At this moment, new neuromonitoring recordings are performed with SSEP, TMEP, and EMG. The EMG is taken with direct stimulation of gearshift inserted into the pedicle trajectory. These data are used to investigate the integrity of pedicle trajectory (see Fig. 36.5).

- The surgeon sensitivity during the penetration of cancellous bone through the pedicle to vertebral body is an important step and depends on appropriate learning curve. Any sudden advancement of the pedicle finder suggests penetration into soft tissue, and thus a pedicle wall violation or vertebral body violation has occurred. Decision of screw diameter and length is based on preoperative assessment but confirmed intraoperatively.

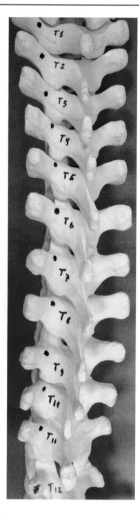

Fig. 36.4 The starting point for each thoracic pedicle

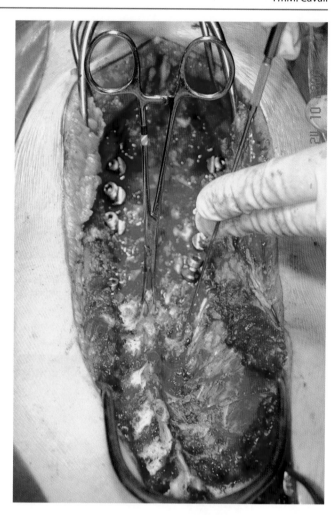

Fig. 36.6 Palpation of five walls of pedicle tract with flexible ball-tipped probe

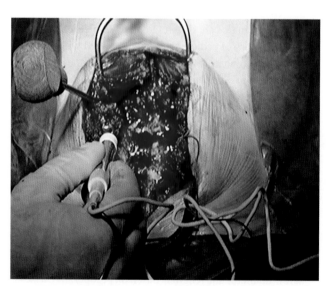

Fig. 36.5 The EMG with direct stimulation of gearshift immediately after complete perforation of pedicle trajectory

- It is important to avoid penetration of the anterior cortex to prevent visceral and vascular injuries. Approximately 90% of strength of the screw comes from the pedicle and posterior half of the vertebral body.
- Once the trajectory of pedicle screw is completed and neuromonitoring data have not demonstrated any signal of wall violation, the pedicle finder (gearshift) is removed. The tract is visualized to make sure that only blood is coming out.
- Excessive bleeding from the pedicle hole may indicate epidural bleeding secondary to medial wall violation, and the presence of cerebrospinal fluid means more medial violation with dural lesion.
- At this point, if any of these situation occurs such as inappropriate neuromonitoring data or signs of violation of pedicle wall, there is an opportunity to redirect the pedicle finder into an appropriate position in the pedicle so that complete intraosseous borders can be obtained.
- Palpation of pedicle tract is the next step. With a flexible ball-tipped probe, the five walls are palpated (see Fig. 36.6).

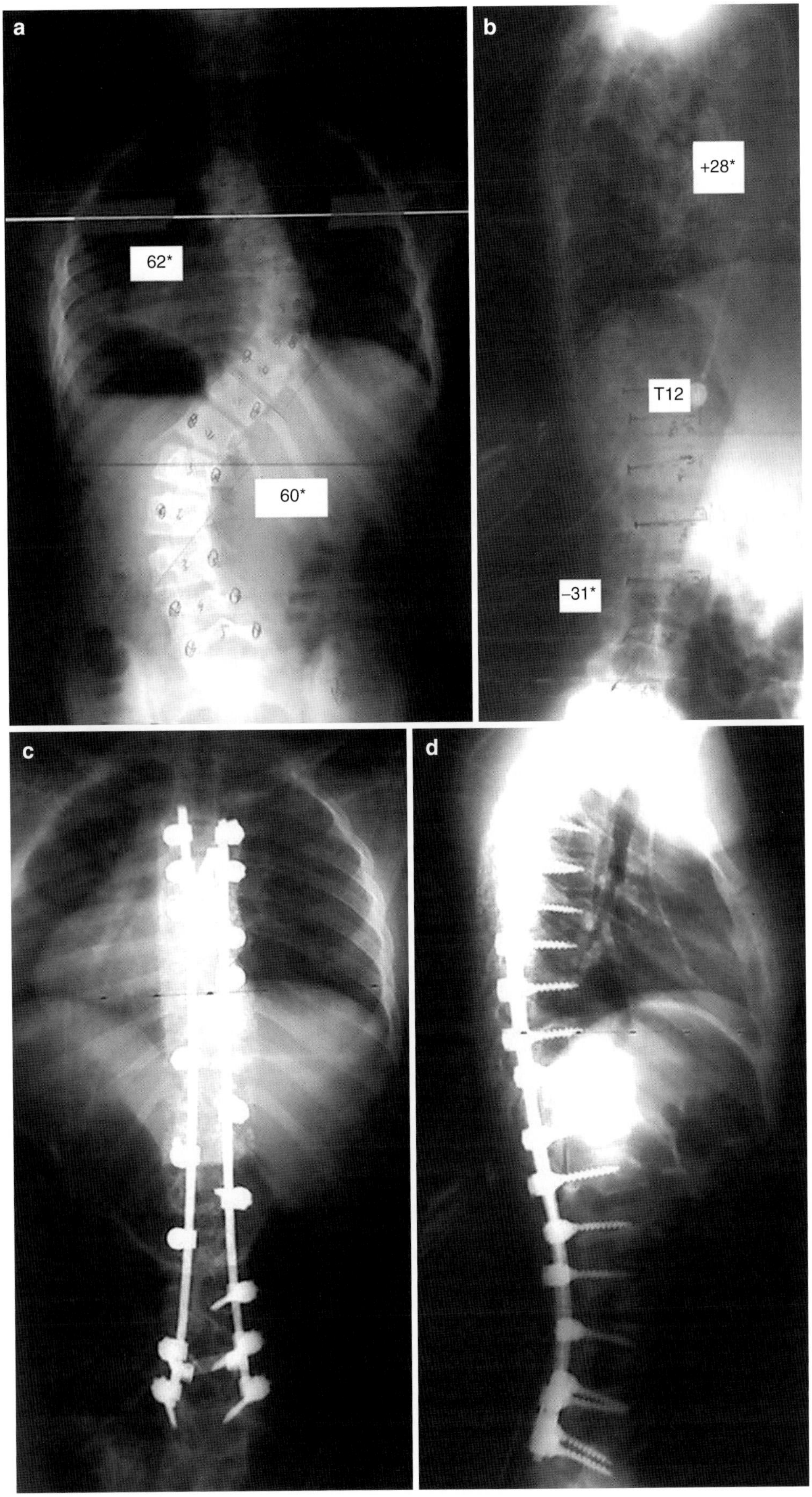

Fig. 36.7 Preoperative assessment of the patient (**a-b**) and intraoperative confirmation and documentation immediately after complete instrumentation (**c-d**)

- The integrity of five walls: medial, lateral, superior (cranial), inferior (caudal), and floor (anterior cortex) is essential to insert the screw. The most important walls are medial and inferior because respectively of the presence of the spinal cord and nerve root. In the literature, the critical violation of any pedicle wall is defined as more than 2 mm, and the most common violated wall is the lateral follow by medial one.
- The measurement of pedicle tract is performed with the same flexible ball-tipped probe after confirmation of integrity of the five walls. Then the tract is tapping, and an adequate screw in length and diameter is inserted into the pedicle.
- The next imperative step is the confirmation and documentation of intraosseous placement of all pedicle screw via images using fluoroscopy or radiography at the end of surgery (Fig. 36.7) and by neuromonitoring data performed after insertion of each screw during the surgery with SSEP, TMEP, and triggered EMG.
- With the screws inserted in appropriated position, the previously rods are placed according to the preoperative plan.

36.7   Tips and Tricks

- In order to prevent violation of the medial wall of pedicle, the half medial part of the superior facet and its caudal projection must be avoided (see Fig. 36.8).
- If the pedicle screw was misplaced and its reposition was not possible in the appropriate place, the screw can be inserted by the in-out-in technique (more lateral and more convergence technique).
- The insertion of pedicle screw in scoliotic spine can be difficult especially on the concave side; then the orientation of the surface of superior facet can be helpful once

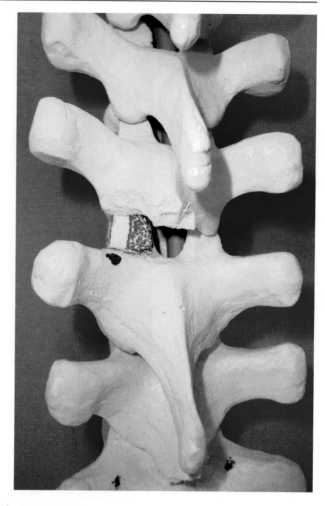

Fig. 36.8 The *red region* is the half medial part of the superior facet (must be avoided), and the *blue landmark* is the entry point of pedicle screw

the direction of pedicle screw has an angle slightly perpendicular with the surface of the superior facet. This is useful for axial and sagittal orientation (see Fig. 36.9).

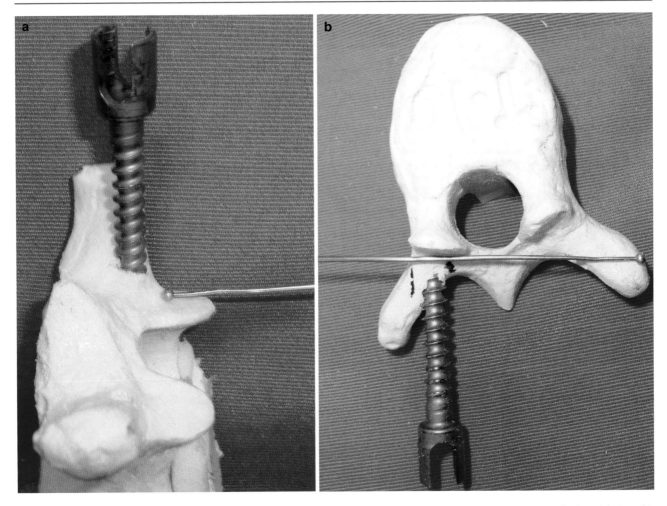

Fig. 36.9 The perpendicular relantionship between axis of pedicle and surface of superior facet, even in sagittal plane (**a**) as in the axial plane (**b**)

References

1. Bergeson RK, Schwend RM, DeLucia T et al (2008) How accurately do novice surgeons place thoracic pedicle screws with the free hand technique? Spine 33(15):E501–E507
2. Chung KJ, Suh SW, Desai S et al (2008) Ideal entry point for the thoracic pedicle screw during the free hand technique. Int Orthop 32:657–662
3. Kim YW, Lenke LG, Kim YJ et al (2008) Free-hand pedicle screw placement during revision spinal surgery. Spine 33:1141–1148
4. Modi HN, Suh SW, Fernandez H et al (2008) Accuracy and safety of pedicle screw placement in neuromuscular scoliosis with free-hand technique. Eur Spine J 17:1686–1696
5. Ofiram E, Polly DW, Gilbert JRTJ et al (2007) Is it safer to place pedicle screws in the lower thoracic spine than in the upper lumbar spine? Spine 32:9–54
6. Schizas C, Theumann N, Kosmopoulos V (2007) Inserting pedicle screws in the upper thoracic spine without the use of fluoroscopy or image guidance. Is it safe? Eur Spine J 16:625–629

Part VII

Anterior Lumbar Spine

Overview of Surgical Techniques and Implants

37

Karsten Wiechert and Felix Hohmann

37.1 Introduction and Core Message

The concept of anterior surgery of the lumbar spine has been well established for decades and addresses all forms of anterior column pathology. There are numerous surgical techniques, most of them standardized, serving specific surgical needs depending on pathology, specific anatomical considerations and the specific implant to be used. The surgical techniques used for the anterior lumbar spine involve combinations of anterior or anterolateral access (open, mini-open or percutaneous) with various forms of instrumentation (plate-screw systems, rod-screw systems, interbody fusion devices, vertebral body replacement devices, artificial disc and nucleus replacement systems).

37.2 Approaches

37.2.1 Classic Open Access

- Thoracolumbar access (transpleural-retroperitoneal T9–L5 as described by Hodgson [6])
- Thoracolumbar access with double thoracotomy T4–L5
- Retroperitoneal-extrapleural access T11–L5 as described by Mirbaha [9]
- Retroperitoneal anterolateral lumbar spinal access L2–5
- Transperitoneal or retroperitoneal access to the lumbosacral junction L4–S1 [2]

These access routes are usually highly invasive. They are used mainly in ventral corrective fusion surgery performed to treat scoliotic and kyphotic deformities and in tumour surgery.

K. Wiechert, M.D. (✉) • F. Hohmann, M.D.
Department of Spine Therapy, Hessingpark Clinic, Hessingstrasse 17, 86199 Augsburg, Germany
e-mail: karsten.wiechert@hessingpark-clinic.de;
felix.hohmann@hessingpark-clinic.de

37.2.2 Mini-Open Access Techniques

There are numerous standardized minimally invasive techniques for reaching the lumbar spine with sufficient exposure of the relevant structures to reach the corresponding pathologies and provide treatment. They are all characterized by limited or minimal surgical trauma and make use of existing anatomical pathways. Most of the techniques allow sufficient exposure of the target structure (disc space, vertebral body/bodies). Anterior mini-open access techniques use various retractor systems, e.g., SynFrame (Synthes) [1], Activ-O (Aesculap). These allow the access routes to be kept as small as possible and the surrounding tissue to be preserved more effectively. Even reconstructive procedures or vertebral body replacements in the lumbar area can be performed using an anterolateral approach. With the aid of endoscopes, it is possible to carry out an instrumented procedure either entirely or partially by endoscopic means, especially anterior interbody fusion [18]. However, some authors instead favour minimalized access without endoscopy (so-called MiniALIF) (ALIF – Anterior Lumbar Interbody Fusion) [4, 8]. Percutaneous procedures are also available. Among the most commonly used are the following:

- MiniALIF anterolateral approach L2–L5
- Mini-open midline approach L2–S1
- Pararectal approach L3–S1
- ALPA – AnteroLateral transPsoatic Approach

MiniALIF Anterolateral Approach to L2–L5

The MiniALIF approach was first described by Mayer [8]. Its key steps are precise positioning, marking of target projection onto the skin and a completely blunt dissection of the muscular planes, the peritoneal sac and exposure of the disc space. It is an entirely universal technique and exposes the disc space and the vertebral bodies. In some cases, the rib cage may restrict access so that certain modifications are necessary. The single steps of the technique are completely standardized, the complications spectrum limited. The MiniALIF technique may be seen as the current gold standard in antero-lateral approaches to the lumbar spine [8].

Mini-Open Midline Approach to L1–S1

This technique is based on the same surgical principles as the anterolateral approach. With the advent of total disc replacement, however, a need for a precise midline placement of the disc prosthesis gained utmost importance. This approach plays a vital role in facilitating minimally invasive surgery in such cases. The planes of the abdominal wall are bluntly dissected and the peritoneal sac exposed. The technique allows for retroperitoneal dissection as well as for transperitoneal exposure of the anterior circumference of the lumbar spine. The approach is easily expandable if necessary and works for the levels L1 to the sacrum. While mono- and bisegmental approaches can easily be carried out, exposure may present limitations for multisegmental surgery.

Pararectal Approach to L2–S1

This approach employs the anatomical pathway lateral to the rectus abdominis muscle. The lumbar spine can be reached safely and elegantly even in multilevel procedures, and there are no limitations on the type of lumbar reconstruction possible. However, midline implantations such as in TDR (total disc replacement) are not ideal because of anatomical and tissue restraints.

ALPA transPsoatic Approach

This approach focuses on a strict lateral approach to the lumbar motion segment and was originally described for implantation of nucleus replacement devices. After blunt dissection of the planes of the abdominal wall, the psoas fibres are exposed and transected up to the disc space. Special attention needs to be given to the fibres of the lumbosacral plexus. The use of neuromonitoring devices is therefore advocated for this approach.

37.2.3 Endoscopic Approaches

There are numerous descriptions of endoscopic techniques for reaching the lumbar spine. A balloon-assisted extraperitoneal technique through an anterolateral approach dissects the peritoneal plane. Critical attention needs to be given to moving the iliac vessels in order to preserve them as the potential for vascular injury is obvious. On the technical side, it must be mentioned that progress during endplate preparation can be nicely monitored with an endoscope. However, a steep learning curve, some medicolegal considerations with regard to general surgical training in access surgery and some limitations in implants and devices have kept these techniques to a niche in anterior spine surgery in the orthopaedic and neurosurgical areas.

37.3 Implants

The implants fulfilling certain tasks in specialized techniques on the lumbar spine are almost without number. This overview can only cover general properties of implants and does not attempt to address every aspect. General implant categories in anterior surgery of the lumbar spine are the following:

- Intersomatic fusion implants
- Total disc replacement devices
- Vertebral body replacements
- Anterior rod systems
- Anterior tension plates

37.3.1 Intersomatic Fusion Implants

This implant category plays a major role in anterior spine surgery. It can be divided into several subgroups, each serving a specific need:

- Intervertebral cages
- Stand-alone implants/cages with additional forms of fixation
- Nucleus replacement devices
- Total disc replacement devices

Intervertebral Cages

These cages are placed in the specially prepared intervertebral disc space and are designed to facilitate fusion of the motion segment. There is a multitude of shapes and designs on the market. The key requirements of these implants are a large contact area for even load distribution and an open-structure facilitating bony ingrowth and subsequent solid bony fusion. It is also important that the design and material are compatible with imaging methods so that fusion status can be assessed. Stable primary fixation of the implant in the vertebral endplate is another important requirement. Most of the intervertebral cages are box-shaped with differences in materials (titanium, PEEK, tantalum) [12]. Some have lordotic angulations; others adapt to the anatomic curvature of the lumbar endplates. Generally, the intersomatic implants used for anterior procedures cover a larger percentage of the endplates than those used for posterior implantation. The radiological results for specific implants may be assessed in the individual literature.

Stand-Alone Implants

The surgical trauma of classic 360° fusion techniques has led to the development of alternatives providing equal biomechanical stability. Minimally invasive anterior approaches involve a standardized surgical technique with a defined risk profile.

The stand-alone implants which incorporate additional fixation with cortical screws and biomechanical tests showed comparable stability to 360° fusion techniques [3, 15, 16]. Anterior stand-alone implant types without fixation show a lack of stability during extension and lateral bending of the motion segment due to incomplete or complete removal of the anterior longitudinal ligament [10, 11]. A combination with anterior plating is necessary to provide anterior tension band stability and additional stiffness in lateral bending and torsional movements.

37.3.2 Nucleus Replacement

The trend in restoring motion and stabilization of the motion segment has led to several nucleus pulposus replacement technologies. Prevention of disc space collapse has been a key goal of nucleus replacement devices. These can be implanted through an anterior, posterolateral or posterior approach. They replace the nucleus and try to mimic its biomechanical properties with regard to axial load and compressive strength, as well as hydration properties. The core material consists of elastic polymers. However, use of most devices is limited to strict study protocols. Long-term results are not yet available.

37.3.3 Total Disc Replacement

Total disc replacement devices are playing an increasingly popular and important role in managing degenerative conditions of the lumbar spine. Their implantation is carried out through an anterior midline or anterolateral approach with special attention to precise implant placement in the midline. The midline total disc implantation may pose a surgical challenge especially at the L4/L5 level due to the position of the venous bifurcation. This potential for complications has led to the development of modified implants and oblique implantation techniques. Precise placement of the total disc device with regard to the centre of rotation and the midline may, however, be equally challenging.

There are numerous design concepts in clinical use. These include constrained, semi-constrained and unconstrained designs with differing bone-implant interfaces, articulating surfaces and centres of rotation. The medium- and long-term superiority of one concept over the other has not yet been proven. However, it has been clinically shown that the devices as such are effective in preserving motion and giving acceptable clinical results. Those implants accounting for the majority of clinical use worldwide are made of alloys and covered with titanium which limits the postoperative MRI compatibility. Another challenge for the coming years is posed by the

revisability of the implant. Early studies show a very high risk of potentially life-threatening complications in revision of total disc replacement. The group of implants in current use can still be considered "first generation".

37.3.4 Vertebral Body Replacement

Numerous indications require the removal of the vertebral body. In the lumbar spine, they generally fall into the categories traumatic deformity, tumours and metastases and infections. Typically, the vertebral body replacements play a key role in a 360° segmental reconstruction with added posterior instrumentation. While the surgical strategy is determined by the underlying indication, reconstruction of the vertebral body generally has the same goals: primary stability and restoration of spinal alignment in all three planes [5]. The implants generally consist of modular elements. Endplates provide secure anchorage and ingrowth into the adjacent bone, as well as lordotic angulations required for proper sagittal alignment. Depending on their main part, vertebral body replacements can be grouped into fixed size and expandable implants. A typical example for the first group is surgical titanium mesh (as used for Harms' cages). The implant is sized intraoperatively and impacted into the gap to be bridged. This implantation may compromise the preliminary segmental correction by a posterior instrumentation in the respective indications. Examples of expandable cages are Synex (Synthes) [14] and Hydrolift (Aesculap) implants. The modular implants are assembled, placed in the gap created by removal of the vertebral body and mechanically expanded after precise placement. This greatly facilitates sagittal correction. Depending on the indication, posterior instrumentation may be added. The surgical principles employed in use of these implants follow the same guidelines in the lumbar spine as in the thoracic spine (see the relevant chapter in this volume).

37.3.5 Single/Double Rod Systems, Anterior Plates [13]

While posterior instrumentation is associated with a certain degree of surgical trauma in 360° fusions, anterior instrumentation plays an important role in stabilizing the motion segment without the necessity of transpedicular screw placement. The indications include idiopathic scoliotic deformity, traumatic kyphotic deformity and reconstruction of the motion segment following partial or total vertebrectomy. The implants consist of small anchoring plates fixed with conventional or hollow screws and a single or double rod system. The anterior plates generally have a trapezoid

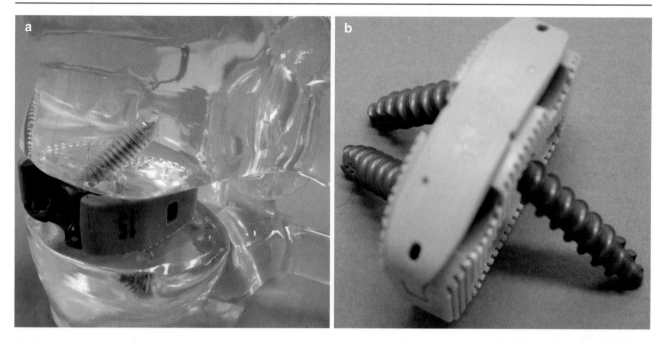

Fig. 37.1 (**a**) Synfix (Synthes) on spine model at L5/S1 level and (**b**) a comparable implant Sovereign (Medtronic)

shape and cover different sizes. Their indication spectrum is the same as those for rod systems except for deformity correction in idiopathic scoliosis. The instrumentations are carried out through an anterolateral approach exposing the lateral surface of the motion segments. In deformity correction, the endplates and anchoring plates are fixed to the motion segment, and the rods play a key role in finalizing the correction. However, in segmental reconstruction, the implant is placed first, correction is archived and the plate or rod system is added subsequently to facilitate fusion in the archived segmental angulations. Biomechanically, equal results to a 360° fusion can be obtained with all implants with special focus on angular stability and transfer of axial load. Anterior tension band plates constitute a subgroup of anterior plates. They are used in addition to an anterior intervertebral instrumentation in spinal fusion and are placed in the anterior midline to restore the stabilizing moment provided by the resected anterior longitudinal ligament. They increase the maximal stability more in flexion and extension than in axial rotation or lateral bending. The plates cover a single motion segment and are fixed with diverging screws in the upper and lower vertebra. With biomechanically comparable results, the anterior tension band plates can make posterior transpedicular instrumentation unnecessary and archive similar fusion rates. Examples of anterior plates or anterolateral plates are the Unity Lumbosacral Fixation System (Blackstone Medical) for L5–S1, Pyramid (Medtronic) and TSLP L5–S1 (Synthes) (see Figs. 37.1, 37.2, 37.3, 37.4 and 37.5).

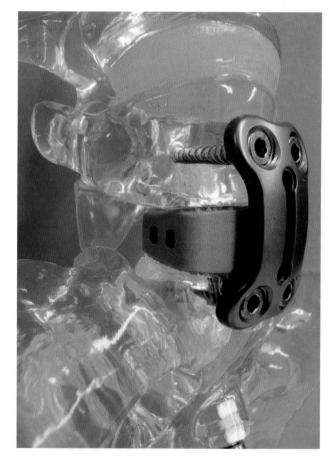

Fig. 37.2 Anterior TSLP plate (Synthes) with ALIF cage L5/S1 on a spine model

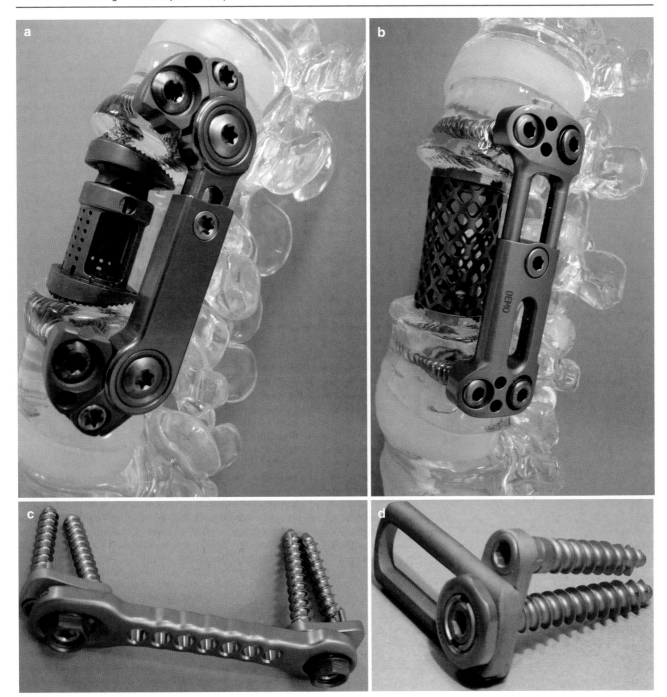

Fig. 37.3 Anterolateral plates (**a**) (Synthes), and (**b**) (Synthes), (**c**) Vantage (Medtronic), (**d**) MACS (Aesculap)

37.4 Special Techniques

One special technique recently introduced is the AxiaLIF technique to provide transvertebral placement of a screw axial to the vertebral body [7]. The indications include disc degeneration at the lumbosacral or the two lowermost lumbar levels. It is advocated that, through a percutaneous approach in the prone position, a presacral axial hole is drilled through the sacrum and the L5 vertebra. Subsequently, a device to curette the disc space and the endplate is introduced, bone graft is placed and the modular screw is placed to facilitate distraction and fusion. While some studies show equal biomechanical results to ALIF, independent medium- and long-term results are yet to be seen. The risk for potentially lethal complications such as intestinal damage and infection is described and is again pointed out hereby.

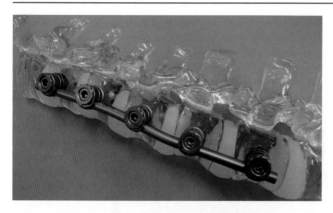

Fig. 37.4 Anterior rod-screw system USS ventral (Synthes)

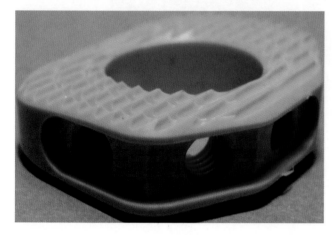

Fig. 37.5 ALIF cage A-Space (Aesculap)

References

1. Aebi M, Steffen T (2000) Synframe: a preliminary report. Eur Spine J 9:44–50
2. Bauer R, Kerschbaumer F, Poisel S (1991) Orthopädische Operationslehre. Band I, Wirbelsäule. Stuttgart/Thieme, New York
3. Cain MJ, Schleicher P, Gerlach R et al (2005) A new stand alone ALIF device: biomechanical comparison with established fixation methods. Spine 30:2631–2636
4. Dewald CJ, Millikan KW, Hammerberg KW et al (1999) An open minimally invasive approach to the lumbar spine. Am Surg 65:61–68
5. Dvorak MF, Kwon BK, Fischer CG (2003) Effectiveness of titanium mesh cylindrical cages in anterior column reconstruction after thoracic and lumbar vertebral body resection. Spine 28:902–908
6. Hodgson AR (1974) Anterior surgical approaches to the spinal column. Advances in orthopedics. Williams & Wilkens, Baltimore
7. Marotta N, Cosar M, Pimenta L et al (2006) A novel minimally invasive presacral approach and instrumentation technique for anterior L5-S1 intervertebral discectomy and fusion: technical description and case presentations. Neurosurg Focus 20(1):E9
8. Mayer HM, Wiechert K (1998) Ventrale Fusionsoperationen an der Lendenwirbelsäule Mikrochirurgische Techniken. Orthopade 27:466–476
9. Mirbaha MM (1971) Anterior approaches to the thoraco-lumbar junction of the spine by retroperitoneal extrapleural technic. Clin Orthop 91:12–18
10. Pellise F, Puig O, Rivas A et al (2002) Low fusion rate after L5-S1 laparoscopic anterior lumbar interbody fusion using twin stand-alone carbon fiber cages. Spine 27:1665–1669
11. Ray CD (2002) Ray threaded titanium cages for stand-alone lumbar interbody fusions: 6-years follow up study. In: Kaech DL, Jinkins JR (eds) Spinal restabilisation procedures. Amsterdam/Elsevier, Boston/London, pp 121–133
12. Spruit M, Falk RG, Beckmann L et al (2005) The in vitro stabilisation effect of polyetheretherketone cages versus a titanium cage of similar design for anterior lumbar interbody fusion. Eur Spine J 14:752–758
13. Thalgott JS, Kabins MB, Timlin M (1997) Four years experience with the AO anterior thoraco-lumbar locking plate. Spinal Cord 35:286–291
14. Vieweg U (2007) Vertebral body replacement system Synex in unstable burst fractures of the thoracic and lumbar spine. J Orthop Traumatol 8:64–70
15. Vieweg U, Liner M, Neurauter A et al (2006) Biomechanical study of a stand-alone cage TOPAZ for the lumbar spine with and without additional posterior fixation. Eur Spine J 15:1561–1562
16. Weber J, Vieweg U (2006) Anterior lumbale interkorporelle Fusion (ALIF) mit einem stabilisierenden Cage. Z Orthop Ihre Grenzgeb 144:40–45
17. Zdeblick TA, David SM (2000) A prospective comparison of surgical approach for anterior L4-L5 fusion. Laparoscopic versus mini anterior lumbar interbody fusion. Spine 25:2682–2687
18. Zuckerman JF, Zdeblick TA, Bailey SA et al (1995) Instrumented laparoscopic spinal fusion. Preliminary results. Spine 20:2029–2034

Ventral Interbody Fusion with Bone or Cage

38

Karsten Wiechert, Felix Hohmann, and Uwe Vieweg

38.1 Introduction and Core Message

First described in 1998 by Mayer [4], the classic mini-ALIF technique still sets the standard for modern anterior access surgery to the lumbar spine. Its universal use is owed in part to a very standardized, stepwise surgical technique resulting in a short learning curve. Another important factor is its complete applicability for the majority of indications requiring anterior lumbar spine surgery. The original publications on the classic miniALIF technique actually describe two different techniques: the minimally invasive anterolateral retroperitoneal approach to the L2/3, L3/4 and L4/5 segments and the anterior trans- or retroperitoneal midline approach to L5/S1 (L4/L5).

38.2 Indications

- Degenerative disc disease
- Degenerative or isthmic spondylolisthesis after posterior instrumentation
- Failed back surgery syndrome including pseudarthrosis
- Fractures
- Posttraumatic kyphotic deformity
- Spondylitis/spondylodiscitis

K. Wiechert, M.D. (✉) • F. Hohmann, M.D.
Department of Spine Therapy, Hessingpark Clinic,
Hessingstrasse 17, 86199 Augsburg, Germany
e-mail: karsten.wiechert@hessingpark-clinic.de;
felix.hohmann@hessingpark-clinic.de

U. Vieweg, M.D., Ph.D.
Clinic for Spinal Surgery, Sana Hospital Rummelsberg,
90593 Schwarzenbruck, Germany
e-mail: uwe.vieweg@yahoo.de

38.3 Contraindications

- Absolute contraindications to this technique do not exist. However, special caution needs to be exercised in cases with previous extensive retroperitoneal surgery or radiation.

38.4 Technical Prerequisites

Where an anterior approach is used, conditions in the hospital must meet a variety of technical requirements such as availability of appropriate positioning aids, standby facilities for general and vascular surgery and a complication management plan for cases of intra-abdominal injury. The approach requires appropriate instruments – especially with regard to length (bipolar forceps, haemoclips) – and suitable implants. Preoperative planning must include clarification of the locations of blood vessels, especially when access is exclusively anterior. CT angiography of the pelvic blood vessels can provide the necessary information. A conventional AP and lateral X-ray overview shows the situation of the iliac crest with regard to the L4/5 level. It should be ensured that appropriate X-ray-transparent operating tables, a C-arm for intraoperative X-ray procedures and Xenon lamps for better illumination are available. Adjustable operating tables and positioning aids facilitate anterior access in the Trendelenburg or da Vinci position and are also helpful for ventrolateral access (Fig. 38.1). For both techniques, a frame-mounted retractor system is helpful (SynFrame, Synthes; activ O retractor, Fig. 38.2, Aesculap; or Miaspas, Fig. 38.3, Aesculap), especially if the surgery is carried out without an assistant [1]. The type of approach can be selected according to the anatomical situation, the position of the major vessels and the indication: lateral retroperitoneal approach, pararectus approach, midline retroperitoneal approach or midline transperitoneal approach (see Fig. 38.4a, b).

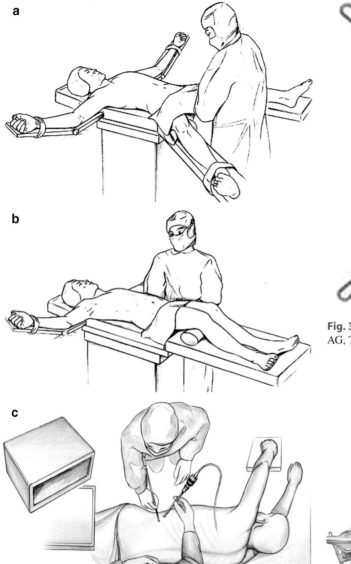

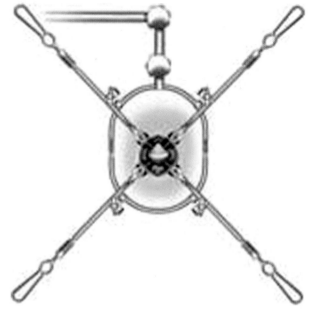

Fig. 38.2 Activ O retractor (Aesculap) (With permission of Aesculap AG, Tuttlingen, Germany)

Fig. 38.1 Different positioning: Da Vinci position for L5/S1 (**a**), conventional supine position for lower lumbar spine (**b**) and lateral position for ventrolateral access to the lumbar spine, here with endoscopic assistance (**c**) (With permission of Aesculap AG, Tuttlingen, Germany)

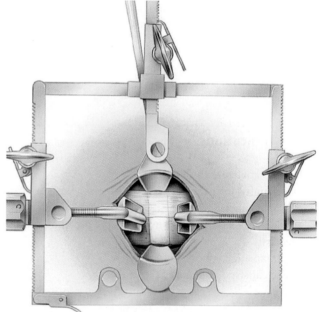

Fig. 38.3 Miaspas ALIF retractor (Aesculap) (With permission of Aesculap AG, Tuttlingen, Germany)

38.5 Planning, Preparation and Positioning

38.5.1 Anterior Midline Retro- or Transperitoneal Approach

Anterior midline access is best carried out in the da Vinci position (see Fig. 38.1a). In total disc replacement surgery, the lumbar spine may not be extended. In the anterior

midline approach, a thorough preoperative assessment of the vascular anatomy is highly recommended, especially with regard to anatomic variations and projection of the bifurcations in relation to the target disc space. In the anterior midline approach, the projection of the disc space needs to be marked in lateral fluoroscopy as well as the midline.

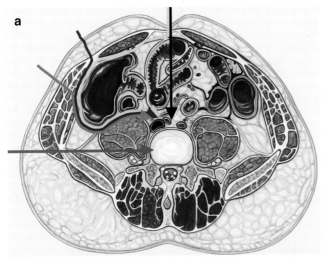

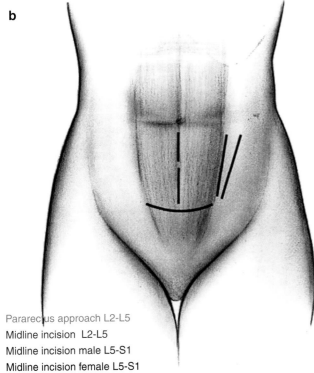

Pararectus approach L2-L5
Midline incision L2-L5
Midline incision male L5-S1
Midline incision female L5-S1

Fig. 38.4 Different anterior lumbar access routes (**a**) (*yellow* midline retroperitoneal approach, *black* midline transperitoneal approach, *blue* pararectal retroperitoneal approach, *green…red..? -*) and the different skin incisions for the various access routes (**b**) (With permission of Aesculap AG, Tuttlingen, Germany)

38.5.2 Lateral Retroperitoneal Approach (L2/3, L3/L4, L4/L5)

The lumbar segments L2/3, L3/4 and L4/5 are reached by a retroperitoneal approach from the left side. For the lateral retroperitoneal approach, the patient is placed in on his or her right side with the operating table tilted backwards depending on the level to be fused. The higher lumbar levels require a

posterior tilt of approx. 40°, while the lower levels (L4/5) require approx. 20° and L3/4 30° of posterior tilt in the axial plane. Dissection of the fibres of the psoas muscle is facilitated if the table is angulated to create a right-sided lateral bend. This also increases the costo-iliac distance. If the left leg is positioned with the knee extended, the tension on the psoas fibres increases, facilitating dissection. The anterolateral approach requires some planning with regard to the rib cage and the iliac crest. If the eleventh rib covers the L2/3 disc space, a more anterior skin incision is necessary. In the lateral approach, it is recommended that the disc space level and the centre of the disc space be marked on the skin. The skin incision should obliquely cross the centre of the disc space.

38.6 Surgical Technique

38.6.1 Approaches

38.6.1.1 Anterior Midline Approaches (L5/S1)

- A midline approach is recommended for the L5/S1 level. Either Pfannenstiel's incision or a linear midline incision may be used (see Fig. 38.4b).
- The projection of the disc space needs to be marked in lateral fluoroscopy as well as the midline. For monolevel fusion surgery, a skin incision approximately 5 cm in length is usually sufficient (see Fig. 38.5), depending on the underlying pathology.
- A linear incision is made in the anterior fascia of the rectus abdominis muscle a few millimetres paramedially (see Fig. 38.6).
- A blunt instrument is used to push the peritoneum away in a medial direction, first from the rear surface of the muscle and then from the lateral abdominal wall (see Fig. 38.7).
- In the anterior midline approach, the dissection is carried out preperitoneally, generally to the left side. The psoas muscle is identified and the anterior edge exposed. Sometimes, the arcuate line needs to be incised for easy exposure. The ureter and the peritoneal sac are then mobilized over the midline.
- Epigastric blood vessels should be coagulated and dissected if necessary.
- The ureter and the presacral plexus are carefully mobilized and retracted together with the peritoneum (coagulation should be avoided).
- The medial sacral vessels are ligated and dissected in the bifurcation of the major vessels (see Fig. 38.8).
- Important landmarks are the lateral edge of the anterior longitudinal ligament, the sympathetic plexus and the lateral edge of the left common iliac vein (especially in L4/5).
- After X-ray verification of the correct target level, the retractor is put in position, and the disc space is prepared for fusion (see Fig. 38.9a, b).

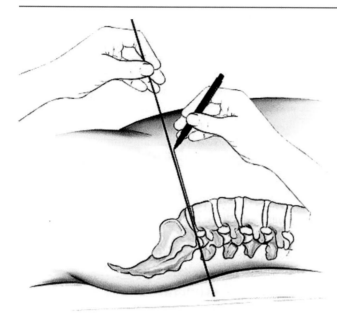

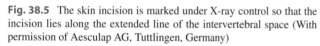

Fig. 38.5 The skin incision is marked under X-ray control so that the incision lies along the extended line of the intervertebral space (With permission of Aesculap AG, Tuttlingen, Germany)

Fig. 38.7 A blunt dissection is used to push the peritoneum away in a medial direction, first from the rear surface of the muscle and then from the lateral abdominal wall (With permission of Aesculap AG, Tuttlingen, Germany)

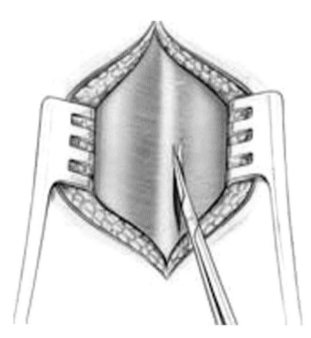

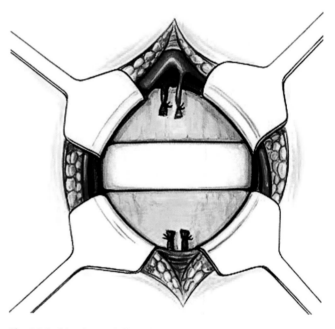

Fig. 38.8 Ligation and dissection of the medial sacral vessels in the bifurcation (With permission of Aesculap AG, Tuttlingen, Germany)

Fig. 38.6 Linear incision of the anterior fascia of the rectus abdominis muscle (With permission of Aesculap AG, Tuttlingen, Germany)

- The muscle fascia is dissected longitudinally where the muscles meet at the lateral margin of the rectus abdominis muscle.
- A blunt instrument is used to push the peritoneum away from the abdominal wall whilst monitoring the epigastric vessels.
- The ureter is mobilized and moved away from the operating site together with the peritoneum.
- The ventrolateral spine is exposed at the anterior margin of the psoas muscle.
- The vessels supplying the neighbouring segment are ligated and dissected, including the ascending lumbar vein if the

38.6.1.2 Anterior Pararectal Approach L2/3, L3/4, L4/5

The anterior pararectus approach is considerably easier in the upper lumbar region of the spine but carries a higher risk of segmental denervation of the abdominal muscles.

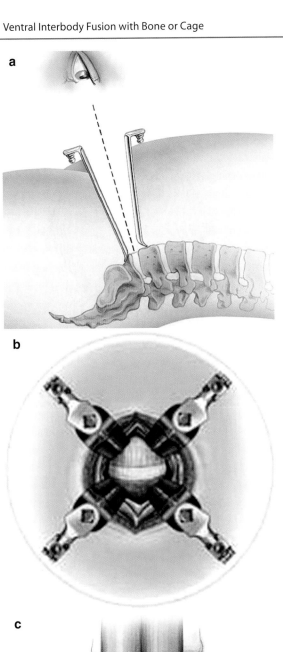

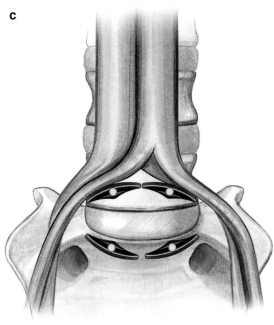

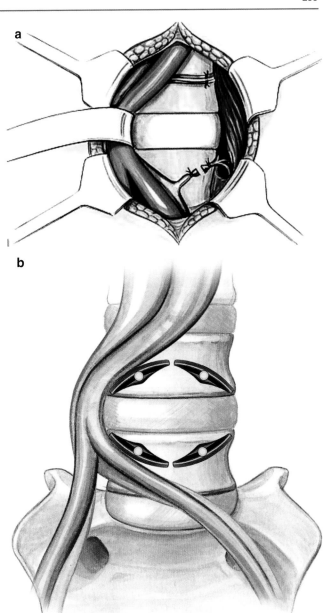

Fig. 38.10 (**a**) The neighbouring segment vessels are ligated and dissected, including the ascending lumbar vein for the approach to the L4/5 segment. (**b**) Preferred retractor placement for exposure of anterior circumference of the disc space (With permission of Aesculap AG, Tuttlingen, Germany)

L4/5 segment is being approached, so that the major vessels can be mobilized to the opposite side (see Fig. 38.10).

- The sympathetic nerve is mobilized in a lateral direction.
- *Note*: In the midline marking process, the lateral inclination of the operating table may have to be adjusted to

Fig. 38.9 Placement of the retractor blades, (**a**) lateral view, (**b**) AP view, (**c**) preferrable relation between retractors and the vascular bifurcations

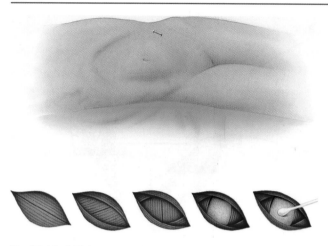

Fig. 38.11 Splitting approach – each muscle layer is dissected in the direction of its fibre orientation (With permission of Aesculap AG, Tuttlingen, Germany)

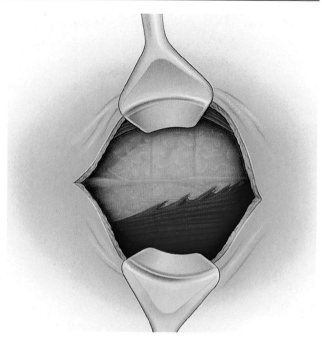

Fig. 38.12 Identification of the psoas muscle (With permission of Aesculap AG, Tuttlingen, Germany)

compensate for any possible turning of the patient caused by retraction of the muscles and abdominal organs.

38.6.1.3 Lateral Approaches

- In the lateral approach, skin marking of the disc space level and the centre of the disc space is recommended, with the skin incision obliquely crossing the centre of the disc space.
- A 5- to 8-cm skin incision is centred above the projection of the centre of the disc space in an oblique direction parallel to the fibres of the external oblique abdominal muscles.
- The lateral approach involves a blunt split of the three abdominal wall muscle sheaths, blunt preparation down to the psoas muscle and exposure of the anterior edge of the psoas muscle.
- Each muscle layer (external oblique, internal oblique, transverse abdominal muscle) is dissected in the direction of its fibre orientation (see Fig. 38.11).
- Care must be taken to preserve the branches of the intercostal nerves 10–12 as well as the iliohypogastric/ilioinguinal nerves which occasionally cross the surgical field between the layers of the internal oblique and transverse abdominal muscle.
- The transverse abdominal muscle should be split as far as possible to avoid opening of the peritoneum. There is more retroperitoneal fat tissue beneath the lateral part of the transverse muscle. Moreover, the peritoneum adheres more to the inner wall of the medial part of this muscle.
- The retroperitoneal space is enlarged by careful, blunt dissection with cottonoids and Langenbeck retractors.
- The psoas muscle is identified as a first anatomical landmark (Fig. 38.12).
- The paravertebral tissues including the ureter and the vascular bundle are gently retracted towards the midline using the blunt hooks. They are incised and sharply dissected from the lateral circumference of the disc space

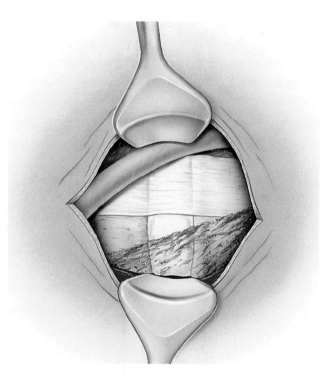

Fig. 38.13 The paravertebral tissue, including the ureter and the vascular bundle, is gently retracted from the midline using blunt hooks (With permission of Aesculap AG, Tuttlingen, Germany)

(see Fig. 38.13). Usually, the lateral border of the left common vein can be identified.

- Dissection should be performed very carefully from the ventrolateral aspect of the vertebral bodies. The segmental vessels of the vertebral body inferior to the disc space can be exposed (see Fig. 38.14).

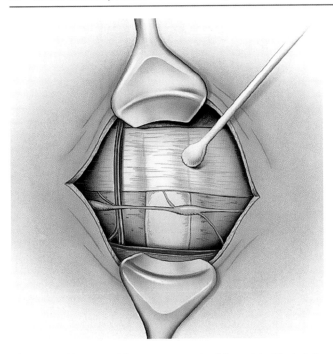

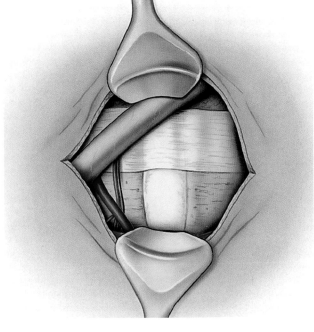

Fig. 38.14 Exposure of the segment vessels of the vertebral body inferior to the disc space

Fig. 38.15 At L4/5, the ascending lumbar vein may obstruct the inferior lateral angle of the surgical field and needs to be ligated with endoclips and dissected (With permission of Aesculap AG, Tuttlingen, Germany)

- The segmental vessels of the inferior vertebral bodies need to be ligated with endoclips and then cut and dissected from the vertebral surface.
- However, dissection is rarely necessary at the L3/4 and L2/3 levels. At L4/5, the ascending lumbar vein may obstruct the inferior lateral angle of the surgical field and needs to be ligated with endoclips and dissected (see Fig. 38.15).
- Dissection should not be extended posterior to the pedicle entrance in order to avoid irritation of the lumbar nerve roots.
- The disc space level is verified under fluoroscopic control.
- The spatial orientation of the disc space is then identified by cutting the annulus fibrosus parallel to the vertebral endplates.

38.6.2 Interbody Fusion and Instrumentation

Instrumentation is completely unlimited in the miniALIF approach. Any intervertebral cages or bone grafts for spinal fusion can be used without specific considerations relating to the approach [3, 5, 6]. Any other type of anterior interbody fusion, including those using homograft or allografts, should be possible with this approach.

38.6.2.1 Interbody Fusion with Autologous Iliac Bone Graft

- With a drill guide, the anterolateral cortex of the adjacent vertebral bodies is drilled in a strictly vertical direction to create the holes for the distraction screws.

- The entry point is about 5–8 mm from the intervertebral space at the lateral border of the anterior longitudinal ligament.
- The drill has a safety range of 10 mm and penetrates only the anterolateral cortex of the vertebral body. Then specially designed anchoring screws are inserted (see Fig. 38.16).
- A retractor frame is put in place. A sharp muscle blade is attached laterally to deflect the psoas muscle, whereas a blunt vascular blade is inserted medially to retract the retroperitoneal vessels (see Fig. 38.17a, b).
- Discectomy and preparation of the graft bed. The endplates are carefully removed with chisels (see Fig. 38.18).
- The subchondral bone is smoothed with a high-speed drill (see Fig. 38.19).
- The height and depth of the iliac crest graft needed are measured with sliding callipers (see Figs. 38.20 and 38.21).
- A tricortical bone graft is harvested through a separate small incision over the lateral iliac crest on the same side. The bone graft is also taken from the middle part of the iliac crest. It is removed using a double saw blade which can be adjusted to the size of the bone graft. The graft is removed with the help of a graft cutter.
- A small hole is drilled into the graft which is then mounted onto a graft holder and impacted into the intervertebral space (see Fig. 38.22).

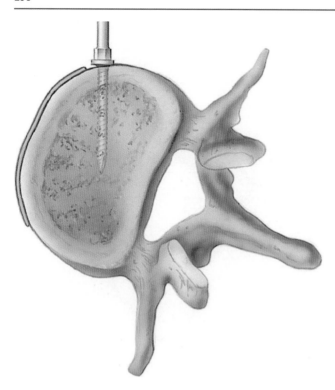

Fig. 38.16 Insertion of specially designed anchoring screws (With permission of Aesculap AG, Tuttlingen, Germany)

38.6.2.2 Interbody Fusion with ALIF Cage Implantation

- The disc space is cleared using disc knives, rongeurs, curettes and bone curettes. Angled instruments are available for the lateral approach. Then bone rasps are used to refresh the cartilage endplates (see Figs. 38.23 and 38.24).
- Determination of implant size using trial implants (see Fig. 38.25). Trial implants are available in heights from 9 to 19 mm in 2-mm increments. The insertion instrument and depth stop are assembled. Before the trial implant is attached, the depth stop must be turned forward to the first line on the depth scale. The trial implant is inserted with the T-handle, and the depth stop is set as appropriate for the implant position. For easier removal of the trial implant, we recommend that the T-handle be replaced with a slap hammer.
- The cage can be filled with bone or bone replacement material in a packing block. The second insertion instrument is preadjusted according to the defined depth stop position. The cage is inserted and corrected with the impactor if necessary (see Fig. 38.26).

a

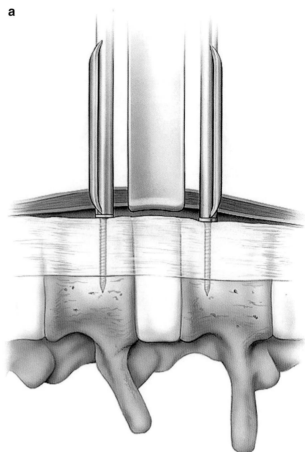

b

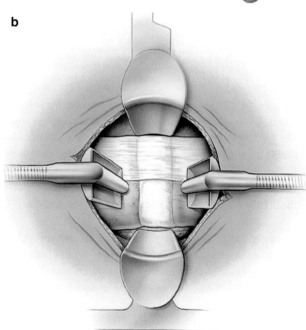

Fig. 38.17 Positioning of the retractor blades in the lateral (**a**) and AP (**b**) view

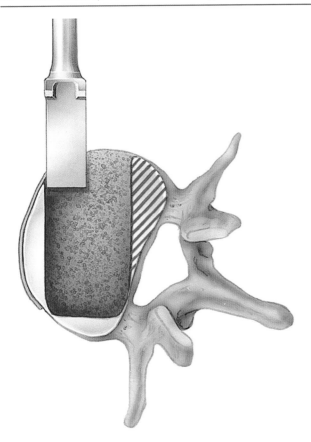

Fig. 38.18 Careful removal of the endplates with chisels (With permission of Aesculap AG, Tuttlingen, Germany)

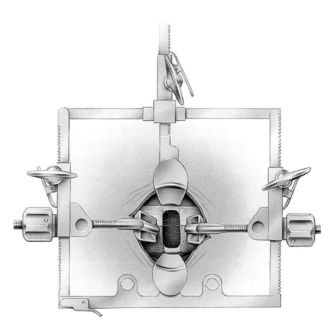

Fig. 38.20 Intraoperative situation after discectomy with Miaspas retractor in position (With permission of Aesculap AG, Tuttlingen, Germany)

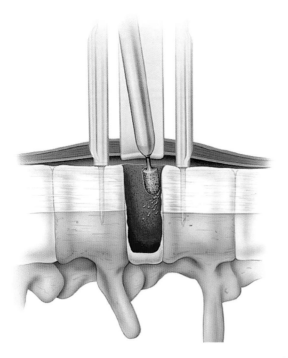

Fig. 38.19 The subchondral bone is smoothed with a high-speed drill (With permission of Aesculap AG, Tuttlingen, Germany)

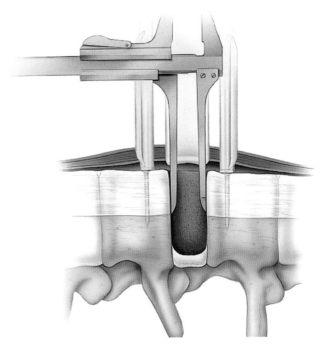

Fig. 38.21 Measurement of the height and depth of the iliac crest graft (With permission of Aesculap AG, Tuttlingen, Germany)

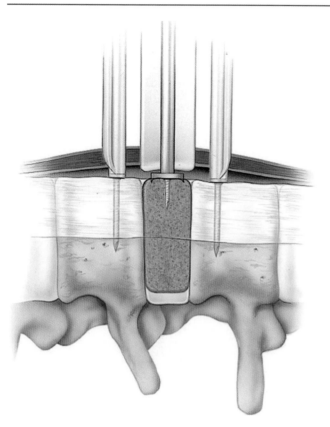

Fig. 38.22 Impaction of the bone piece with a graft holder into the intervertebral space (With permission of Aesculap AG, Tuttlingen, Germany)

38.6.2.3 Anterior and Anterolateral Plating

Various systems are available to stabilize the anterior or anterolateral lumbar spine. They include plate-screw systems (e.g., TSLP, Synthes; MACS, Aesculap; Pyramid, Medtronic), rod-screw systems (e.g., VentroFix, Synthes) and cages with an integrated plate (e.g., SynFix, Synthes). For a less invasive procedure, it is essential that a retractor system (e.g., activ O, Aesculap; SynFrame, Synthes) be used for anterior and anterolateral plating of the lumbar spine. The preparation and fixing of the retractor blades make instrumentation much easier. For example, the blades of the activ O retractor are placed at the cranial and caudal ends of the segment and fixed with pins. The other blades hold the abdominal viscera and

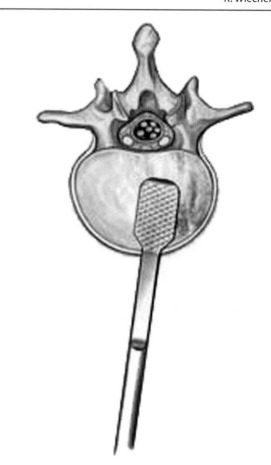

Fig. 38.23 Cleaning of the disc space using disc knives, rongeurs, curettes and bone curettes. Then bone rasps are used to refresh the cartilage endplates (With permission of Aesculap AG, Tuttlingen, Germany)

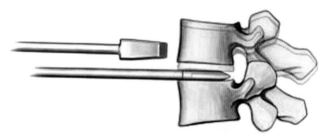

Fig. 38.24 After discectomy, a distractor should be inserted horizontally and then rotated (With permission of Aesculap AG, Tuttlingen, Germany)

Fig. 38.25 Determination of implant size using trial implants. The trial implant is inserted with the slap hammer (With permission of Aesculap AG, Tuttlingen, Germany)

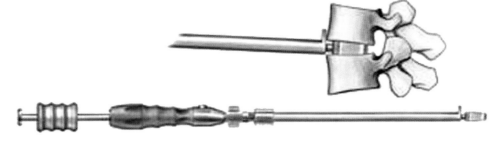

Fig. 38.26 The cage is inserted and corrected with the impactor (With permission of Aesculap AG, Tuttlingen, Germany)

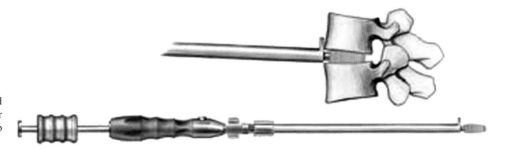

the psoas muscle to the side (see Fig. 38.27a, b). With the aid of the retractor blades, the psoas muscle is pushed from ventral to dorsal. The authors do not recommend direct entry through the psoas muscle as in the transmuscular XLIF approach. The use of the TSLP (Synthes) is made easier by temporary fixation pins. The appropriate plate is fixed to the ventral spine with the pins. After intraoperative X-ray checks of the position of the plate with respect to the spine, the plate is anchored at a stable angle using four screws [2, 7, 8]. The access route can be kept smaller when cages with an integrated plate (SynFix, Synthes; Topaz, Ulrich) are used. The operating time is reduced because some of the instrumentation steps are rendered unnecessary.

38.7 Tips and Tricks

- A preoperative colour-coded 3D CT angiogram is recommended in all cases where the vascular anatomy cannot be precisely identified or where there seem to be anatomic variations.
- Once the patient has been positioned, it is mandatory that an X-ray check of the target level be carried out in two planes prior to surgery.
- Sometimes, the operating table or its base obscures the visual plane. A preoperative check after the final tilt can save trial-and-error X-rays during the operation, thereby reducing radiation exposure for patient and surgeons.

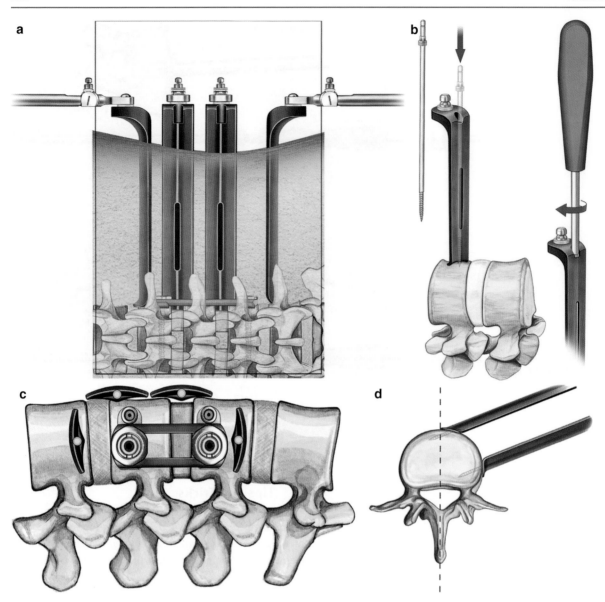

Fig. 38.27 (**a–d**) Ventrolateral plating of the lumbar spine using a retractor system (activ O, Aesculap). Retractor blades are positioned at the cranial and caudal ends of the segment and fixed with pins. The other blades hold the abdominal viscera and psoas muscle to the side

References

1. Aebi M, Steffen T (2000) Synframe: a preliminary report. Eur Spine J 9:44–50
2. Cain MJ, Schleicher P, Gerlach R, Pflugmacher R et al (2005) A new stand alone ALIF device: biomechanical comparison with established fixation methods. Spine 30:2631–2636
3. Dvorak MF, Kwon BK, Fischer CG (2003) Effectiveness of titanium mesh cylindrical cages in anterior column reconstruction after thoracic and lumbar vertebral body resection. Spine 28:902–908
4. Mayer HM, Wiechert K (1998) Ventrale Fusionsoperationen an der Lendenwirbelsäule. Mikrochirurgische Techniken. Orthopade 27: 466–476
5. Thalgott JS, Giuffre JM, Klezl Z, Timlin M (2002) Anterior lumbar interbody fusion with titanium mesh cages, coralline hydroxyapatite, and demineralised bone matrix as part of a circumferential fusion. Spine J 2:63–69
6. Spruit M, Falk RG, Beckmann L et al (2005) The in vitro stabilisation effect of polyetheretherketone cages versus a titanium cage of similar design for anterior lumbar interbody fusion. Eur Spine J 14:752–758
7. Vieweg U, Liner M, Neurauter A et al (2006) Biomechanical study of a stand-alone cage TOPAZ for the lumbar spine with and without additional posterior fixation. Eur Spine J 15:1561–1662
8. Weber J, Vieweg U (2006) Anterior lumbale interkorporelle Fusion (ALIF) mit einem stabilisierenden Cage. Z Orthop Ihre Grenzgeb 144:40–45

Total Lumbar Disc Replacement

39

Christoph J. Siepe

39.1 Introduction and Core Messages

Fusion of lumbar motion segments for the treatment of intractable low-back pain (LBP) has been associated with a variety of negative side effects. Perceived disadvantages such as accelerated adjacent level morbidities, iatrogenic superior segment facet joint violation, symptomatic complaints from facet, and sacroiliac joints or facet joint hypertrophy with consecutive narrowing of the spinal canal have previously been reported [1–12]. In an attempt to avoid these previously published and fusion-related negative side effects, a variety of new motion preserving technologies including total lumbar disc replacement procedures (TDR) have been introduced. This chapter outlines the technique of TDR with ProDisc II (Synthes, Paoli, PA; Fig. 39.1).

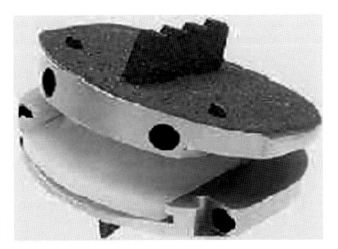

Fig. 39.1 Total lumbar disc replacement with a modular, ball-and-socket-type prosthesis (ProDisc II, Synthes, Paoli, PA). The convex polyethylene inlay is locked into the bottom endplate (© by Synthes)

C.J. Siepe, M.D., Ph.D.
Head of Department of Spine Surgery,
Schön Klinik München Harlaching, Spine Center,
Harlachinger Str. 51, 81547 Munich, Germany
e-mail: csiepe@schoen-kliniken.de

39.2 Indications

The primary indication for TDR is the treatment of predominant and intractable LBP from lumbar degenerative disc disease (DDD) with or without Modic changes. Favorable outcomes have similarly been reported in candidates following previous minimally invasive discectomy as well as in candidates with DDD and accompanying central to mediolateral disc herniations with predominant LBP [13]. The procedure can be performed mono- or bisegmentally. However, inferior results must be expected in multilevel procedures [14]. Although technically more challenging, better outcomes have been reported for TDR at the level above the lumbosacral junction in comparison to TDRs performed at the lumbosacral junction [14]. Due to increasing and additive destabilizing effects [15–17], the authors do not recommend to perform TDR for more than 2-level pathologies.

39.3 Contraindications

Stringent preoperative decision making is crucial in order to achieve satisfactory outcomes following TDR. The commonly agreed upon indications and contraindications for this procedure have been thoroughly outlined previously [13, 18–23]. Due to an extensive list of contraindications which have previously been published, it is estimated that only about 3–5% of fusion candidates are potential candidates for TDR [18, 20]. The most common contraindications include:

- Central or lateral spinal stenosis
- Predominant radiculopathy
- Facet joint arthrosis/symptomatic facet joint complaints
- Spondylolysis/spondylolisthesis
- Spinal instability (iatrogenic/altered posterior elements, e.g., following laminectomy)
- Major deformity/curvature deviations (e.g., scoliosis)
- Metabolic bone disease (e.g., manifest osteoporosis/osteopenia)
- Previous operation with severe scarring and radiculopathy
- Compromised vertebral body (irregular endplate shape)
- Previous/latent infection
- Metal allergy
- Spinal tumor
- Posttraumatic segments

39.4 Technical Prerequisites

The disc spaces are approached through means of a miniopen laparotomy using a retroperitoneal approach [24, 25]. Technical prerequisites include:

- Radiolucent and adjustable operating table
- X-ray
- Access equipment for retroperitoneal approach (i.e., retractor blades, retractor frame)

- Monitoring of oxygen saturation in the left lower extremity with pulse oximeter attached to the left toe

39.5 Planning, Preparation, and Positioning

- For preoperative planning, it is recommended to analyze the corridor line to the disc space, the sacral tilt, and the vascular anatomy on preoperative X-ray (standing lateral images) as well as on sagittal and axial MRI images (Fig. 39.2a, b).
- The patient is placed in a supine position; the surgeon is positioned in between the legs of the patient (Fig. 39.3).
- The corridor line to the disc space (lateral X-ray fluoroscopy), the anterior midline (AP fluoroscopic control), as well as the skin incision are marked on the patient's skin surface (Fig. 39.4a, b).
- For TDR at the lumbosacral junction, the table is slightly tilted in a head-down position to alleviate the access as well as the preparation toward the disc space.
- Any kind of lumbar hyperextension on the operating table should be avoided.

39.6 Surgical Technique

39.6.1 Approach

- Midline horizontal skin incision across the target region. For bisegmental TDRs at the last two lumbar motion segments, the surgeon can either choose to perform a horizontal skin incision in between the two target disc spaces, or alternatively opt for an oblique skin incision.
- Subcutaneous preparation and longitudinal incision of the linea alba.
- Levels above the lumbosacral junction should be approached via a left retroperitoneal approach due to the vascular anatomy of the prevertebral vessels.
- For TDRs at L5/S1, a right retroperitoneal approach is recommended in order to enable anterior midline access to upper lumbar levels, i.e., if another TDR procedure is intended at a later stage.
- Exposure of the linea arcuata and dissection in a craniolateral direction should be performed after the peritoneal sac has been identified and bluntly mobilized away from the fascia.
- The preparation is continued medially, exposing the psoas muscle as well as the iliac vessels adjacent to the medial

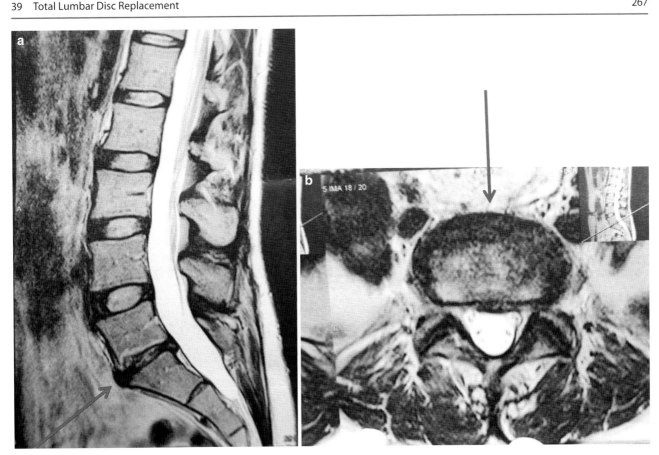

Fig. 39.2 MRI images of an adequate, "perfect" candidate for total lumbar disc replacement with single-level degenerative disc disease. The *arrow* delineates the projected access corridor to the disc space L5/S1. (**a**) Demonstrates a regular sagittal alignment which facilitates an anterior approach to the disc space L5–S1. (**b**) Demonstrates a large-access corridor ("safe zone," *arrow*) to the disc space L5–S1 without the need of extensive mobilization of the iliac vessels or the vascular bifurcation. The axial images furthermore serve to exclude any advanced degenerative changes in the facet joints. Preoperative fluoroscopically guided spine infiltrations are helpful in an attempt to rule out any clinically relevant facet or sacroiliac joint complaints

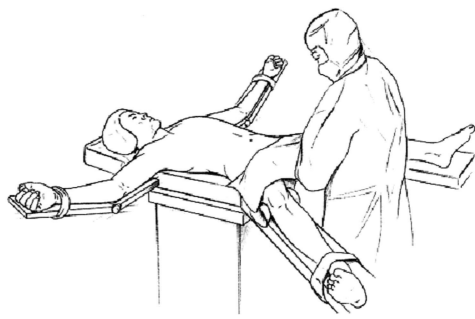

Fig. 39.3 The patient is positioned in a supine position (Modified da Vinci position). The surgeon is positioned in between the legs of the patient (© by Synthes)

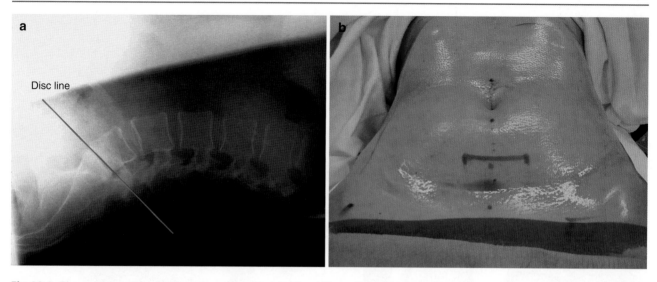

Fig. 39.4 The projection of the disc line (**a**) as well as the anatomic midline are marked on the patient's skin surface (**b**) under lateral fluoroscopic control

border of the M. psoas. The ureter is identified and carefully protected behind retractors.

- For TDRs at the level L4/5 or above, exposure and identification of the ascending lumbar vein is recommended. Ligation of the ascending lumbar vein may be required to avoid intraoperative vascular complications in this area before mobilization of the major prevertebral vessels [26].
- Exposure and identification of the disc space.
- Intraoperative fluoroscopic control should confirm the adequate level as well as the precise midline marking of the spine in the AP view. Previous studies have reported that the medial border of both pedicles may be used as a more reliable anatomic landmark for precise midline identification in comparison to the projection of the spinous processes.
- At L5/S1, the median presacral vessels should be identified and ligated. In the majority of cases, bipolar coagulation is sufficient; otherwise, clipping of the vessels may be required.
- Blunt lateral mobilization of the prevertebral vessels. The vessels are retracted laterally with self-retaining retractors which are mounted to an operating frame, attached to the operating table.

39.6.2 Preparation of the Disc

- Excision of the anterior annulus is followed by a complete discectomy.
- Meticulous endplate preparation. Care should be taken not to violate the integrity of the cortical endplates.
- Distraction of the disc space (Fig. 39.5a, b). Previous biomechanical studies have recommended to leave the PLL

intact wherever possible. In cases of advanced stages of disc space collapse, however, it may be required to partially resect or incise the posterior annulus as well as the posterior longitudinal ligament (PLL) in order to achieve adequate disc space height restoration.

39.6.3 Instrumentation

- Insertion of a trial implant (Fig. 39.6a, b).
- An adjustable stopper which is attached to the insertion device prevents excessive posterior placement of the trial implant.
- The metallic implant endplates should cover the largest possible surface area of the adjacent vertebral bodies.
- Overdistraction of the disc space should be avoided. In the majority of cases, an implant height of 10 mm is sufficient.
- Similarly, avoid excessive lordosis of the implant. The prostheses tend to shift into a more lordotic position postoperatively, which may result in a segmental hyperlordosis and possible impingement of the facet joints [27–31]. In general, 6° of overall implant lordosis is sufficient. For TDRs performed at the lumbosacral junction, it may be advisable to shift some of the lordosis to the caudal endplate, particularly in patients with a steeper sacral inclination.
- Confirmation of adequate trial implant positioning in both AP and lateral plane with X-ray (Fig. 39.6a, b). The implant should be precisely positioned in the midline. Posterior implant positioning is crucial. The posterior projection of the prosthesis should be in line with the posterior wall of the adjacent vertebral bodies. In order to achieve adequate posterior implant positioning, removal of posterior osteophytes may be required (Fig. 39.7).

Fig. 39.5 (**a**) Following a complete discectomy, distraction of the collapsed segments can be achieved with a straight or curved spreader forceps (© by Synthes). (**b**) Intraoperative verification of the disc space distraction under image intensifier

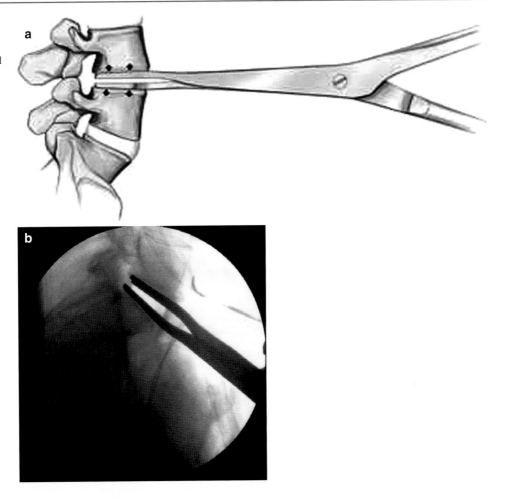

Fig. 39.6 Insertion of the trial implant. A strict midline positioning of the implant should be confirmed under AP fluoroscopic control (**a**). Lateral X-ray images should confirm the largest possible prosthesis surface area as well as an adequate posterior positioning of the implant (**b**). An adjustable stopper which is attached to the insertion device prevents excessive posterior placement of the trial implant (© by Synthes)

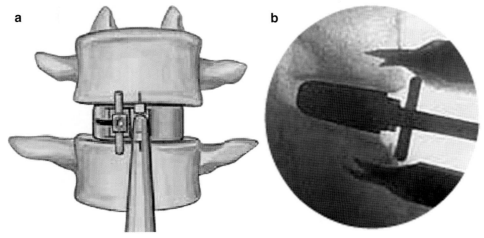

- The keel bed is prepared with custom-made chisel instruments which are available in 10, 12, and 14 mm heights, respectively. The chisel device is securely guided through openings along the midline of the trial implant (Fig. 39.8a). The trial implant serves as a guide for the chisel and sets the direction and the chisel depth (Fig. 39.8b). The chisel cut should be checked under image intensifier (Fig. 39.8c).

- Trial implant and chisels are left in place until the implant is fully assembled ex vivo to avoid bleeding following their removal from the cancellous bone.
- The trial implant is removed and replaced by the actual endplates of the implant which are mounted to the insertion device. The bottom endplate is locked to the inserter by turning the inserter arms (Fig. 39.9). Previous chiseling of the keels serves as guidance for adequate implant

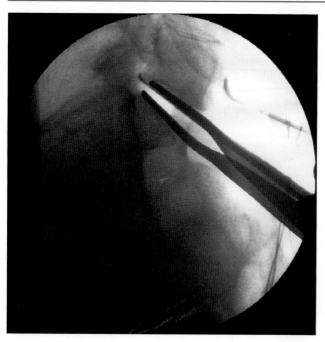

Fig. 39.7 Intraoperative removal of posterior osteophytes

insertion. Posterior implant positioning is confirmed under lateral fluoroscopic control. Care should be taken that no surrounding soft tissues are impinged during the process of implant insertion. This step is furthermore preformed without segmental distraction.

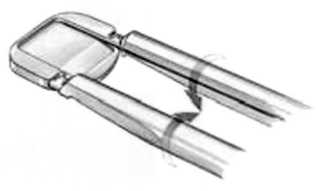

Fig. 39.9 Connection and locking between the bottom implant endplate and the inserter arms

Fig. 39.8 Preparation of the keel bed. The chisel device is securely guided through openings along the midline of the trial implant (**a**). The trial implant serves as a guide for the chisel and sets the direction and the chisel depth (**b**). The chisel cut should be checked under image intensifier (**c**)

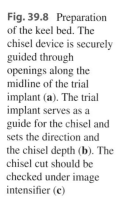

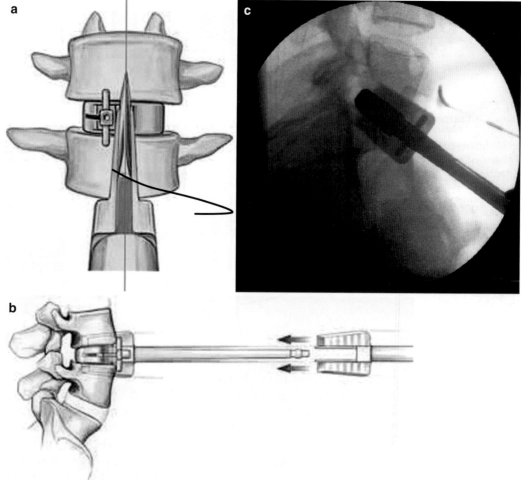

- The insertion device now serves to guide the UHMWE-PE (ultra high molecular weight polyethylene) inlay into the caudal endplate. The PE inlay is inserted into the slots of the insertion device ("dome up"). An adequately sized and corresponding distracter is attached to the inserter. The wing nut is used to screw the distracter down to the mechanical stop. During this process, the PE inlay should be easily advanced. Excessive resistance may be a sign of inlay impingement which should be strictly avoided.

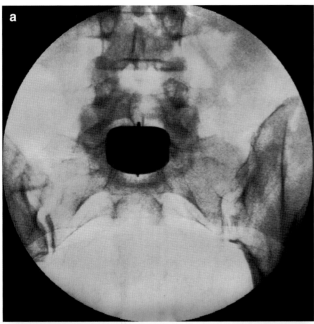

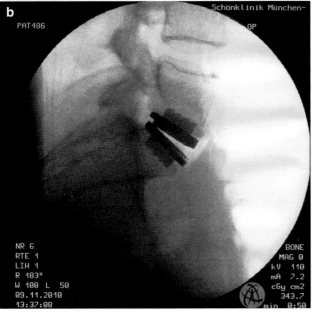

Fig. 39.10 Final AP (**a**) and lateral (**b**) fluoroscopic images demonstrate an adequate implant positioning in both planes

- This process is finalized with a "pusher," until the inlay easily snaps into the caudal endplate. This is usually confirmed by a "click" sound. Macroscopic inspection must confirm that the anterior border of the inlay as well as the caudal endplate is in line with no visible steps or gaps between both components.
- Removal of all insertion instruments and final X-ray control to confirm adequate implant positioning (Fig. 39.10a, b).
- Careful removal of the retractor blades and final inspection of the operating site to confirm that no intraoperative complications, i.e., from vascular structures or the ureter, have occurred.
- Insertion of a drain is generally not required.
- Closure of the linea alba, subcutaneous tissue adaptation, as well as skin closure.

39.7 Postoperative Care

During the immediate postoperative period, supervision of wound healing, regular checkups of the abdomen, as well as the neurological status are paramount and regularly monitored. The patients are generally discharged within a few days following the operative intervention.

One of the advantages of TDR in comparison to fusion candidates is an early, brace-free mobilization of the patients, as well as an early resumption of sporting and professional activities. The postoperative treatment and mobilization regime in patients with an uneventful intraoperative TDR procedure has been outlined previously [32]:

- Mobilization from the first postoperative day with physiotherapeutic assistance.
- External stabilization/brace not required.
- Early resumption of physical activities is encouraged on a moderate level in noncontact sports (e.g., swimming, cycling) within the first 3 months following a short rehabilitation period.
- Solid osteointegration of the implants allows for further load increase and participation in preoperative sporting activities from 3 to 6 months postoperatively.
- In an uneventful postoperative course, participation even in highly demanding physical contact sports/extreme sports has been shown to be accessible and may be resumed from 4 to 6 months postoperatively.

39.8 Complications and Pitfalls

39.8.1 Surgery-Related Complications

- Injury to ureter and vascular lesions (high risk in TDR revision surgery)
- Deep vein thrombosis and arterial pulmonary embolism

- General surgery-related complications such as postoperative ileus, retroperitoneal hematoma, lymphocele, seroma, or urinoma [33]
- Infections
- Retrograde ejaculations/sexual dysfunction [34]
- Postsympathectomy-related complaints

39.8.2 Implant-Related Complications

- Implant subsidence/dislocations
- PE extrusions
- Postoperative pedicle or isthmus fractures
- Spinal cord and/or nerve root injury
- Persisting complaints from facet and iliosacral joints

39.9 Tips and Tricks

- For all TDRs at the level L4/5 and above and for selected cases of TDRs at the lumbosacral junction, 3-dimensional CT color-coded reconstruction of the prevertebral vessels provides valuable information about the vascular topography (Fig. 39.11) [13, 35]. In selected cases, the vascular anatomy can pose a contraindication against TDR.
- Avoid hyperextension of the lumbar spine on the operating table.
- Carefully prevent and avoid any kind of soft tissue impingement during the process chiseling, trial implant, or implant placement.

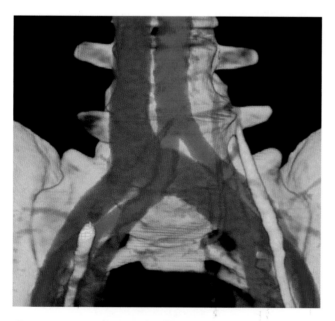

Fig. 39.11 Color-coded, 3D-CT angiography with a reconstruction of the prevertebral vessels

- When bleeding from the epidural venous plexus is encountered, it can be managed by the use of hemostatic agents such as Floseal® (Baxter).
- In cases of TDR above the lumbosacral junction, or all cases of TDR at the lumbosacral junction which required significant mobilization of vascular structures, it is advisable to attach a Gore© membrane to the anterior circumference of the disc space, behind the prevertebral vessels. In cases of anterior TDR revision surgery later than 2 weeks after the primary intervention, which has been associated with a high rate of intraoperative vascular lesions [36], the membrane may facilitate better mobilization of the vascular structures due to avoidance of scar tissue formation between the vascular structures and the anterior circumference of the vertebral body.
- A variety of oblique disc replacement implants have recently been developed. The availability of these oblique implants reduces the risk of vessel mobilization in comparison to TDRs that require a straightforward, midline implantation. These oblique disc replacement implants can therefore be recommended for TDRs performed at the level above the lumbosacral junction in selected cases.

References

1. Gillet P (2003) The fate of the adjacent motion segments after lumbar fusion. J Spinal Disord Tech 16:338–345
2. Goulet JA, Senunas LE, DeSilva GL et al (1997) Autogenous iliac crest bone graft. Complications and functional assessment. Clin Orthop Relat Res:76–81
3. Kumar MN, Jacquot F, Hall H (2001) Long-term follow-up of functional outcomes and radiographic changes at adjacent levels following lumbar spine fusion for degenerative disc disease. Eur Spine J 10:309–313
4. Lee CK (1988) Accelerated degeneration of the segment adjacent to a lumbar fusion. Spine 13:375–377
5. Park P, Garton HJ, Gala VC, Hoff JT et al (2004) Adjacent segment disease after lumbar or lumbosacral fusion: review of the literature. Spine 29:1938–1944
6. Umehara S, Zindrick MR, Patwardhan AG et al (2000) The biomechanical effect of postoperative hypolordosis in instrumented lumbar fusion on instrumented and adjacent spinal segments. Spine 25:1617–1624
7. Katz V, Schofferman J, Reynolds J (2003) The sacroiliac joint: a potential cause of pain after lumbar fusion to the sacrum. J Spinal Disord Tech 16:96–99
8. Maigne JY, Planchon CA (2005) Sacroiliac joint pain after lumbar fusion. A study with anesthetic blocks. Eur Spine J 14:654–658
9. Ha KY, Lee JS, Kim KW (2008) Degeneration of sacroiliac joint after instrumented lumbar or lumbosacral fusion: a prospective cohort study over five-year follow-up. Spine 33:1192–1198
10. Moshirfar A, Jenis LG, Spector LR et al (2006) Computed tomography evaluation of superior-segment facet-joint violation after pedicle instrumentation of the lumbar spine with a midline surgical approach. Spine 31:2624–2629

11. Shah RR, Mohammed S, Saifuddin A et al (2003) Radiologic evaluation of adjacent superior segment facet joint violation following transpedicular instrumentation of the lumbar spine. Spine 28:272–275

12. Cardoso MJ, Dmitriev AE, Helgeson M et al (2008) Does superior-segment facet violation or laminectomy destabilize the adjacent level in lumbar transpedicular fixation? An in vitro human cadaveric assessment. Spine 33:2868–2873

13. Siepe CJ, Mayer HM, Wiechert K et al (2006) Clinical results of total lumbar disc replacement with ProDisc II: three-year results for different indications. Spine 31:1923–1932

14. Siepe CJ, Mayer HM, Heinz-Leisenheimer M et al (2007) Total lumbar disc replacement: different results for different levels. Spine 32:782–790

15. McAfee PC, Cunningham BW, Hayes V et al (2006) Biomechanical analysis of rotational motions after disc arthroplasty: implications for patients with adult deformities. Spine 31:S152–S160

16. Sariali el-H, Lemaire JP, Pascal-Mousselard H et al (2006) In vivo study of the kinematics in axial rotation of the lumbar spine after total intervertebral disc replacement: long-term results: a 10–14 years follow up evaluation. Eur Spine J 15:1501–1510

17. Ching AC, Birkenmaier C, Hart RA (2010) Short segment coronal plane deformity after two-level lumbar total disc replacement. Spine (Phila Pa 1976) 35:44–50

18. Huang RC, Lim MR, Girardi FP et al (2004) The prevalence of contraindications to total disc replacement in a cohort of lumbar surgical patients. Spine 29:2538–2541

19. McAfee PC (2004) The indications for lumbar and cervical disc replacement. Spine J 4:177S–181S

20. Wong DA, Annesser B, Birney T et al (2007) Incidence of contraindications to total disc arthroplasty: a retrospective review of 100 consecutive fusion patients with a specific analysis of facet arthrosis. Spine J 7:5–11

21. Chin KR (2007) Epidemiology of indications and contraindications to total disc replacement in an academic practice. Spine J 7: 392–398

22. Blumenthal S, McAfee PC, Guyer RD et al (2005) A prospective, randomized, multicenter Food and Drug Administration investigational device exemptions study of lumbar total disc replacement with the CHARITE artificial disc versus lumbar fusion: part I: evaluation of clinical outcomes. Spine 30:1565–1575; discussion E1387–E1591

23. Zigler J, Delamarter R, Spivak JM et al (2007) Results of the prospective, randomized, multicenter Food and Drug Administration investigational device exemption study of the ProDisc-L total disc replacement versus circumferential fusion for the treatment of 1-level degenerative disc disease. Spine 32:1155–1162; discussion 1163

24. Mayer HM, Wiechert K (2002) Microsurgical anterior approaches to the lumbar spine for interbody fusion and total disc replacement. Neurosurgery 51:S159–S165

25. Mayer HM, Wiechert K, Korge A et al (2002) Minimally invasive total disc replacement: surgical technique and preliminary clinical results. Eur Spine J 11(Suppl 2):S124–S130

26. Jasani V, Jaffray D (2002) The anatomy of the iliolumbar vein. A cadaver study. J Bone Joint Surg Br 84:1046–1049

27. Cakir B, Richter M, Kafer W et al (2005) The impact of total lumbar disc replacement on segmental and total lumbar lordosis. Clin Biomech (Bristol, Avon) 20:357–364

28. Liu J, Ebraheim NA, Haman SP et al (2006) Effect of the increase in the height of lumbar disc space on facet joint articulation area in sagittal plane. Spine 31:E198–E202

29. Rohlmann A, Zander T, Bergmann G (2005) Effect of total disc replacement with ProDisc on intersegmental rotation of the lumbar spine. Spine 30:738–743

30. Siepe CJ, Hitzl W, Meschede P et al (2009) Interdependence between disc space height, range of motion and clinical outcome in total lumbar disc replacement. Spine 34:904–916

31. Adams MA, Roughley PJ (2006) What is intervertebral disc degeneration, and what causes it? Spine 31:2151–2161

32. Siepe CJ, Wiechert K, Khattab MF et al (2007) Total lumbar disc replacement in athletes: clinical results, return to sport and athletic performance. Eur Spine J 16:1001–1013

33. Patel AA, Spiker WR, Daubs MD et al (2008) Retroperitoneal lymphocele after anterior spinal surgery. Spine (Phila Pa 1976) 33:E648–E652

34. Flynn JC, Price CT (1984) Sexual complications of anterior fusion of the lumbar spine. Spine 9:489–492

35. Datta JC, Janssen ME, Beckham R et al (2007) The use of computed tomography angiography to define the prevertebral vascular anatomy prior to anterior lumbar procedures. Spine 32:113–119

36. Brau SA, Delamarter RB, Kropf MA et al (2008) Access strategies for revision in anterior lumbar surgery. Spine 33:1662–1667

Part VIII

Posterior Lumbar Spine

Overview of Surgical Techniques and Implants

40

Uwe Vieweg

40.1 Introduction and Core Messages

Posterior lumbar spine surgery uses various access routes (midline, lateral, far-lateral paracoccygeal) and can employ classic open, mini-open (microscopic or video assisted) or percutaneous access techniques. Decompression operations can be performed by using these access methods, and there are various possibilities of instrumentation as can various forms of instrumentation. The implants are divided into the following groups: rigid systems (internal fixator systems such as rod-screw or screw-plate systems, screws, pedicle screw-hook systems, cages and spacers for interbody fusion); different dynamic or semirigid systems; and so-called nonfusion systems (pedicle-based systems, interspinous spacers, facet replacements). The following are types of posterior stabilisation systems available: tulip screw–type systems, side-loading systems and plate systems. For the interbody fusion, there are cages in titanium as well as in PEEK on the market. Also, there are implants for the motion preservation available. The spectrum of those implants rises from dynamic pedicle screw systems, interspinous spacers and facet replacement implants.

40.2 Approaches (see Fig. 40.1)

- *Midline posterior approach*
A midline approach to the lumbar region is most frequently used for posterior lumbar spine surgery. The exposure of the deeper layer of muscles, however, is imprecise and can entail substantial tissue damage and blood loss. Besides providing access to the cauda equina and the intervertebral discs, the midline approach can expose the posterior elements of the spine: the spinous processes, laminae, facet joints and pedicles. The midline approach can be extended proximally and distally. The skin incision is made straight along the midline, even in scoliosis cases. For fusion cases, the incision should be one to two segments longer than the section to be fused. The preparation has to be performed strictly subperiosteally to preserve the blood vessels and nerves, which supply the muscles, and to prevent bleeding. In this approach technique, the lumbar spine is prepared from cranial to caudal.

- *Mediolateral posterior approaches*
Transmuscular paramedian approach and intermuscular Wiltse approach
The paramedian approach, as well as the intermuscular Wiltse approach, allows a good exposure of the nerve roots at the lumbar levels [16]. The Wiltse technique is a paramedian approach to the lumbosacral junction. Unlike a midline incision, where the exposure is created by cutting through the muscle planes, a Wiltse approach utilises a blunt dissection of the muscles, this means between the fascial planes of the multifidus and longissimus muscles to create the exposure. In the 1960s, Wiltse et al. described the sacrospinalis-splitting approach to the lumbar spine [20]. This procedure was accomplished by making a

U. Vieweg, M.D., Ph.D.
Clinic for Spinal Surgery, Sana Hospital Rummelsberg,
90593 Schwarzenbruck, Germany
e-mail: uwe.vieweg@yahoo.de

U. Vieweg, F. Grochulla (eds.), *Manual of Spine Surgery*,
DOI 10.1007/978-3-642-22682-3_40, © Springer-Verlag Berlin Heidelberg 2012

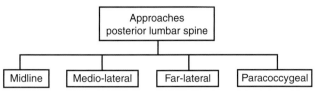

Fig. 40.1 Approaches for the posterior lumbar spine

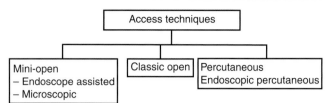

Fig. 40.2 Access techniques

paraspinous incision through the deep fascia and developing the plane between the multifidus and longissimus muscles. A paramedian skin incision is made to perform the transmuscular approach.

The intramuscular Wiltse approach allows the surgeon to approach the spine in a less-invasive way in comparison to a midline incision. It is known as a mini-open approach, invasive because it preserves the posterior musculature of the spine and it is performed unilaterally. In 1953, Watkins described a far-lateral approach, a route between the erector spinae (iliocostalis) and the quadratus lumborum, which requires some resection of the ilium for proper muscle reflection. Another option is the lateral intramuscular planar approach to the lumbar spine described by Newman [17].

- *Transforaminal approach*
  The transforaminal approach to the L5–S1 interspace provides a minimally invasive corridor through which discectomy and interbody fusion can safely be performed. It may provide an alternative route of access to the L5–S1 interspace in those patients who have unfavourable anatomy for, or contraindication to, the traditional open anterior approach to this level [1].

40.3   Access Techniques (see Fig. 40.2)

The access techniques used can be subdivided into classic open, mini-open and percutaneous techniques. The access routes can be made considerably smaller if special retractors are used [14]. These include: MLD-retractor, Caspar retractor (Aesculap); METRx or Quadrant (Medtronic); and ProView Minimal Access Portal System (Blackstone Medical) MaXcess (Nuvasive). These techniques are subsumed under the heading of mini-open access. To optimise visualisation, especially in minimally invasive and less-invasive spine surgery, either an operating microscope or an optic is used. The techniques are referred to with reference to the visualisation method employed (microscopic

or video assisted) [5, 14]. Combinations of percutaneous, microscopic, endoscopic and mini-open access techniques can be used (see Fig. 40.2) [5].

40.4   Implants (see Fig. 40.3)

Rigid Systems

- Screws and pins
  For the posterior approach, there are several translaminar screws or translaminar pins (ECF Peek from Signas) available. This translaminar pin is a further development of the translaminar facet screw fixation (TLPF). The implantation is performed by using a percutaneous paracoccygeal approach. A reduction and stabilisation of minor spondylolisthesis can be achieved by direct screwing as described by Buck [2].

  With a special-designed interbody fusion device (AxiaLIF), a transsacral approach can be achieved, for example, with the transsacral screw of TranS1.

  Examples: Multiple fragment screw–translaminar screw, transsacral screw (TranS1 Inc.) and ECF PEEK translaminar pin (Signus). Using a percutaneous paracoccygeal approach, axial fluoroscopically guided interbody fusion (AxiaLIF) is possible with a special transsacral screw (TranS1 Inc.) [1]. Translaminar pin fixation (TLPF) is a further development of translaminar facet screw fixation (TFSR). Compression and stabilisation of minor spondylolisthesis can be achieved by direct screwing, as described by Buck [2].

- Hook-screw systems
  Example: Hook-screw construct described by Morscher [12].

  This surgical procedure is to reconstruct and stabilise the fractured pars interarticularis in minimal spondylolytic spondylolisthesis. It allows compression of the defect without crossing the defect with the screw. Direct repair is indicated only in the absence of disc degeneration.

Fig. 40.3 Implants for the posterior lumbar spine

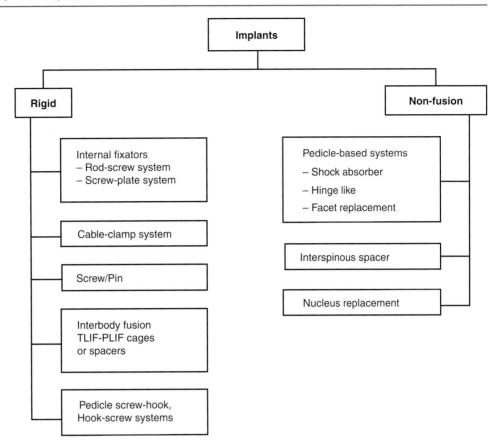

After the age of 25 years, this procedure should not be carried out.

• Internal fixator (screw-rod or screw-plate systems)
  Dorsal stabilisation procedures employ transpedicularly positioned implants with stable angle fixation. From the internal fixator as described by Dick, further development led to the fixator described by Kluger and the Universal Spine System USS (Synthes) and MOSS System (DePuy). The rigid internal fixator systems can be grouped in different ways according to their design details, for example, top-loading and side-loading systems, polyaxial screw, monoaxial screw, reduction screws, augmentation screws and cannulated screws [3, 4, 9].

Internal Fixator Systems for Open Implantation (Current and Older Systems)

Examples: TSRH (Texas Scottish Rite Hospital) 3D Spinal Instrumentation (Medtronic), CD HORIZON LEGACY (Medtronic), MOSS-MIAMI Family (DePuy), SFS Spinal Fixation System (Blackstone Medical), Monarch Spine system (Zimmer Spine), ST 360° Spinal Fixation System (Zimmer Spine), Synergy Spinal System (Interpore Cross International), USS-Universal Spinal System (Synthes), Click'X (Synthes) (see Fig. 40.4), SOCON (Aesculap), Silhouette Spinal Fixation System (Zimmer Spine), Sequoia (Zimmer Spine), Instinct Java (Zimmer Spine), Xia (Stryker), ConKlusion (Signus), SSE Spine System Evolution (Aesculap) and S^4 Spinal System (Aesculap) (see Fig. 40.5).

Systems for Less-Invasive Percutaneous Implantation

Silverbolt (VertiFlex), CD Horizon Longitude System (Medtronic), CD Horizon Sextant System I/II (Medtronic), Pathfinder (Zimmer Spine), MANTIS (Stryker), SpheRx (Nuvasive), SpiRIT (Synthes), ProView, ICON (Blackstone Medical) and Expedium Viper (DePuy Spine).

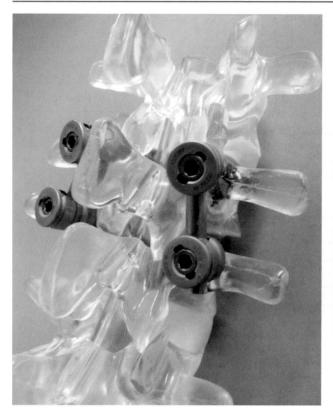

Fig. 40.4 Click'X, internal fixator system (Synthes)

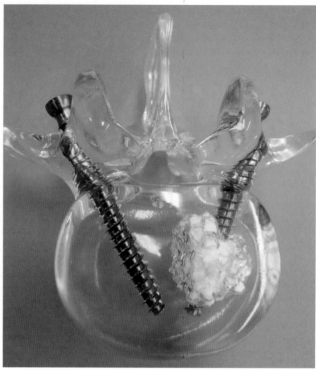

Fig. 40.6 Cannulated pedicle screw click'X for augmentation (Synthes)

Pedicle Screw Systems for Augmentation

SOCON (Aesculap), S⁴ Spinal System (Aesculap) and Click'X (Synthes) (see Figs. 40.4 and 40.6)

- Cable-clamp systems
  Example: Universal Clamp System (Zimmer Spine)
- The universal clamp is a polyester band passed under the lamina and connected to a rod by a titanium clamp. This is an alternative for replacing screws and hooks for thoracolumbar spinal diseases
- Screw-plate systems
  Monarch plate or rod system (DePuy Spine)
      It is about a combination of pedicle bolt and in-line polyaxial screw technology. Modular polyaxial washers can be added to provide an angulation at any position
  Example: Monarch plate or rod system (DePuy Spine)
- Rod-cable systems
  Luque rod and rectangle with wire fixation (Surgicraft), ISOLA (DePuy Spine)
      It is used in deformity cases and employs screws, wires, slotted connectors, hooks and rods to correct the thoracolumbar spine
  Examples: Luque rod and rectangle with wire fixation (Surgicraft), ISOLA (DePuy Spine)
- Interbody implants (cages, spacers)
  - *Titanium net cylinders*
  Examples: Harms titanium net cylinder (DePuy Spine), SynMesh (Synthes)
  NGage Surgical Mesh System (Blackstone Medical)

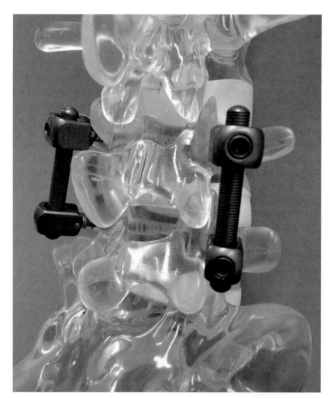

Fig. 40.5 Cosmic internal fixator (Ulrich) with mobile (hinged) screwhead

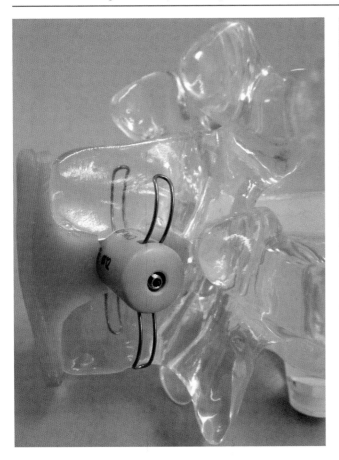

Fig. 40.7 Inspace (Synthes)

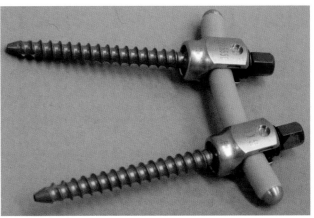

Fig. 40.8 Semirigid PEEK rod system (Medtronic)

- *PLIF Cages* (box like)
  Examples: Ardis PEEK implant (Zimmer Spine), Trabecular Metal PLIF (Zimmer Spine), OIC Cage (Stryker), ProSpace PEEK or titanium cages/spacers (Aesculap), Tetris PEEK (Signus) and Pillar PL (Blackstone Medical).
- *TLIF* cages (kidney-shaped design)
  Trabecular Metal TLIF and TraXis TLIF Peek (Zimmer Spine), CAPSTONE (Medtronic), Devex/Leopard (DePuy Spine), Mobis PEEK (Signus), Pillar TL (Blackstone Medical) and T-Space (Aesculap).

Semirigid or Dynamic Systems (Nonfusion Systems)

Semirigid or dynamic types of instrumentation for motion preservation have been developed for the lumbar spine. Dynamic stabilisation describes the treatment method employed to achieve stabilisation by maintaining the disc with controlled motion of the segment [7]. The implants for dynamic stabilisation are either fixed in the pedicle or secured between the spinous processes.

Nucleus replacements, which are implanted posteriorly, are another option.

- Interspinous implants
  Examples: The principle of implanting a spacer between adjacent spinous processes was used by Knowles to relieve the posterior annulus in patients with disc herniation [18].

  Most implants act in the sagittal plane to inhibit extension. They cause a reduction in lordosis of the motion segment [11] which is visible on X-rays and a reduction in pressure within the disc, thus reducing the load on the facet joint surfaces [19]. They also cause an increase in the subarticular diameter and a widening of the neural foramina. The Wallis implant, for example, is made of PEEK (polyetheretherketone). In addition, the implant includes two ligaments made of woven Dacron that are wrapped around the spinous processes and fixed under tension to the blocker. The Wallis interspinous implant is fixed to the spine by two polyester bands looped around the proximal and distal spinous processes [10, 16]. The DIAM (Medtronic) was designed to dynamically support the vertebrae while at the same time maintaining distraction of the foramina. Other recently developed dynamic stabilisation systems are the X-Stop interspinous process decompression system (St. Francis Medical Technologies), the Coflex (Paradigm Spine) and Inspace (Synthes) (see Fig. 40.7 and 40.8).

  However, there exist today no international contents about indications for interspinous devices. Actually, there are controversies about effectiveness of interspinous devices.

- Pedicle screw–based systems
  Examples: Graf Band (SEM Co.), Dynesys (Zimmer Spine), Cosmic (Ulrich Medical), Isobar TTL (Scient'x) and TOPS – Total Posterior Arthroplasty device (Implant).

  Dynamic stabilisation with pedicle screw–based systems presents an alternative to instrumented immobilisation and relief of spine segments [20]. The Graf Band, which first became available in 1992, was the first pedicle screw–based system [7].

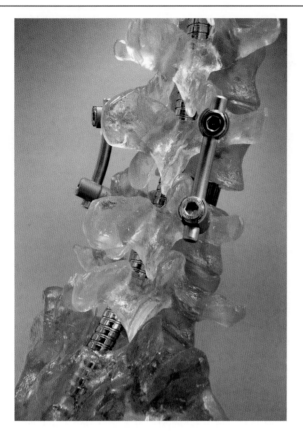

Fig. 40.9 Rigid S⁴ internal fixator (Aesculap)

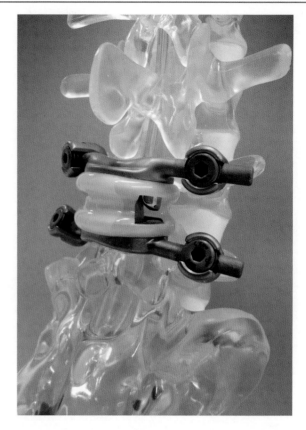

Fig. 40.10 TOPS – total posterior arthroplasty device (Implaint)

The Dynesys Dynamic Stabilization System (DSS) (Zimmer Spine) was developed by Dubois [15]. Extensive scientific results have been published for Dynesys [8]. Figure 40.8 demontrates a semirigid PEEK rod system. The cosmic system (see Fig. 40.9) is a stable and nonrigid system. The screw features a hinged joint between the head and threaded part, which causes the load to be shared between the implant system and the anterior vertebral column. Other options are facet replacement devices, which are designed to replace degenerative facet joints with a prosthetic implant like the TOPS – Total Posterior Arthroplasty device (Implaint) (see Fig. 40.10).

- Nucleus replacements
  Examples: Prosthetic Disc Nucleus (PDN) (Raymedica) and DASCOR Disc Arthroplasty System (Disc Dynamics).

Some nucleus replacement devices can be implanted using a dorsal access route, for example, PDN (Raymedica) or, in part, DASCOR (Disc Dynamics). The PDN devices are constructed from two components: an inner copolymer hydrogel pellet and an outer, superstrong woven jacket of high molecular weight polyethylene fibres [13].

References

1. Aryan HE, Newman CB, Gold JJ et al (2008) Percutaneous axial lumbar interbody fusion (AxiaLIF) of the L5-S1 segment: initial clinical and radiological experience. Minim Invasive Neurosurg 51:225–230
2. Buck JE (1970) Direct repair of the defect in spondylolisthesis. J Bone Joint Surg Br 52:432–437
3. Cui Y, Lewis G, Qi G (2002) Numerical analysis of models of standard TSRH spinal instrumentation: effect of rod cross-sectional shape. Comput Methods Biomech Biomed Engin 5:75–80
4. Dick W (1989) Intercorporelle spondylodese L4/L5 und L5/S1. Oper Orthop Traumatol 1:43–47
5. Foley KT, Smith MM (1997) Microendoscopic discectomy. J Neurosurg 3:301–307
6. Gillet P, Petit M (1999) Direct repair of spondylolisis without spondylolisthesis, using a rod-screw construct and bone grafting of the pars defect. Spine 24:1252–1256
7. Grevitt MP, Gardner AD, Spilsbury J et al (1995) The Graf stabilisation system: early results in 50 patients. Eur Spine J 4:169–175
8. Grob D, Benini A, Junge A et al (2005) Clinical experience with the Dynesys semirigid fixation system for the lumbar spine. Surgical and patient-oriented outcome in 50 cases after an average of 2 years. Spine 30:324–331
9. Kluger P (1989) Das Fixateurprinzip an der Wirbelsäule. In: Stuhler T (ed) Fixateur externe – Fixateur interne. Springer, Berlin
10. Korovessis P, Repantis T, Zacharatos S et al (2009) Does Wallis implant reduce adjacent segmental degeneration above lumbosacral instrumented fusion? Eur Spine J 18:830–840

11. Lindsey DP, Swanson KE, Fuchs P et al (2003) The effect of an interspinous implant on the kinematics of the instrumented and adjacent levels in the lumbar spine. Spine 28:2192–2197

12. Morscher E, Gerber B, Fasel J (1984) Surgical treatment of spondylolisthesis by bone grafting and direct stabilization of spondylolysis by means of a hook screw. Arch Orthop Trauma Surg 103: 175–178

13. Ray CD (2002) The PDN prosthetic disc-nucleus device. Eur Spine J 11(Suppl 2):S137–S142

14. Roh SW, Kim DH, Cardoso AC et al (2000) Endoscopic foraminotomy using MED system in cadaveric specimens. Spine 25:260–264

15. Stoll TM, Dubois G, Schwarzenbach O (1999) The dynamic neutralization system for the spine: a multi-center study of a novel non-fusion system. Eur Spine J 11(Suppl 2):S170–S178

16. Vialle R, Harding I, Charosky D et al (2007) The paraspinal splitting approach: a possible approach to perform multiple intercostolumbar neurotisations: an anatomic study. Spine 32:631–634

17. Newman EW (2007) Lateral intramuscular planar approach to the lumbar spine and sacrum. Technical note. J Neurosurg Spine 7:270–273

18. Whitesides TE Jr (2003) The effect of an interspinous implant on intervertebral disc pressures. Spine 28:1906–1907

19. Wilke HJ, Magerl F, Nelter S, et al. (2000) Biomechanical in vitro comparison of translaminar pins versus translaminar screws for instrumentation of spinal segments. Poster, Eurospine

20. Wiltse LL, Bateman JG, Hutchinson RH et al (1968) The paraspinal sacrospinalis-splitting approach to the lumbar spine. J Bone Joint Surg Am 50:919–926

Microsurgical Intra- and Extraspinal Discectomy

41

Luca Papavero

41.1 Introduction and Core Messages

Three microsurgical approaches are presented to deal with lumbar herniated discs. The intraspinal approaches include the "interlaminar" (ILA) and the "translaminar" (TLA) ones. The interlaminar route is indicated when the extruded disc fragment and/or contained herniation is located between the midline and the medial border of the pedicle (roughly 70%). The translaminar approach is valuable for removing a cranially extruded disc fragment impinging the exiting root. This herniation is commonly within the root canal, i.e., between the medial and lateral rim of the pedicle (roughly 20%). The extraspinal approach, or more precisely the transmuscular paraspinal route, deals with disc fragments extruded with at least two-thirds of the volume laterally to the lateral border of the pedicle (roughly 10%). Features common to all the tree techniques are: (1) a carefully preoperative planning, mostly by MRI, for choosing the most convenient approach; (2) the use of the microscope from skin to skin; (3) the application of soft tissue and facet joint sparing techniques, requiring the insertion of miniaturized retractors; and (4) whenever possible, the solely removal of the offending disc fragment leaving the disc space alone.

L. Papavero, M.D., Ph.D.
Clinic for Spine Surgery, Schön Clinic Hamburg,
Dehnhaide 120, 22081 Hamburg, Germany
e-mail: lpapavero@schoen-kliniken.de

41.2 Interlaminar Approach (ILA) [3]

41.2.1 Indications

- All "pure" contained disc herniations and extruded disc fragments between the midline and the medial border of the pedicle. Referring to the disc space, the fragments may be caudally or cranially extruded. In the latter case, the translaminar approach is more selective.
- Disc herniations combined with central/recess stenosis or with asymptomatic segmental instability.
- Recurrent disc herniations.

41.2.2 Contraindications

- Disc herniations which bulk is located laterally to the lateral border of the pedicle.

41.2.3 Technical Requirements

- Intraoperative fluoroscopy.
- Microscope. Following features are useful: long holding arm of the *stative* in order to place the micro behind the surgeon, "in front" stereoscopic oculars, powerful illumination (e.g., 300W Xenon), and external video-line for ORP.
- Positioning device allowing reduction of lumbar lordosis (e.g., Wilson frame, Fig. 41.1).
- Small retractor to be introduced through a 2–3-cm skin incision.
- Microsurgical instruments, better if bayoneted (Fig. 41.2).
- Optional: high-speed drill with angled handpieces, cutting *burrs*, and diamond dust–coated *burrs*.

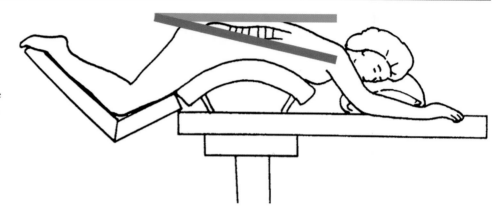

Fig. 41.1 Wilson frame: note that the lumbar spine should be parallel to the floor and straightened. Hip, knee, and ankle are only moderately flexed. Positioning for a translaminar approach should consider that the lumbar laminae "dive" (red line), therefore tilting the table a bit head-up wards will bring the laminae in a horizontal plane (green line): this makes drilling of the translaminar hole easier

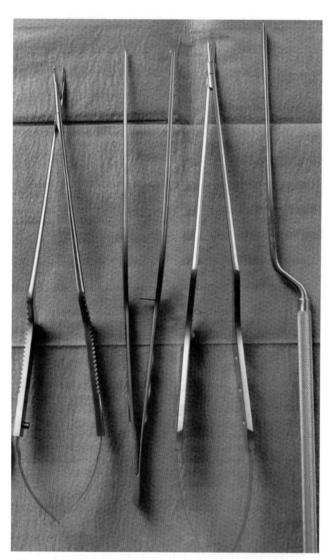

Fig. 41.2 Bayoneted instruments prevent the fingers from obstructing the microsurgical field

41.2.4 Preparation, Planning, and Positioning

- *Plain X-rays in AP and lateral view*: Optional in first surgery cases, provided that the MRI investigation encloses a coronal slice (scoliosis!). Obligatory (1) in recurrent disc surgery for evaluating the bone defect (2) whenever the MRI leads to suspect a bony anormality (spina bifida, defect of pars interarticularis).
- *MRI*: the first choice investigation! *Sagittal slices*: contained disc herniation (DH) or extruded fragment? Caudal or cranial fragment dislocation (suitable for translaminar approach)? Midvertebral body herniation (on halfway between two disc spaces)? Foraminal slice: black neuroforamen? Extraforaminal slice: disc fragment still apparent? *Axial slices*: intra-axillary disc fragment? How much of the DH is underneath the thecal sac, intraforaminal, or extraforaminal? Pseudomeningocele in recurrent disc surgery? *Coronal slices*: which approach for combined intra- and extraforaminal DH? *Gadolineum*: amount of scar tissue on the way to and into the spinal canal? Differentiation between recurrent DH and scar tissue?
- *CT-scan*: second choice whenever MRI is contraindicated or not available. Disco-CT (discography+CT): helpful in suspected extraforaminal DH. CM-enhanced CT: indicated for recurrent disc, differentiation between intraforaminal DH vs. neurinoma.
- *Myelography*: as third option.
- We recognize that several positionings could provide good clinical results, especially with experienced ORP. The features of our favorite positioning are described below:
  - The patient is placed prone on the Wilson frame. Advantages: hip and knee joints are not flexed, especially important in obese patients! The lordosis of the lumbar spine can be reduced as required by increasing the height of the arches. The distance between the arches can be adjusted according to the size of the patient in order to allow a free hanging abdomen (Fig. 41.1).
  - The head is positioned into the ProneView mask (manufacturer: Dupaco, Oceanside, California, USA). Eyes, nose, and chin are protected: the anesthesiologist is enabled to check them anytime by a mirror (Fig. 41.3)!
  - For safety reasons, the patient is secured with a belt on the gluteal area: this becomes helpful when the OR table has to be tilted away from the surgeon, e.g.,

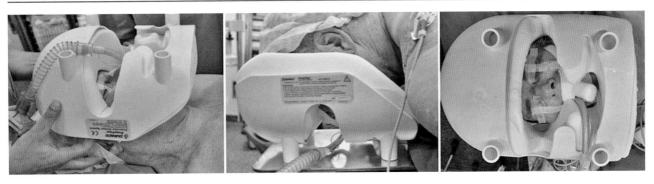

Fig. 41.3 The mask fits to the face before turning the patient (*left*), patient prone with the mask resting on a mirror (*center*), mirror for checking eyes, nose, chin, and airways (*right*)

in dealing with extraforaminal disc herniations (EFDH).

- The OR table is tilted to get the lumbar spine parallel to the floor.

- *X-ray labeling*: A 2–3-cm skin incision does not allow a "seek and find" surgery. Therefore, the correct X-ray labeling of the surgical target area is of paramount importance.

- The needle is always inserted contralateral to the intended surgical side in order to avoid subcutaneous or intramuscular hematoma and off the midline in order to prevent CSF leakage. The needle is perpendicular to the target area (and to the floor): soft tissue dissection is easier straight forward down! Even small oblique deviations can lead to the wrong level, especially in obese patients.

- The needle should point to the equator of the target disc. With increasing experience, it may point to the extruded disc fragment.

41.2.5 Surgical Technique

The interlaminar space can be approached via a subperiosteal (SP) or a transmuscular (TM) route. Although the use of the microscope "skin to skin" is optional, its advantages will be quickly appreciated dealing with a miniaturized surgical corridor. The most relevant steps are described below: single-shot antibiotic (e.g., cephazoline, 2 g) 30 min before skin incision.

- *Skin* (SP and TM): 2-cm incision, 5 mm off the midline.

- *Fascia*: semicircular incision toward the midline. Five holding sutures on the medial lip secured to a clamp with weights (SP). Straight incision with one holding suture on each side (TM).

- *Muscle*: retraction of the paravertebral muscles with a Langenbeck from the interspinal ligament. Sharp

dissection of the rotators from the lower rim of the superior lamina and from the facet joint capsule. Insertion of a miniaturized Caspar-type speculum-counter-retractor system ("piccolino," manufacturer: Medicon, Tuttlingen, Germany, Fig. 41.4a) (SP). Blunt splitting with the index finger until the laminofacet junction can be palpated. Opening of the muscular corridor with miniaturized Langenbecks or with a dilator. Insertion of an expandable tubular retractor ("Microdisc XS," manufacturer Medicon, Tuttlingen, Germany) with 15 mm diameter. The tube is secured with a "snake," a self-holding arm, to the OR table (Figs. 41.5 and 41.6) (TM).

- *Interlaminar space*: from this step onward, the surgical technique is identical. The lower rim of the cranial lamina, the medial border of the facet joint, and the yellow ligament should be the area of interest. A fluoroscopic control of the level is performed. Following a lateral flavectomy or flavotomy with suspension sutures, the epidural fat is exposed. The medial border of the inferior articular process is undercut or drilled off until the lateral border of the root is palpated.

- *Epidural dissection*: up-down dissection of the epidural fat performed with a microdissector and a flat sucker (so-called mole-technique, Fig. 41.4c), along with prudent bipolar coagulation of veins, opens the access to the root-DH complex.

- *Management of the DH*: the local anatomy will dictate the necessary steps. Usually, a gentle separation of the cleavage plane between root and disc material is accomplished first. In our experience, the root retraction is performed intermittently with the flat sucker instead of with a conventional root retractor. Free disc fragments are removed with miniaturized forceps (manufacturer: Medicon, Tuttlingen, Germany, Fig. 41.4b). If indicated, the annulus is split bluntly with the dissector, and further disc material is removed. In the authors' experience, additional discectomy is performed in 20–30% of the cases.

Fig. 41.4 (**a**) Miniaturized speculum, (**b**) miniaturized forceps (*black*), and (**c**) flat sucker

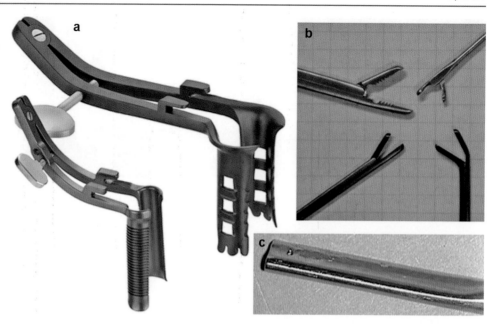

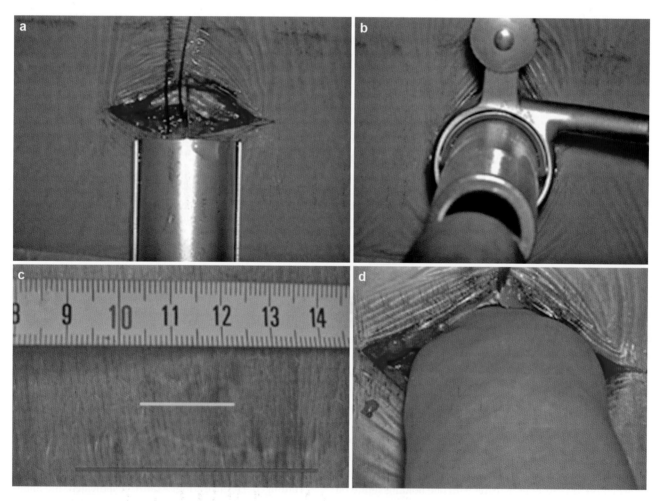

Fig. 41.5 Transmuscular approach: (**a**) 20-mm skin incision, blunt muscle splitting with a dilator (**b**) or with the index finger (**d**), (**c**) scar of transmuscular approach (*yellow line*) for a recurrent disc following previous conventional subperiosteal approach (*red line*)

Fig. 41.6 Close-up view (**a**) of the expandable tubular retractor in situ; the tubular retractor is fixed with a self-holding adjustable arm, "the snake" (**b**); and intraoperative fluoroscopy of the closed (**c**) and opened (**d**) tube

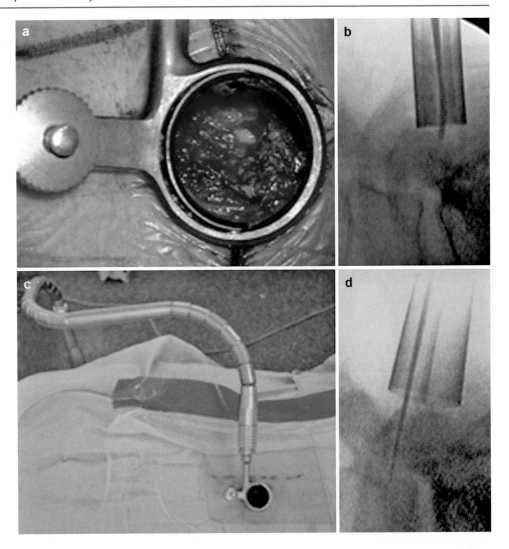

- *Closure*: the disc space, when opened, is rinsed with Ringer solution. The opening of the annulus is closed with a collagen sponge coated with fibrinogen and thrombin (TachoSil, manufacturer: Behring, Marburg, Germany). The epidural fat is mobilized in order to cover the root. Careful hemostasis goes along with closure by layers.

41.2.6 Postoperative Care

The patient is encouraged to leave the bed 6 h after surgery. Sitting is allowed starting from the first postoperative day. Physiotherapy starts the morning after surgery. Hospital staying is usually 3 days.

41.2.7 Complications

The literature lists several "generic" complications such as deep venous thrombosis, pulmonary embolism, urinary infections, missed pathology, retroperitoneal vessel injury, and postoperative segmental instability which fortunately became more than exceptional events. However, even the refined microsurgical techniques are still burdened by complications such as root injury (0.5%), dural tears (1.5%), spondylodiscitis (>1%), and "recurrent DH" (5%).

41.3 Translaminar Approach (TLA) [1, 2, 4, 6, 8]

41.3.1 Indications

- Cranially extruded disc fragments pushing the exiting root against the lower rim of the pedicle. Usually they are also located intraforaminally (Fig. 41.7a, b).
- Recurrent cranially extruded disc fragments of disc herniations previously addressed by an interlaminar approach.

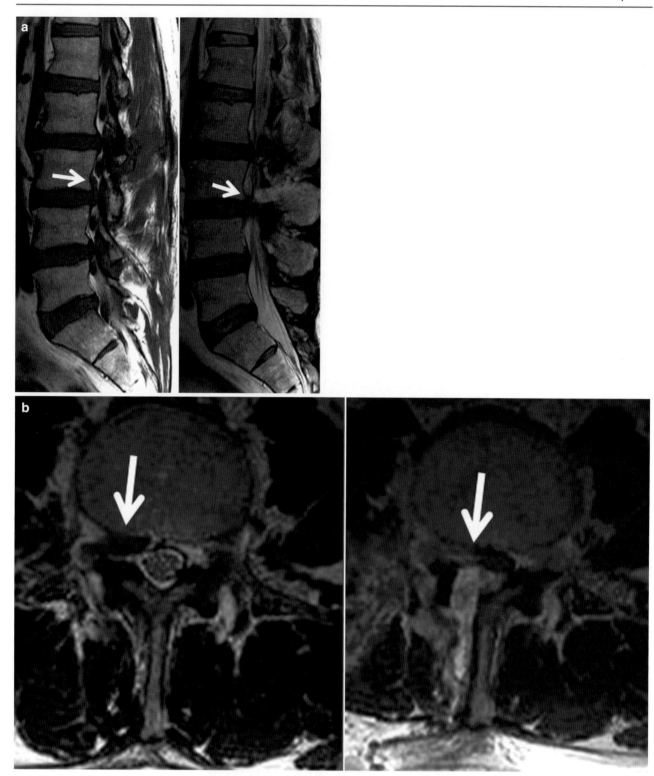

Fig. 41.7 (**a**) Cranially extruded disc fragment L3/L4 (*arrow*, *left*), which has been removed via a translaminar approach (*arrow*, *right*). (**b**) The axial slice shows that the disc fragment (*arrow*) impinges the exiting L3 root on the right side (*left*). The postoperative picture confirms the removal through the lamina (*right*)

41.3.2 Contraindications

- Severe spinal canal stenosis and spina bifida lack of an adequate lamina.
- In case of a foraminal DH, the bulk of the fragment should be between two lines, marking the medial and lateral borders of the superior facet: disc material located more laterally should be approached through a paraspinal approach.

41.3.3 Technical Requirements

- The same as for ILA.
- A must: drill with angled handpieces, cutting *burrs*, and diamond dust–coated *burrs*.

41.3.4 Preparation, Planning, and Positioning

- *MRI*: *sagittal slices*: measure the distance between upper border of the disc space and cranial rim of the fragment! The translaminar hole will be centered on the halfway of this distance. *Axial slices*: look at how much of the bulk of the DH is underneath the thecal sac and how much is lateral of it or even intraforaminal. The translaminar hole is centered on the lateral border of the thecal sac.
- Basically the same as for ILA.
- Important: the target lamina should be parallel to the floor! This may require to tilt the OR table a little bit head upward. The advantages of a horizontal target lamina are twofold: the placement of the retractor blade and the drilling of the hole become easier (Fig. 41.1).
- *X-ray labeling*: the needle should point to the maximum bulk of the DH which is usually halfway between the upper border of the target disc space and the lower rim of the cranial pedicle.
- At the beginning of the learning curve, the upper border of the target disc space and the lower rim of the cranial pedicle may be labeled separately and the skin incision centered in between (Fig. 41.8).

41.3.5 Surgical Technique

The lamina can be approached via a subperiosteal (SP) or a transmuscular (TM) route. The soft tissue approach mirrors exactly that to the interlaminar space and has been already described. Remember, the width and the overlapping of the lamina in relation to the disc space increase in the caudal-cranial direction, whereas the width of the isthmus decreases. This means that the translaminar hole will be more medially and more ovale-shaped in the cranial direction (Fig. 41.9).

- *Lamina*: irrespective of the kind of speculum used, the lateral border of the lamina should be visible underneath the

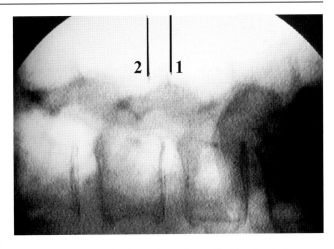

Fig. 41.8 Intraoperative fluoroscopy: the needle (*1*) points to the upper rim of the target disc, whereas the needle (*2*) points to disc fragment just underneath the lower rim of the cranial pedicle

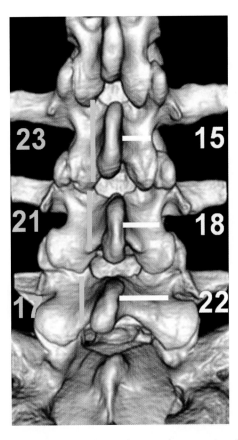

Fig. 41.9 *White numbers*: distance between the upper rim of the disc space and the lower border of the correspondent lamina; *black numbers*: width of the lamina

retractor valve. A dissector is placed onto the lamina where the bulk of the DH is suspected and a fluoroscopic control is performed. At this point, the lamina should have been tilted parallel to the floor so that the cutting burr can be held more easily perpendicular to the lamina. With slow circular movements, a round (L5) or oval-shaped (L4 and cranially) hole of about 10 mm in diameter is performed

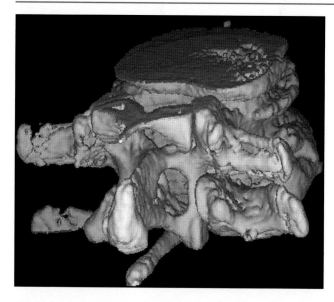

Fig. 41.10 Postoperative 3D-CT which shows a translaminar hole L3 on the right side

(Fig. 41.10). Three layers, "white" (outer cortical bone), "red" (spongy bone), and "white" (inner cortical bone), will be drilled off. For the sake of safety, the inner cortical bone should be drilled with a diamond burr. Remarks: (1) At least 3 mm of the lateral border should be spared in order to avoid a fracture of the pars interarticularis (Fig. 41.11). (2) Usually, the translaminar hole is located just cephalad to the cranial insertion of the yellow ligament. So, after removal of the thin shell of inner cortical bone with small punches, epidural fat will appear.

- *Epidural dissection*: up and down dissection of the fat along the lateral border of the thecal sac. That should be continued cranial up to the axilla of the exiting root.
- *Management of the DH*: Usually, an extruded or subligamentous disc fragment/s can be mobilized. After decompression, the root slips caudally into the visible field (Fig. 41.12). The root canal is probed with a double-angled hook. If an extensive annular perforation is detected, the disc space should be cleared. In our experience, that was

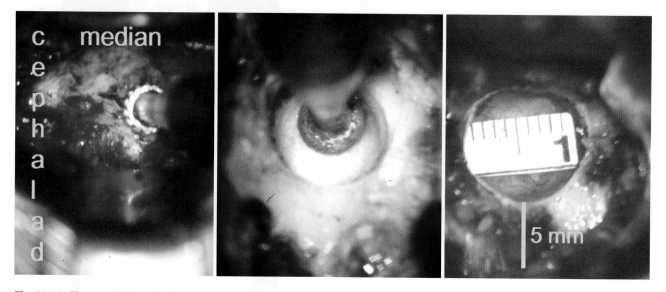

Fig. 41.11 The superficial cortical bone of the lamina is drilled off with a cutting burr (*left*), the inner cortical bone with a diamond dust–coated burr (*center*), keep at least 3 mm safety zone at the lateral border of the pars interarticularis (*right*)

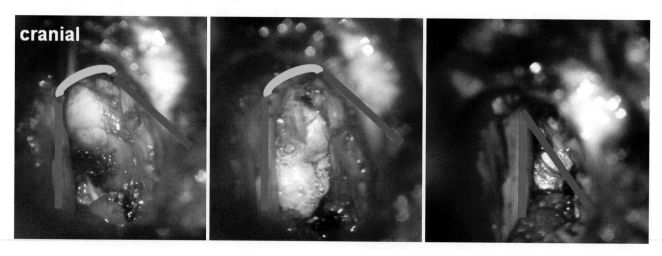

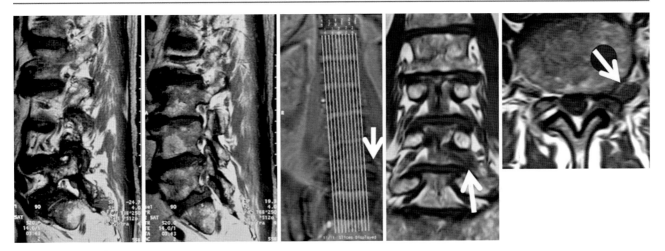

Fig. 41.13 (From *left to right*) Inapparent paramedian slices due to faulty scanning (*center*) omitting the extraforaminal areas, especially on the *left side* (*arrow*); the coronal view shows that the left-sided L4 root is severely impinged by an extraforaminal DH (*arrow*). The disc fragment is also clearly visible on the axial slice (*right, arrow*): compare the different distribution of the extraforaminal fat

required in merely 20% of the cases. The rate of recurrence was 7%.

- *Closure*: Gelfoam soaked with long-acting steroid to fill in the hole is optional, but it should be avoided if the disc space has been cleared.
- *Postoperative care*: same as for ILA.

41.3.6 Complications

Tilting of the OR table in order to direct the lamina quite parallel to the floor minimizes the risk of wrong level surgery.

The particularly thin axillary dura should be handled very carefully during dissection of adherent disc fragments. Due to the narrow access, gluing a patch on accidental durotomy is the best solution.

Although not a complication, enlarging the hole to conventional laminotomy becomes necessary whenever a significant annular perforation is detected on the caudal half of the disc space, especially at the L5/S1 level.

41.4 Extraforaminal Approach (EFA) [5, 7]

41.4.1 Indication

- Disc fragment located at least two-thirds lateral to the pedicle.

41.4.2 Contraindication

- Foraminal disc herniations located more than two-thirds inside the root canal.

41.4.3 Technical Requirements

- The same as for TLA.

41.4.4 Preparation, Planning, and Positioning

- MRI: sagittal slices: cave! Usually, they are not scanned lateral enough, i.e., lateral to the root canal, and miss the EFDH. Axial slices: compare the amount and distribution of the extraforaminal fat tissue on both sites. Coronal slices: although rarely performed, they are of invaluable help to show the spatial relationship between exiting root, root canal, and extraforaminal compartment (Fig. 41.13).
- Basically the same as for ILA.
- For safety reasons, the patient should be belted on the gluteal region: the OR table has to be tilted 20–30° away from the surgeon in order to get a better oblique view of the extraforaminal compartment. Especially, obese patients may risk to "roll over" on their own fat.
- *Lateral view* (*X-ray labeling*): insert a spinal needle one finger's breadth lateral to the spinous process, perpendicularly to the skin, and projecting toward the lower border

---

Fig. 41.12 Epidural dissection on the *right side*: the intra-axillary disc fragment pushes the root upward to the lower rim of the pedicle (*left*); the epidural capsule has been removed from the DH (*center*); after the removal of the space occupying disc fragment, the root becomes visible in the surgical field (*left*). *Red line*: lateral border of the thecal sac; *yellow line*: axilla of the exiting root; *blue line*: lower border of the exiting root

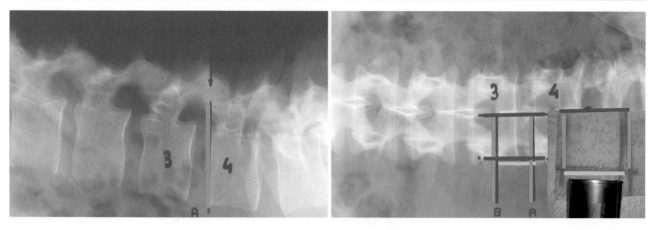

Fig. 41.14 Labeling of the lines of reference on the intraoperative lateral (*Left*) and AP (*right*) view

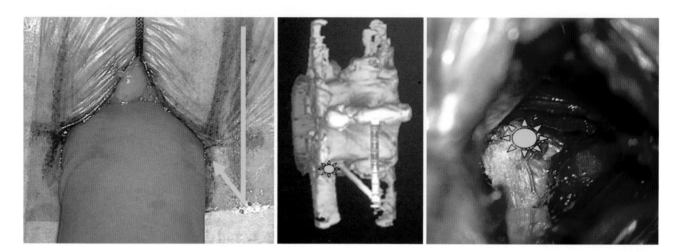

Fig. 41.15 Blunt splitting of the muscles pointing to the medial third of the transverse process cranial to the target disc (*left*), 3D-CT depicting the access (*center*), target point (*asterisk*) of the transverse process (*right*)

of the affected disc space. Draw a horizontal line at this level (A). Switch the C-arm into the AP-view: Two horizontal lines are drawn: (1) the lower border of the affected disc space should be identical with the previous marking in the lateral view (A) and (2) the lower border of the transverse process above the affected disc (B). Two vertical lines are also drawn: (1) the midline (row of the spinous processes) (C) and (2) a line about 4 cm off to the midline, marking the lateral boundary of the pedicle above and below the affected disc (D). The distance between the two horizontal lines (AB) is the skin incision and will be 3–4 cm in length and about 4 cm paramedian (Fig. 41.14).

41.4.5 Surgical Technique

- The transmuscular blunt splitting approach to EFDH at the level L4/L5 or more cranially can be performed with an expandable tubular retractor or with a miniaturized

speculum combined with medial and lateral counterretractor blades (Fig. 41.15). At the level L5/S1, the author recommends the use of two counterretractors inserted perpendicular to each other. That allows to choose four blades of different lengths matching with the following structures: facet joint (medial), transverse plane (lateral), transverse process (cranial), and ala (caudal) (Figs. 41.16 and 41.17). Furthermore, the use of the microscope "skin to skin" is advised.

- *Skin*: 3 cm in length, 4 cm off the midline.
- *Transmuscular route*: after incision of the fascia of m. erector spinae, the muscle is dissected bluntly using the index finger along the cleavage plane between the multifidus and the longissimus muscle (Fig. 41.15). If this fibrous separation cannot be palpated, the muscle is split downward to the medial third of the transverse processes. The selected retractor is then introduced so that the tips rest firmly on the lower half of the upper transverse process and on the upper half of the lower one. The lateral surface of the pars interarticularis represents the medial border of

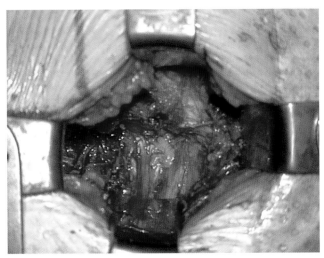

Fig. 41.16 Surgical field to approach L5/S1 on the *left side*: the upper blade rests on the facet joint, the left one on the transverse process L5

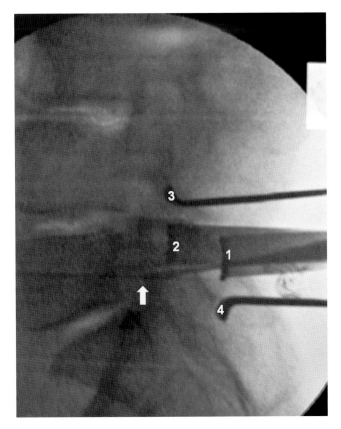

Fig. 41.17 Intraoperative fluoroscopic control L5/S1: (*1*) medial blade on the facet joint, (*2*) lateral blade, (*3*) cranial blade a bit cephalad to the transverse process L5, (*4*) blade on the ala sacri, dissector pointing to the DH (*arrow*)

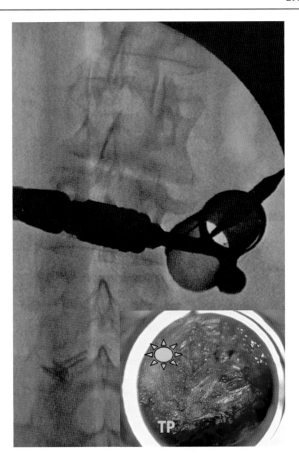

Fig. 41.18 Intraoperative fluoroscopic control in AP view for approaching a left-sided extraforaminal DH L3/L4. Note the concave curve of the degenerative scoliosis. Close-up view of the medial third of the transverse process (*asterisk*) (*bottom right*)

the surgical exposure. A fluoroscopic check at this point of the procedure is essential (Fig. 41.18).

- *Extraforaminal compartment*: tilting the OR table by 15–20° away from the surgeon gives a better view of the area lateral of the pedicle. Drilling off bone is usually not necessary, except in the case of an extremely hypertrophied facet joint or at the L5/S1 level. The medial half of the intertransverse muscle is incised and pushed laterally, thereby exposing the intertransverse membrane, also called the "intertransverse ligament." After its incision, the fat surrounding the nerve appears. Because of the proximity of the nerve, the accompanying vessels, and DH, the sucker should also be used as a nerve retractor. However, beware of an excessive retraction of the dorsal ganglion in order to minimize the incidence of postoperative burning dysesthesias! Branches of the radicular artery should be dissected carefully and spared whenever possible. The accompanying veins can be cauterized if they hinder the access to the disc fragment.

- *Management of the DH*: Typically, we find the nerve and the ganglion pushed laterally and cranially by the mostly free disc fragment. As a rule, removal of the fragment alone is sufficient. If an extensive perforation of the annulus is evident, clearing of the disc space should be considered. After probing the root canal with a double-angled blunt hook for residual fragments, the nerve may be covered with a Gelfoam soaked with crystalline steroid.

- *Closure*: placing a drain is optional and in our experience seldom necessary. Musculature requires no suturing.
- *Special considerations for the L5/S1 level*: because of the particular anatomical relationship between disc space, transverse process L5, and ala, the microsurgical muscle-splitting approach at the lumbosacral level should be practiced by a surgeon who is already familiar with the technique at the more cranial levels. Repeated intra-operative fluoroscopic checks may also be necessary. If difficulties should arise, switching to the conventional "macroapproach" should be considered.
- *Postoperative care*: as previously described.

41.4.6 Complications

Reflex sympathetic dystrophy occurs in 1–2% of the patients, mostly within 1 week after surgery, especially at the L5/S1 level. It is characterized by burning discomfort of the shiny leg which becomes very sensitive to touch. Due to the intracanalicular location of the ganglion, every manipulation of the nerve in the extraforaminal compartment stretches the ganglion which may cause postoperative causalgic disturbances. Therapy: codeine, sympathetic block (Marcaine 1%), and physiotherapy.

References

1. Bernucci C, Giovanelli M (2007) Translaminar microsurgical approach for lumbar herniated nucleus pulposus (HNP) in the "hidden zone": clinical and radiologic results in a series of 24 patients. Spine 32(2):281–284
2. Di Lorenzo N, Porta F, Onnis G et al (1998) Pars interarticularis fenestration in the treatment of foraminal lumbar disc herniation: a further surgical approach. Neurosurgery 42:87–90
3. Mayer HM (2005) Lumbar disc herniations: the microsurgical inter-laminar, paramedian approach. In: Mayer HM (ed) Minimally invasive spine surgery. Springer, Heidelberg, pp 284–296
4. Papavero L (2005) Lumbar disc herniations: the translaminar approach. In: Mayer HM (ed) Minimally invasive spine surgery. Springer, Heidelberg, pp 304–314
5. Papavero L (2005) Lumbar disc herniations: the extraforaminal approach. In: Mayer HM (ed) Minimally invasive spine surgery. Springer, Heidelberg, pp 297–303
6. Soldner F, Helper BM, Wallenfang Th et al (2002) The translaminar approach to canalicular and cranio-dorsolateral lumbar disc herniations. Acta Neurochir (Wien) 144:315–320
7. Tessitore E, de Tribolet N (2004) Far-lateral lumbar disc herniation: the microsurgical transmuscular approach. Neurosurgery 54(4): 939–942
8. Vogelgesang JP (2007) The translaminar approach in combination with a tubular retractor system for the treatment of far cranio-laterally and foraminally extruded lumbar disc herniations. Zentralbl Neuro-chir 68(1):24–28

Microsurgical Decompression

42

Frank Grochulla

42.1 Introduction and Core Messages

Degenerative lumbar spinal canal stenosis is a frequent disease of the "aging spine," leading to mono- or bilateral leg symptoms that are often described as spinal claudication [2, 9, 10]. The primary goal in treatment is to relieve the patients' leg symptoms. Surgery for lumbar spinal stenosis is generally accepted when conservative treatment has failed or if progressive neurological deficits occur [1]. In the past, laminectomies are considered to be the treatment of choice in lumbar spinal stenosis without instability [3, 8, 10]. Due to the risk of destabilization after laminectomy, limited approaches and less-invasive techniques for decompression have been proposed by several authors [4–7]. Today, laminotomy under microscopic guidance is the preferred surgical technique in lumbar spinal stenosis presenting without additional deformity or segmental instability. During the past decade, approaches and techniques for laminotomy have been modified in different manners. In this chapter, the ipsilateral interlaminar approach for microsurgical decompression of the ipsi- and contralateral spinal canal in the so-called over the top technique is described.

42.2 Indications

- Acquired degenerative central and lateral spinal canal stenosis with clinical symptoms (e.g., spinal claudication), verified by MRI or CT scan
- Failed conservative treatment
- No symptoms/signs for segmental instability

42.3 Contraindications

- Unstable lumbar degenerative scoliosis
- Spondylolisthesis grade I or higher with dominant low-back pain
- Severe and/or dominant low-back pain
- Absolute contraindications for general anesthesia

42.4 Technical Prerequisites

- Microscope
- Microsurgical instruments (e.g., Bayonet-shaped instruments)
- Tubular retractor system (e.g., Caspar retractor)
- High-speed drill
- Fluoroscopy

42.5 Planning, Preparation, and Positioning

The patient is placed prone for this procedure on a Wilson frame or alternatively placed on a special operating table in the knee-chest position (mecca position) (see Fig. 42.1). In this positioning, the abdomen is free, thus relieving pressure on the abdominal venous system and decreasing venous backflow into the spinal canal through Batson plexus. Furthermore, the amount of lumbar lordosis is decreased, and the interlaminar spaces are widened. Thus, it is easier to enter the spinal canal for decompression.

F. Grochulla, M.D.
Department for Spinal Surgery, Hospital for Orthopaedics, Trauma Surgery and Spinal Surgery, Euromed Clinic, Europa-Allee 1, Fürth 90763, Germany
e-mail: frank.grochulla@euromed.de

Fig. 42.1 (**a**) Knee-chest (mecca) position, situation in the OR and illustration (**b**), and as an alternative prone positioning (**c**)

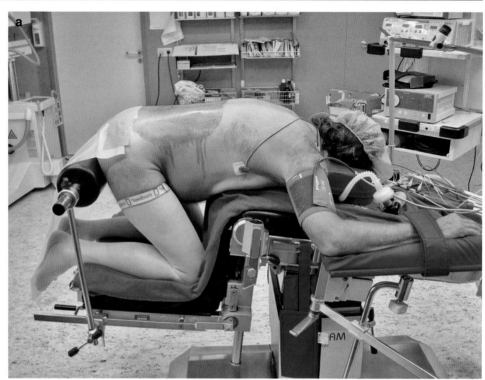

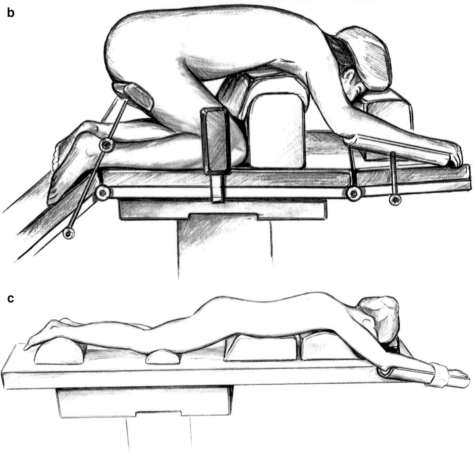

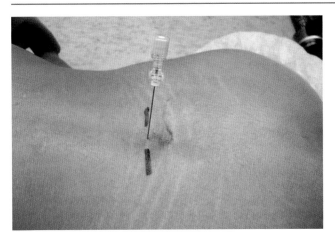

Fig. 42.2 The target level is localized with an inserted needle under lateral fluoroscopy control

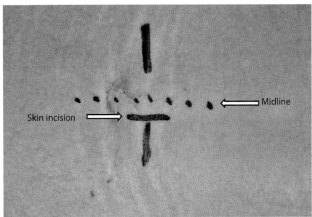

Fig. 42.3 Skin incision 5–10 mm lateral to the spinous process on the affected side and typically 2–3 cm in length for one level

For positioning, some special aspects have to be considered in (mostly elderly) patients with acquired spinal canal stenosis: patients can have limited mobility of the joints (shoulder, hip, knee) and of the cervical spine (avoid head rotation!).

Localization: The target level(s) is localized with an inserted needle under lateral fluoroscopy control, and the approach is planned and marked (see Fig. 42.2). It is important to place the superficial approach exactly over the lumbar segment of interest because of the limited extent of the microsurgical approach.

42.6 Surgical Techniques

- The author recommends the application of the surgical microscope from the beginning of the surgical procedure.
- The skin incision is up to 5–10 mm lateral to the spinous process on the affected side and typically 2–3 cm in length for one level. In the presence of bilateral symptoms, a left-sided approach is preferred for right-handed surgeons.
- A semicircular paramedian incision is made in the thoracolumbar fascia. The length of this incision can be longer than the skin incision (see Fig. 42.3).
- Subperiosteal dissection of the paravertebral muscles is carried out, and a self-retraining speculum retractor (Caspar, Aesculap,- or metrx retractor, Medtronic) is inserted (see Fig. 42.4). It is necessary to control the force of the retractor during surgery to avoid pressure necrosis of the surrounding cutaneous and musculature tissue.
- The laminae of the adjacent vertebrae and the interlaminar space are exposed.
- With a high-speed burr (see Fig. 42.5a, b), the decompression of the ipsilateral spinal canal is started with the

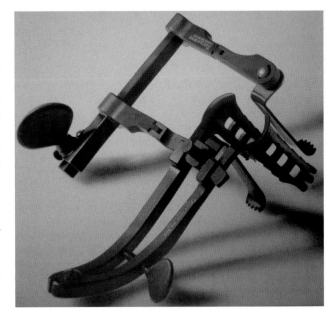

Fig. 42.4 Caspar tubular retractor system

removal of lower half of the cephalad lamina until the origin of the ligamentum flavum is exposed (see Fig. 42.6). The ligamentum flavum will be seen to thin out at the cephalad lamina and is detached from the lamina with a dissector. At this point, epidural fat and the dura can be identified (see Fig. 42.7). The extension of the interlaminar space is completed by resection of the cephalad part of the caudal lamina and by resection of a portion of the medial part of the facet joint (medial facetectomy).

- After complete exposure of the ipsilateral ligamentum flavum, it can be removed with rongeurs. Adhesions of the dura to the ligamentum flavum are dissected carefully in order to avoid dural laceration.

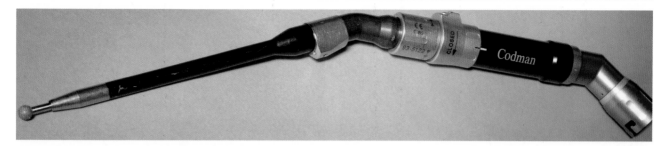

Fig. 42.5 Angular handpiece for high-speed drill

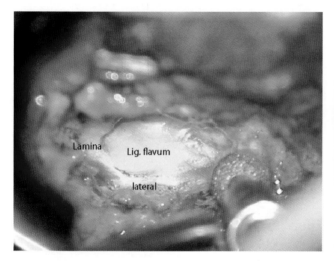

Fig. 42.6 Partial removal of the lamina and exposure of the ligamentum flavum

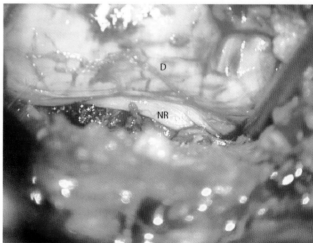

Fig. 42.8 Exposure of dura and nerve root after ipsilateral decompression. *D* dura, *NR* nerve root

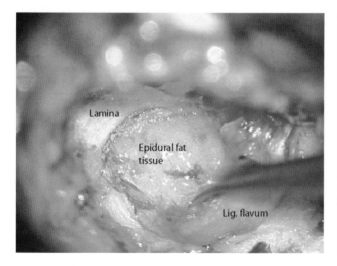

Fig. 42.7 The ligamentum flavum is detached from the lamina with a dissector. Epidural fat and the dura can be identified

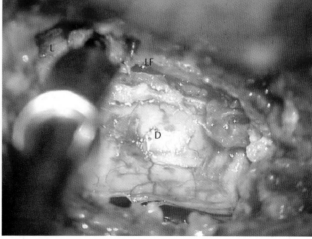

Fig. 42.9 Undercutting of the lamina with a high-speed burr. *L* lamina, *LF* ligamentum flavum, *D* dura

- An adequate ipsilateral subarticular decompression has been accomplished when the medial part of the pedicle and the lateral border of the nerve root are identified – and when the traversing nerve root can be easily mobilized (Fig. 42.8).

- The contralateral decompression is initiated by a tilting of the table away from the surgeon, and the microscope is adjusted to obtain a clear field of vision across the midline. Utilizing a high-speed burr, the undercutting of the adjacent laminae and the part of the base of the spinous process is performed (Fig. 42.9).

- The next step is the resection of the contralateral ligamentum flavum and the subarticular decompression until the lateral border of the dura and the medial border of the contralateral inferior pedicle is identified. In cases with severe stenosis, the dura should be separated from the ligamentum flavum with blunt dissection before resection to avoid cerebrospinal fluid leak.
- The adequate decompression should be checked with a blunt probe.
- Check the bone margins with a blunt dissector to be certain that no sharp bony spicules remain (which can penetrate the dura postoperatively).
- Meticulous hemostasis and wound closure.

42.7 Postoperative Care

- Bed rest for 6 h in supine position with elevated chest (30°) to elevate lumbar CSF pressure for compression of epidural veins.
- We recommend bracing only in cases with more than two-level decompression.

References

1. Amundsen T, Weber H, Nordal HJ et al (2000) Lumbar spinal stenosis: conservative or surgical management? A prospective 10-year study. Spine 25:1425–1435
2. Berney J (1994) Epidemiology of narrow spinal canal. Neurochirurgie 40:174–178
3. Herkowitz HN, Kurz LT (1991) Degenerative lumbar spondylolisthesis with spinal stenosis. A prospective study comparing decompression with decompression and intertransverse process arthrodesis. J Bone Joint Surg Am 73:802–808
4. Hopp E, Tsou PM (1988) Postdecompression lumbar instability. Clin Orthop Relat Res 227:143–151
5. McCulloch JA (1998) Microsurgery for lumbar spinal canal stenosis. In: McCulloch JA, Young PH (eds) Essentials of spinal microsurgery. Lippincott-Raven, Philadelphia, pp 453–486
6. Poletti CE (1995) Central lumbar stenosis caused by ligamentum flavum: unilateral laminotomy for bilateral ligamentectomy. Preliminary report of two cases. Neurosurgery 37:343–347
7. Senegas J, Etchevers JP, Vital JM, Baulny D, Grenier F (1988) Recalibration of the lumbar canal, an alternative to laminectomy in the treatment of lumbar canal stenosis. Rev Chir Orthop Reparatrice Appar Mot 74:15–22
8. Silvers HR, Lewis PJ, Ash HL (1993) Decompressive lumbar laminectomy for spinal stenosis. J Neurosurg 78:695–701
9. Verbiest H (1954) A radicular syndrome from developmental narrowing of the lumbar vertebral canal. J Bone Joint Surg Br 36-B:230–237
10. Verbiest H (1975) Pathomorphologic aspects of developmental lumbar stenosis. Orthop Clin North Am 5:177–196

Endoscopic Lumbar Disc Surgery

43

Sebastian Ruetten

43.1 Introduction and Core Messages

Minimally invasive techniques can reduce tissue damage and its consequences. Endoscopic operations are now considered standard in certain areas. The most common full endoscopic technique for patients with lumbar disc afflictions is the posterolateral transforaminal operation. Laser and bipolar radiofrequency current can be used. Removal of intra- or extraforaminal disc herniations is technically possible. Resection of herniations within the spinal canal – in the sense of a retrograde removal from intradiscal through the existing annulus defect – has been described. Nevertheless, difficulties in the resection of herniated discs located within the spinal canal cannot always be completely ruled out. Using the lateral transforaminal access, the spinal canal can be more sufficiently reached under continuous visualization. Even so, the bony borders of the foramen and the exiting nerve may limit mobility and thus the resection of dislocated disc material. In addition, the pelvis and abdominal organs may hinder access. Thus, there may be limitations for the transforaminal procedure. The full endoscopic interlaminar access was developed to enable operation of pathologies outside the indication spectrum for the transforaminal procedure. The combination of new operative accesses with the technical advances now enables for the first time a full endoscopic procedure with visual control which is equal to conventional operations when the indication criteria are heeded. Basically, the transforaminal procedure

has more limitations than the interlaminar, but at the same time, it less tissue traumatic.

43.2 Indication

43.2.1 General Indication

The indication for operation corresponds to current valid standards [1]. The greatest experience has been gained in the therapy of herniated discs and lateral spinal canal stenoses [2–6]. Existing secondary pathologies, such as instabilities, must possibly be treated at the same time with other procedures. The following indications are currently unequivocal (Figs. 43.1, 43.2, and 43.3):

- Sequestered or nonsequestered lumbar disc herniations, independent of localization
- Recurrent disc herniations after conventional or full endoscopic operations
- Lateral bony and ligamentary spinal canal stenoses
- In special cases, cysts of the zygoapophyseal joint
- In special cases, positioning of implants in the intervertebral space
- In special cases, intervertebral debridement and draining in spondylodiscitis

43.2.2 Indication for Transforaminal Approach

All intra- and extraforaminal disc herniations are taken as indications for the transforaminal approach. In disc herniations within the spinal canal, the following inclusion criteria must be heeded due to the limited mobility [3–6]:

- Sequestration toward cranial maximal to the start of the pedicle above, toward caudal maximal to the middle of the pedicle below the level in question

S. Ruetten, M.D., Ph.D.
Center for Spine Surgery and Pain Therapy, Center for Orthopaedics and Traumatology, St. Anna-Hospital,
Hospitalstr. 19, 44649 Herne, Germany
e-mail: spine-pain@annahospital.de

U. Vieweg, F. Grochulla (eds.), *Manual of Spine Surgery*,
DOI 10.1007/978-3-642-22682-3_43, © Springer-Verlag Berlin Heidelberg 2012

Fig. 43.1 Posterolateral
transforaminal approach

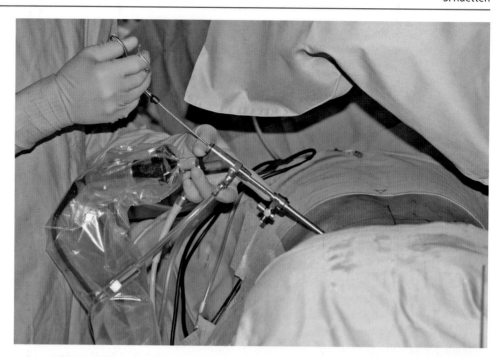

Fig. 43.2 Lateral transforaminal
approach

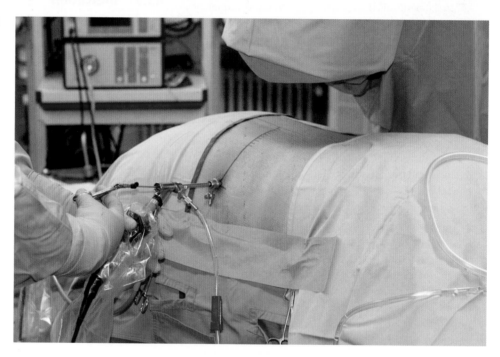

- In orthograde lateral ray path, pelvic overlay of the level
  in question maximal to the middle of the pedicle
  Note: In lateral spinal canal stenoses, the craniocaudal
  extension should reach maximal from the upper edge of
  the pedicle below to the lower edge of the pedicle above
  the level in question. In applying the usually necessary
  lateral approach, the access pathway may not be shifted
  by abdominal structures. This is especially to be heeded
  in the levels cranial to L3/4. If the finding is not entirely

clear, a single abdominal CT scan should be made through
the disc for evaluation and preoperative planning.

43.2.3 Indication for Interlaminar Approach

- All disc herniations located within the spinal canal which
  cannot be operated technically in the transforaminal
  approach because of the criteria cited are taken as indications for the interlaminar approach [2–5].

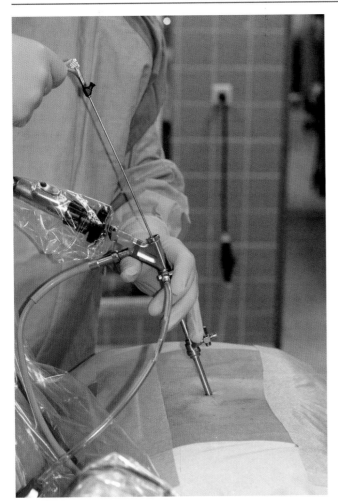

Fig. 43.3 Interlaminar approach

43.3 Contraindications

- All criteria which generally apply as contraindications to decompressing operations, taking into consideration the specific technical possibilities and the inclusion criteria of each surgical procedure, are considered contraindications.

43.4 Technical Prerequisites

An X-ray permeable, electrically adjustable operation table and a C-arc are necessary. In addition to the surgical instruments and optics, general equipment for endoscopic operations under fluid flow are needed, such as monitor, camera unit, light source, documentation system, fluid pump, shaver system, or radiofrequency generator. Equipment available for arthroscopy or endoscopy can be used.

43.5 Planning, Preparation, and Positioning

As with all microsurgical techniques, the intraoperative procedure must be planned preoperatively based on imaging findings. The goal is to perform the resection of spinal canal structures as sparingly as possible depending on the pathology. Full endoscopic operations can usually be performed under general anesthesia. This is more comfortable for both the patient and the surgeon, enables positioning as needed, and also makes extensive work within the spinal canal possible. The operations are performed with the patient in prone position on an X-ray permeable table, under orthograde radiological control at two levels. The patient lies on a hip and thorax roll to relieve the abdominal and thoracic organs. The operation table can be adjusted intraoperative lumbar either lordotic or kyphotic depending on the anatomy and pathology. A single-shot antibiosis is applied for infection prophylaxis.

43.6 Operating Technique

43.6.1 Transforaminal Approach [3–6]

- First, the skin incision is localized. The goal is to reach the spinal canal as tangentially as possible. At levels L4/5 and L3/4, in lateral ray path, the dorsal line of the descending facet usually serves as the boundary which should not be crossed toward ventral. To avoid injury to abdominal organs, a single abdominal CT scan through the individual disc should be made for evaluation and preoperative planning, especially in the cranial levels when findings are not unequivocal. Depending on the scan, an individual, less-lateral approach should be selected.
- A 1.5-mm atraumatic spinal needle is inserted through the skin incision orthograde to the disc space in the target area (Fig. 43.4). After a 0.8-mm target wire is inserted and the cannula removed, the cannulated dilator is inserted.
- The target wire is removed, and the 7.9-mm operation sheath with beveled opening is pushed through the dilator (Figs. 43.5 and 43.6). From this point on, decompression is made under visualization and continuous irrigation with isotonic saline without any special additives.
- Further entry into the epidural space which may be required is made under visual control. If the bony diameter of the foramen does not permit passage, the foramen is widened with a burr and instruments.
- If the position of the exiting nerve is not clear, for example, in intra- or extraforaminal herniation or foraminal stenosis, an extraforaminal access is created

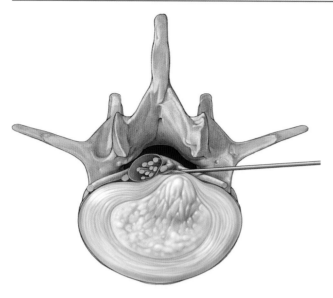

Fig. 43.4 Example of the end position of the operation sheath *AP* in the spinal canal

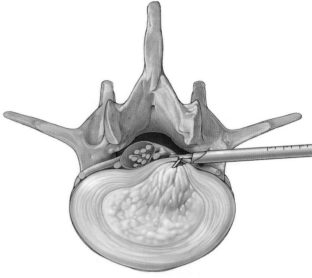

Fig. 43.6 Full endoscopic transforaminal operation

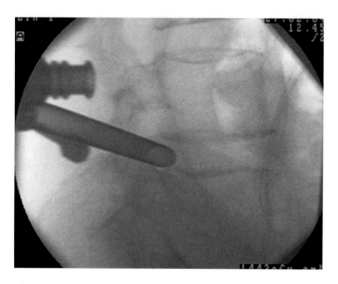

Fig. 43.5 The opening of the operation sheath is in the epidural space

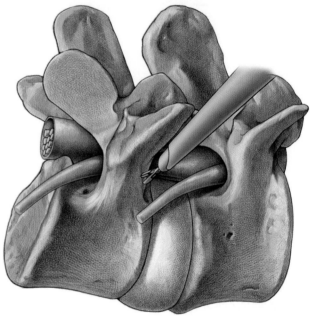

Fig. 43.7 Start of the extraforaminal operation on the caudal pedicle outside the foramen

on the caudal pedicle as a safe zone, and further preparation toward the pathology is made under visual control (see Fig. 43.7).

- The precise performance of decompression depends on the finding in each case.

43.6.2 Interlaminar Approach [2–5]

- The skin incision is made as medial as possible over the interlaminar window. The craniocaudal localization depends on the findings of the pathology in question.
- The dilator is inserted bluntly on the lateral edge of the ligamentum flavum or on the descending facet of the zygoapophyseal joint.

- The 7.9-mm operation sheath with beveled opening is inserted via the dilator in the direction of the ligament (see Fig. 43.8).
- From this point on, the further procedure is performed under visualization and continuous irrigation with isotonic saline solution without any special additive. To reach the spinal canal, the ligamentum flavum is incised lateral to ca. 3–5 mm.
- The further procedure is enabled by the elasticity of the ligament (see Figs. 43.9 and 43.10).

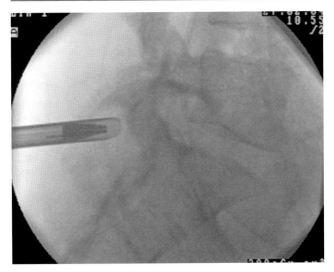

Fig. 43.8 Inserted dilator with operation sheath

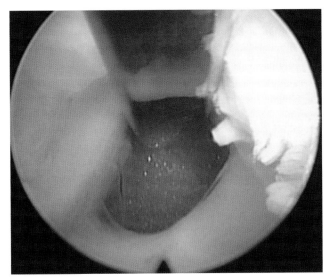

Fig. 43.9 Lateral incision of the ligamentum flavum

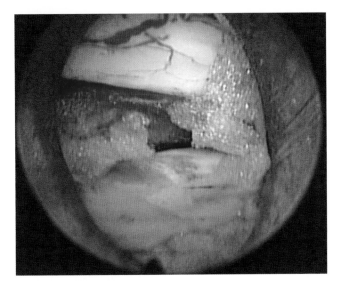

Fig. 43.10 Identification of the anatomical structures

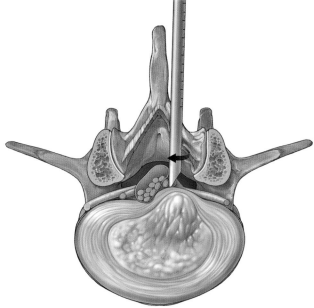

Fig. 43.11 Rotation of the operation sheath

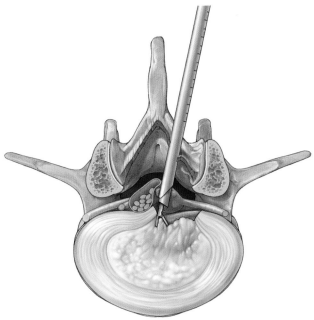

Fig. 43.12 Full endoscopic interlaminar operation

- The operation sheath with beveled opening can be used as a second instrument by rotation and serves, for example, as a nerve hook in shifting the neural structures toward medial (see Figs. 43.11 and 43.12).
- If the bony diameter of the interlaminar window does not permit passage or in the operation of a spinal canal stenosis, the window is enlarged using a burr and instruments.
- In cases of clearly dislocated sequesters which cannot be completely reached from a level without more extensive

bone resection, consideration can be given to creating another access later via the neighboring interlaminar window.

- The precise performance of the decompression depends on the findings in each case.

43.7 Possible Complications

Possible complications during microsurgical procedures are known, and there are numerous publications [7–10]. A minimally invasive procedure can reduce the complication rate, though statistically it cannot be completely avoided [11, 12]. In principle, all of the complications are possible which are known in conventional operating procedures [2–6]. With respect to the full endoscopic procedures, it must be emphasized that a one- or two-sided switch to an open procedure may be necessary for the therapy of a complication. Especially, endoscopic suture of a dural injury is technically not possible. Theoretically, in long operating times and overlooked blockage of the outflow of irrigation fluid, the consequences of increased pressure within the spinal canal and the attached and neighboring structures cannot be completely ruled out. In the interlaminar approach, a long-lasting and uninterrupted excessive retraction of the neural structures with the working sheath toward medial must be avoided or made only intermittently in order to avoid the risk of neurological damage. In the transforaminal approach, the risk of injury to the exiting nerves cannot be completely ruled out. In using the lateral access, it must be ruled out that abdominal organs block the path of access. Especially during the learning curve, experience has shown that there is an increased risk that complications will occur, as is the case in any new technique.

References

1. Andersson GBJ, Brown MD, Dvorak J et al (1996) Consensus summary on the diagnosis and treatment of lumbar disc herniation. Spine 21:75–78
2. Ruetten S, Komp M, Merk H et al (2009) Surgical treatment for lumbar lateral recess stenosis with the full-endoscopic interlaminar approach versus conventional microsurgical technique: a prospective, randomized, controlled study. J Neurosurg Spine 10:476–485
3. Ruetten S, Komp M, Merk H et al (2009) Recurrent lumbar disc herniation following conventional discectomy: a prospective, randomized study comparing full-endoscopic interlaminar and transforaminal versus microsurgical revision. J Spinal Disord Tech 22:122–129
4. Ruetten S, Komp M, Merk H et al (2008) Full-endoscopic interlaminar and transforaminal lumbar discectomy versus conventional microsurgical technique: a prospective, randomized, controlled study. Spine 33:931–939
5. Ruetten S, Komp M, Merk H et al (2007) Use of newly developed instruments and endoscopes: full-endoscopic resection of lumbar disc herniations via the interlaminar and lateral transforaminal approach. J Neurosurg Spine 6:521–530
6. Ruetten S, Komp M, Godolias G (2005) An extreme lateral access fort the surgery of lumbar disc herniations inside the spinal canal using the full-endoscopic uniportal transforaminal approach – technique and prospective results of 463 patients. Spine 30:2570–2578
7. Ramirez LF, Thisted R (1989) Complications and demographic characteristics of patients undergoing lumbar discectomy in community hospitals. Neurosurgery 25:226–231
8. Rompe JD, Eysel P, Zollner J (1999) Intra- and postoperative risk analysis after lumbar intervertebral disk operation. Z Orthop Ihre Grenzgeb 137:201–205
9. Stolke D, Sollmann WP, Seifert V (1989) Intra- and postoperative complications in lumbar disc surgery. Spine 14:56–59
10. Wildfoerster U (1991) Intraoperative complications in lumbar intervertebral disc operations. cooperative study of the spinal study group of the German Society of Neurosurgery. Neurochirurgica 34:53–56
11. Schick U, Doehnert J, Richter A et al (2002) Microendoscopic lumbar discectomy versus open surgery: an intraoperative EMG study. Eur Spine J 11:20–26
12. Weber BR, Grob D, Dvorak J et al (1997) Posterior surgical approach to the lumbar spine and its effect on the multifidus muscle. Spine 22:1765–1772

Translaminar Screw Fixation

44

Stefan Schären

S. Schären, M.D.
Department of Orthopaedic Surgery/Spine,
University Hospital, Spitalstrasse 21,
4031 Basel, Switzerland
e-mail: sschaeren@uhbs.ch

44.1 Introduction and Core Messages

Translaminar screws (TLS) were developed by F. Magerl in 1980 as an evolution to the transarticular screws first published by D. King 1948 and later modified by H. Boucher 1959 [1, 5, 6]. Compared to these precursors, TLS have a longer trajectory in bone blocking the facet joints as setscrews more efficiently [3, 7]. Since the screw directory runs tangentially to the exiting nerve root, the risk for injury is minimal. Compared to pedicle screws, TLS yield inferior biomechanical stability especially in flexion and rotation [2, 4]. With pedicle screws nowadays being the gold standard for posterior instrumentation, TLS remain an elegant and cost-effective method for selected cases. The translaminar screw fixation is a safe and effective method for posterior stabilization of one or two motion segments. It is mostly used supplementary to anterior fusion techniques and can effectively stabilize one or two motion segments in conjunction with anterior instrumentation [8, 9]. This technique is contraindicated in anterior column defect.

44.2 Indications

Stabilization in degenerative disorders with mainly intact posterior elements:

- Posterior fusion of one or two motion segments from T12 to S1
- Supplementary to anterior interbody fusion

- In combination with pedicle instrumentation for long-range fusion (see Fig. 44.7)

44.3 Contraindications

- Missing posterior elements, e.g., after laminectomy
- Missing anterior support, e.g., fracture and tumor
- Fusion of three and more levels
- Severe osteoporosis

44.4 Technical Prerequisites

Fluoroscopy, positioning device (e.g., Relton Hall frame), 4.5-mm cortical screws in various lengths (usually 45–55 mm), preferably in titanium for better MRI compatibility (e.g., Synthes GmbH, Solothurn, Switzerland), long 3.2-mm drill and drill sleeve, and long tab. Alternatively, carbon/PEEK pins can be used (Signus GmbH, Alzenau, Germany) (see Fig. 44.1).

44.5 Surgical Technique

44.5.1 Approach

A standard midline posterior approach is performed with subperiosteal exposure of the spinous processes, laminae, and transverse processes. The joint capsules of the motion segments to be fused are resected, and the bony elements are thoroughly cleaned using a chisel. In order not to compromise the bony elements which are important for the TLS, a formal decortication should not be performed. In case of spinal stenosis or disc hernia, decompressive laminotomy or discectomy is added, preserving the lamina.

U. Vieweg, F. Grochulla (eds.), *Manual of Spine Surgery*,
DOI 10.1007/978-3-642-22682-3_44, © Springer-Verlag Berlin Heidelberg 2012

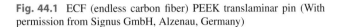

Fig. 44.1 ECF (endless carbon fiber) PEEK translaminar pin (With permission from Signus GmbH, Alzenau, Germany)

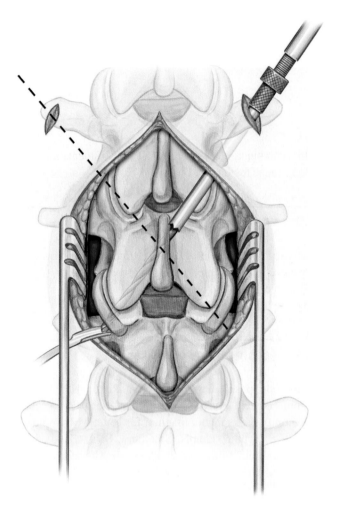

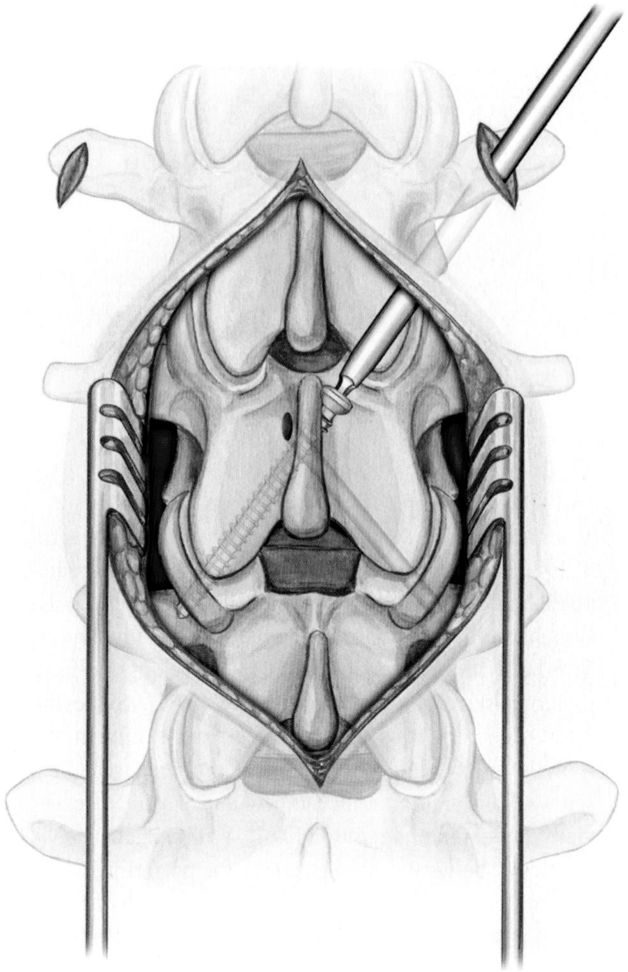

Fig. 44.3 Insertion of the 4.5-mm cortical screw of appropriate length

Fig. 44.2 Direction of a long 3.2-mm drill bit, protected with a drill sleeve

44.6   Instrumentation

- The first screw hole is drilled starting cranially from the base of the spinous process aiming toward the inferior border of the opposite transverse process. The drill subcortically passes the contralateral lamina, crosses the facet joint, and penetrates the cortex of the transverse process (Fig. 44.2).

- After measuring the screw length, the hole is tabbed shortly across the facet joint taking care not to penetrate the outer cortex.
- The corresponding 4.5-mm titanium cortical screw is inserted until the screw head has contact with the spinous process (Fig. 44.3).
- The second screw hole is drilled running posterior to the first screw through the opposite lamina.
- After measuring and tabbing, a second screw is inserted (Figs. 44.4–44.6).
- In case of posterior fusion, the posterior elements are covered with bone graft (e.g., from the iliac crest).

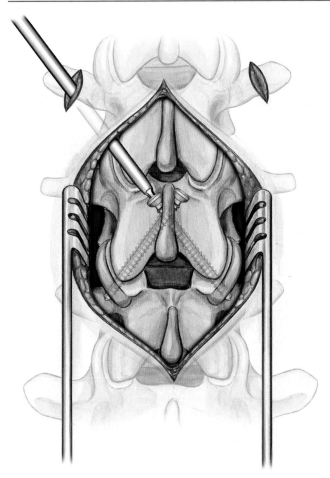

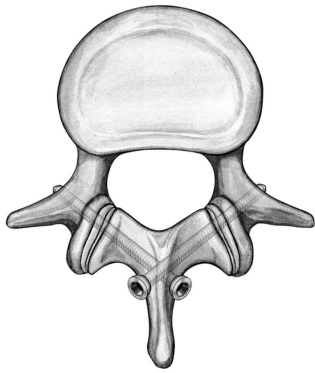

Fig. 44.5 Screws seen in the axial plane

Fig. 44.4 Insertion of the second translaminar screw

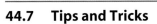

44.7   Tips and Tricks

- In the event of a deep situs and abundant soft tissues, it is possible to drill and insert the screw percutaneously using a troikar system.
- Similarly, in case of anterior fusion, a minimized posterior approach can be performed, exposing only the spinous process, lamina, and facet joint, and inserting the screws percutaneously.

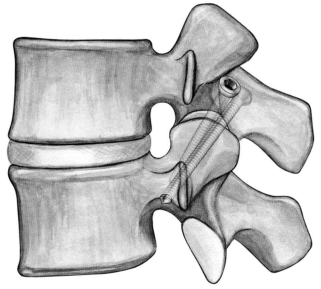

Fig. 44.6 Lateral view of the two-inserted screws

Fig. 44.7 (**a, b**) A 47-year-old
woman with candida spondylodiscitis L4/5 with severe destruction
of the adjacent end plates was
treated with posterior transpedicular stabilization L3/S1, anterior
debridement, and fusion L4/5 using
iliac crest autograft followed by
antimycotic treatment.
Translaminar screws L3/4 and L4/5
were used, avoiding the insertion of
transpedicular screws penetrating
into the infected vertebral bodies of
L4 and L5. AP and lateral
radiographs 24 months postoperatively show solid fusion and stable
implants

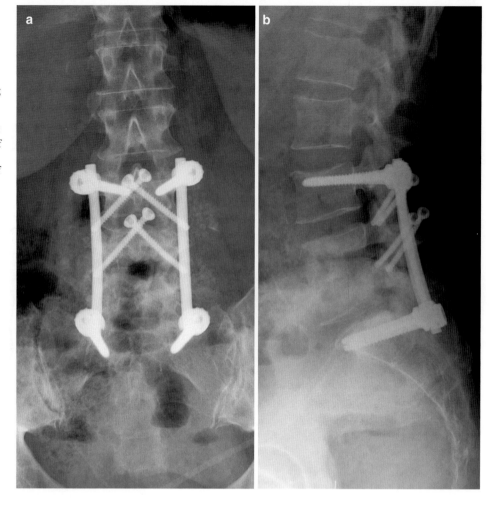

References

1. Boucher H (1959) A method of spine fusion. J Bone Joint Surg 41-B:248–259
2. Heggenes MH, Esses SI (1991) Translaminar facet joint screw fixation for lumbar and lumbosacral fusion. A clinical and biomechanical study. Spine 16S:266–269
3. Jeanneret B, Kleinstück F, Magerl F (1995) Translaminar screw fixation of the lumbar facet joints. Oper Orthop Traumatol 4:37–53
4. Kandziora F, Schleicher P, Scholz M et al (2005) Biomechanical testing of the lumbar facet interference screw. Spine 30:E34–E39
5. King D (1944) Internal fixation for lumbosacral fusion. Am J Surg 66:357–361
6. Magerl F (1980) Verletzungen der Brust- und Lendenwirbelsäule. Langenbecks Arch Chir 352:427–433
7. Montesano PX, Magerl F, Jacobs RR et al (1988) Translaminar facet joint screws. Orthopedics 11:1393–1397
8. Phillips FM, Cunningham B, Carandang G et al (2004) Effect of supplemental translaminar facet screw fixation on the stability of stand-alone anterior lumbar interbody fusion cages under physiologic compressive preloads. Spine 29:1731–1736
9. Rathonyi GC, Oxland TR, Gerich U et al (1998) The role of supplemental translaminar screws in anterior lumbar interbody fixation: a biomechanical study. Eur Spine J 7:400–407

Vertebroplasty and Kyphoplasty

45

Khalid Saeed, Edward Bayley, and Bronek Boszczyk

45.1 Introduction and Core Messages

Vertebroplasty and kyphoplasty are described including indications, contraindications, surgical technique and complications. Both vertebroplasty and kyphoplasty achieve good pain relief in appropriately selected patients with osteoporotic compression fractures and those with spinal metastases, multiple myeloma and some traumatic fractures as discussed further in the chapter. The main technical point to remember is never to cross the projection of medial pedicle cortex in AP view before posterior vertebral wall has been reached in the lateral view.

45.2 Indications

- Painful osteoporotic vertebral compression fractures (VCFs) which have failed conservative treatment or show unacceptable progressive collapse. Patients most likely to benefit have fractures that demonstrate bone marrow oedema on MRI or radiotracer uptake on a nuclear medicine bone scintigram. Two recent randomized trials have concluded that they found no beneficial effect of vertebroplasty as compared with a sham procedure in patients with painful osteoporotic vertebral fractures [1, 7].

- Vertebral metastases with painful pathological fractures unsuitable for curative resection. Patients with spinal metastases and multiple myeloma can be treated with vertebral augmentation, and a biopsy can be obtained at the same time [3].

- Traumatic fractures
  Balloon kyphoplasty is principally suitable for treatment of vertebral fractures that have a localized fragmented zone within the spongiosa and a kyphotic deformity or for treatment of endplate impression fractures. These criteria are met by fractures of type A1.1 (endplate impression fracture), A1.2 (wedge fracture) and A3.1 (incomplete burst fracture) [1-6] (see Fig. 45.1a–d). According to current knowledge, split fractures (A2), burst fractures (A3.2) and complete burst fractures (A3.3) are not suitable for balloon kyphoplasty, as the splitting component of these fractures cannot be stabilized by the augmentation. However, a complete burst fracture type A3.3 must be distinguished from an osteoporotic collapse of a vertebral body type A1.3 as the latter is suitable for balloon kyphoplasty, as the endplates are hardly fragmented or not fragmented at all, unlike in a complete burst fracture.

K. Saeed, MBBS, FRCSI (Neurosurgery) (✉)
Department of Spinal Surgery, New Cross Hospital,
The Royal Wolverhampton Hospitals NHS Trust,
Wednesfield Road, Wolverhampton WV10 0QP, UK
e-mail: drksaeed@hotmail.com

E. Bayley
Department of Spinal Surgery, The Centre for Spinal Studies and Surgery, Queens Medical Centre, University Hospital NHS Trust, Nottingham, UK

B. Boszczyk, M.D., DM
The Centre for Spinal Studies and Surgery, Queens Medical Centre, University Hospital NHS Trust, Nottingham NG7 2UH, UK
e-mail: bronek.boszczyk@nuh.nhs.uk

U. Vieweg, F. Grochulla (eds.), *Manual of Spine Surgery*,
DOI 10.1007/978-3-642-22682-3_45, © Springer-Verlag Berlin Heidelberg 2012

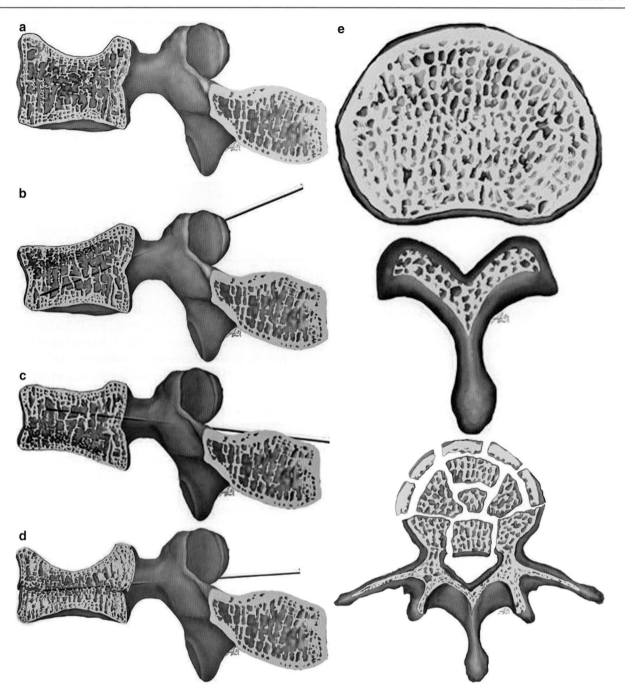

Fig. 45.1 Schematic drawing of various fracture types and the appropriate needle trajectories. (**a**) Endplate impression fracture A1.1. (**b**) Superior wedge fracture A1.2.1. (**c**) Inferior wedge fracture A1.2.3. (**d**) Vertebral body collapse A1.3. (**e**) Axial views of an incomplete burst fracture below the level of the pedicles (*upper image*) and at the level of the pedicles (*lower image*) demonstrating disruption of the posterior wall only at the level of the pedicles

- Vertebral haemangiomas

  VP is an effective treatment option in this category if the pain is the main presenting feature. It is not suitable for cases with neurological deficit [8]. VP can achieve pain relief as well as stabilization, reducing the risk of secondary vertebral collapse. This treatment must be reserved only in vertebral haemangiomas which are symptomatic and resistant to common conservative treatments, with radiological evidence of aggressiveness and/or epidural extension [5].

  Balloon kyphoplasty (KP) is indicated if vertebral height restoration or cavity formation is the aim, e.g., in correcting the kyphotic deformity associated with osteoporotic VCFs, or traumatic vertebral fractures as mentioned before in the indications section or for situations where cavity formation might help, e.g., in difficult indications for tumourous lesions. In order to achieve this aim, procedure should be performed relatively early on after the fracture (literature recommending periods of under 3 weeks to under 3 months).

45.3 Contraindications

- Coagulation disorders.
- Patient unfit for general anaesthetic or local anaesthetic with sedation or unable to lie prone on the operating table for the duration of the procedure.
- Pregnancy (relative contraindication).
- Hypersensitivity to cement components.
- Local infection.
- Relative: pulmonary hypertension (exacerbation through fat embolism).
- Neurological compromise through posterior wall fracture or tumour mass extension.
- Precaution: posterior wall disruption (increased leakage rate).
- Adequate preoperative imaging is also an essential prerequisite to do the procedure and if for some reason, the relevant landmarks cannot be visualized on AP and lateral imaging, then it is not possible to proceed.

45.4 Technical Prerequisites Planning, Preparation and Positioning

Preoperative workup should include MR scan with STIR sequences (fat suppression sequences that identify oedema) for proper identification of the painful vertebral level, and clinical and radiological correlation is required as the collapsed vertebra may not always be the source of the pain and the pathology may reside in another noncollapsed vertebra. A chest x-ray is essential as well to count the ribs when dealing with thoracic spine. Adequate imaging quality and proper positioning of the patient on the table is essential, and before draping the patient, one must ensure that appropriate landmarks can be seen on AP and lateral fluoroscopy. On AP image, pedicles should be seen to lie in the upper lateral quadrant of the vertebral body; spinous processes should lie midway between the pedicles, and both the endplates and the posterior wall must come to lie parallel (superimposed so that double image is eliminated) on the AP and lateral images. The procedure can be performed

either under general anaesthetic or with local anaesthetic and sedation depending on patient/anaesthetist/surgeon preference and anticipated duration of procedure. The patient is positioned prone on pillows on a radiolucent operating table. A single C-arm fluoroscopy is usually used which can be easily switched between AP and lateral orientation, although some surgeons prefer biplanar imaging with two image intensifiers.

45.5 Surgical Technique

45.5.1 Vertebroplasty

- After prepping and draping, under image intensifier in AP view, and after local anaesthetic infiltration, transverse 1–2-cm stab incisions are made over the entry points which in the lumbar spine is over the tip of the transverse process and in the thoracic spine, for the extrapedicular approach, immediately superior to the costal angle of the relevant rib [2] (see Fig. 45.2).
- The entry point can be adjusted also based on the fact whether unilateral or bilateral approach is being done and how much convergence is required (in unilateral approach, more convergence is required and hence more lateral starting point on the skin).
- Central placement of the needle usually results in sufficient cement distribution in the smaller vertebrae of the thoracic spine.
- The vertebral body can be either directly penetrated by the Jamshidi needle or first Kirschner (K)-wires are placed into the relevant vertebral bodies and then Jamshidi needle can be passed over the K-wires.
- The vertebrae can be accessed through transpedicular approach in lumbar spine and transcostovertebral approach in the thoracic spine [2].
- Once K-wire is advanced 2–2.5 cm into the pedicle without breaching the medial cortex on the AP view, switch to lateral view to see if the posterior vertebral cortex has been penetrated.
- If the needle/K-wire is in the vertebral body, then this can be advanced further and converged more at this stage. One must never breach the medial pedicle cortex on AP view without penetrating the posterior vertebral cortex on the lateral view. Jamshidi needles are then passed over the K-wires.
- Once the surgeon is satisfied with the position of the Jamshidi needles, that lateral image is saved on the screen as a reference image (this helps identify leakages through comparing the current image with the reference image without cement).
- Cement is mixed and, when of appropriate consistency, injected under live screening, (lateral view) watching for

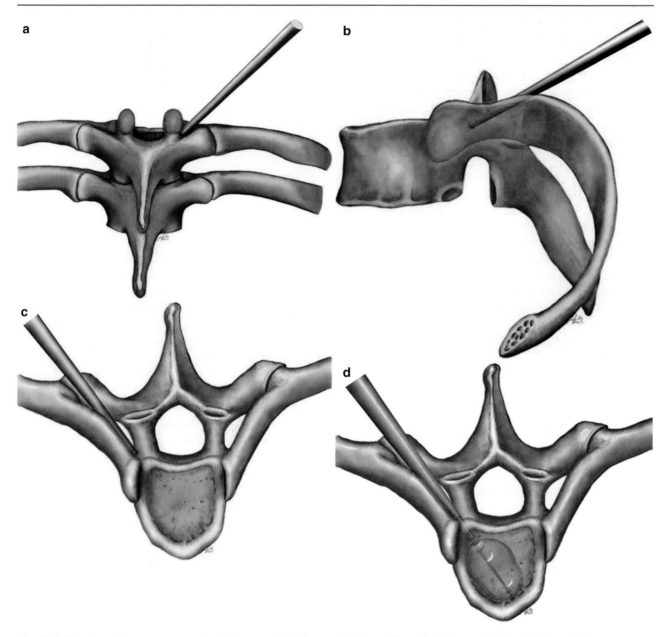

Fig. 45.2 Drawing of the transcostovertebral placement of the bone biopsy needle with the tip just penetrating the lateral pedicle at its base. In the view from posterior (**a**), the needle passes above of the transverse process and meets the pedicle at the craniolateral circumference. The lateral view (**b**) confirms the placement of the tip of the needle close to the base of the pedicle. In an axial view (**c**), the needle is seen to pass through the costovertebral gap, between the neck of the rib and the lateral pedicle circumference, towards the base of the pedicle (**d**) balloon inflated within the vertebral body

any leak either posteriorly into the spinal canal or anteriorly into the veins.

- *Note*: We try not to exceed 20–30 ml of cement injection in one sitting because of the risk of fat embolism resulting in pulmonary hypertension. Close collaboration with the anaesthetist is essential, and if the cardiorespiratory state is compromised, injection should stop. Also, if there is any leakage of cement into canal or vessels, injection should be aborted.

45.5.2 Balloon Kyphoplasty

- The relevant anatomy (pedicles, posterior vertebral wall, endplates, spinous processes, etc.) should be clearly identifiable on image intensifier before proceeding.
- In KP, it is essential to place the balloon in an optimum position in the middle of the vertebral body to achieve best possible reduction of the fracture without injuring the lateral margins of the vertebral body.

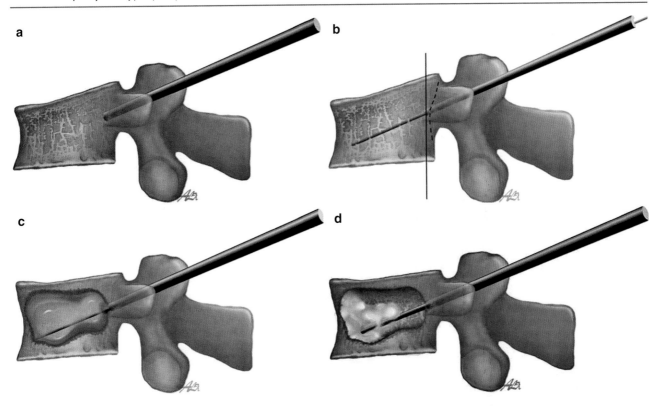

Fig. 45.3 Lateral view of balloon kyphoplasty (**a**). The tip of the working cannula lying just within the posterior vertebral cortex (**b**), the K-wire and then the drill passed to the anterior third of the vertebral body where balloon is going to be sited (**c**). Balloon seen inflated and see the height restoration (**d**) cement being injected into the cavity created by the balloon

- The principles and tool introduction are similar to the technique for PV described earlier.
- The K-wire is inserted first on AP view so that the needle tip appears to lie just outside the pedicle ring on AP view when bone contact is made. It is then advanced so that it does not breach the medial pedicle cortex on AP view until it penetrates the posterior vertebral wall on the lateral view.
- On AP view, tip of the needle should not cross the midline. On lateral view, K-wire is advanced to the anterior third of the vertebral body.
- Jamshidi needle is passed over the K-wire.
- Bone biopsy can be taken with the biopsy bone filler, and a hand drill bit can be used to drill the area where the balloon is going to lie and smoothen the bone edges.
- A special curette can be used as well; the angle at the tip can be changed to 30°, 60° and 90°. Then, Jamshidi needle is withdrawn and working cannula passed over the K-wire, the tip of the cannula lying only about 3 mm ventral to the posterior wall of the vertebra (to give space for the balloon) (see Fig. 45.3).
- Bilateral approach is used and balloons are then passed bilaterally so that they lie in the middle next to each other, making sure that both markings of the balloons should lie outside the working cannula (Fig. 45.3).

- The balloons are then simultaneously inflated keeping an eye on the pressure and the volume of the balloon and also frequently checking with imaging.
- The inflation of the balloons is continued until the maximum volume or maximum pressure is reached or the pressure keeps dropping indicating that further elevation of the endplate is not possible.
- Cement is then mixed, and once of appropriate viscosity, balloons are deflated and removed and the cavity in the bone filled with bone cement using bone fillers through the working cannulae under live fluoroscopy.
- The bone fillers and the working cannulae are removed once the cement is fully hardened and stab incisions are sutured.
- Final AP and lateral images are obtained.

45.6 Complications and Their Avoidance

Listing all the possible complications is beyond the scope of this chapter; however, few salient learning points are mentioned: Both PV and KP are deceptively "easy" techniques and should only be performed by properly trained surgeons who can also deal with complications, e.g., able to do open surgery (decompression/stabilization), if needed.

Cement leakage: Cement should be viscous enough before injecting. Good-quality imaging is essential to recognize the leaks at the very early stage. In difficult cases where fluoroscopy is suboptimal, CT-guided procedure combined with fluoroscopy can be done. Cement with an adequate radiopacity must be used.

Pulmonary emboli: Both VP and KP procedures will expel a volume of marrow equal to that of the cement injected. Although this is asymptomatic in most patients, those with pre-existing pulmonary disease, e.g., COPD, are particularly at risk and should be monitored accordingly. They should be informed of the high risk preoperatively and amount of cement injected in one sitting should be limited in such patients.

Disc space leaks: In case of large leaks into the disc space, consideration should be given to augmenting the adjacent vertebra or careful follow-up of this, as there has been some speculation that this leads to higher incidence of adjacent vertebral fracture.

Acknowledgement   Illustrations courtesy of spinegraphics@gmx.net.

References

1. Buchbinder R, Osborne RH, Ebeling PR et al (2009) A randomized trial of vertebroplasty for painful osteoporotic vertebral fractures. N Engl J Med 361:557–568
2. Boszczyk BM, Bierschneider M, Hauck S et al (2005) Transcostovertebral kyphoplasty of the mid and high thoracic spine. Eur Spine J 14:992–999
3. Mendel E, Bourekas E, Gerszten P, Golan JD (2009). Percutaneous techniques in the treatment of spine tumors: what are the diagnostic and therapeutic indications and outcomes? Spine (Phila Pa 1976). 2009 Oct 15;34(22 Suppl):S93–100
4. Jensen ME, Evans AJ, Mathis JM et al (1997) Percutaneous polymethylmethacrylate vertebroplasty in the treatment of osteoporotic vertebral body compression fractures: technical aspects. AJNR Am J Neuroradiol 18:1897–1904
5. Guarnieri G, Ambrosanio G, Vassallo P et al (2009) Vertebroplasty as treatment of aggressive and symptomatic vertebral hemangiomas: up to 4 years of follow-up. Neuroradiology 51:471–476
6. Magerl F, Aebi M, Gertzbein SD et al (1994) A comprehensive classification of thoracic and lumbar injuries. Eur Spine J 3:184–201
7. Kallmes DF, Comstock BA, Heagerty PJ et al (2009) A randomized trial of vertebroplasty for osteoporotic spinal fractures. N Engl J Med 361:569–579
8. Acosta FL Jr, Dowd CF, Chin C, Tihan T, Ames CP, Weinstein PR (2006) Current treatment strategies and outcomes in the management of symptomatic vertebral hemangiomas. Neurosurgery. Feb;58(2):287–95; discussion 287–95

Transpedicular Stabilization with Internal Fixation in the Thoracolumbar and Lumbar Spine

Robert Morrison and Uwe Vieweg

46.1 Introduction and Core Messages

The preparation of the pedicle requires knowledge of the following points: anatomical structures marking the entry point, pedicle orientation, and desired screw length. Performing an adequate preoperative planning (radiographs, CT-scan) and planning of the instrumentation based on these diagnostics are elemental for a good surgical result. The instrumentation of the lumbar spine allows stabilization and reduction using the posterior implants. For biomechanical reasons, an additional anterior procedure can be necessary to achieve a lasting stability.

46.2 Indications

- Fractures of the thoracolumbar or lumbar spine
- Degenerative disorders
- Tumors or infections of the spine

46.3 Contraindications (Relative)

- Osteopenia and osteoporosis
- Ongoing infection within the instrumented vertebra
- Poor medical condition of the patient

46.4 Technical Prerequisites

Fluoroscopy, special cushions (e.g., Wilson Frame), internal fixator (rod-screw system) or screw plate system, and radiolucent operating table.

46.5 Planning, Preparation, and Positioning

Preoperative measurement includes the pedicle diameter and especially the transverse diameter. This can be done either with AP radiographs or, more correctly, with a CT scan. If the transverse diameter is large enough to carry the screws, the preoperative planning can take place. The correct *entry point* can be found after identifying the necessary landmarks. These include the facet joint with its boarders and the transverse process. (*Note*:

R. Morrison, M.D. (✉)
Department of Spine Surgery, Sana Hospital Rummelsberg,
Rummelsberg 71, 90592 Schwarzenbruck, Germany
e-mail: dr.r.morrison@googlemail.com

U. Vieweg, M.D., Ph.D.
Clinic for Spinal Surgery,
Sana Hospital Rummelsberg,
90593 Schwarzenbruck, Germany
e-mail: uwe.vieweg@yahoo.de

U. Vieweg, F. Grochulla (eds.), *Manual of Spine Surgery*,
DOI 10.1007/978-3-642-22682-3_46, © Springer-Verlag Berlin Heidelberg 2012

Table 46.1 Average pedicle diameters and angulations within the lumbar spine. Adapted from Olsewski et al. [2]

Vertebra	Gender	Transversal pedicle diameter (mm)	Transversal angle of the pedicle (°)	Inclination angle of the pedicle (°)
L1	M	9.5	7	5
	F	7.7	5	6
L2	M	9.6	7	6
	F	7.9	6	5
L3	M	11.7	8	6
	F	9.6	7	6
L4	M	14.7	11	6
	F	12.5	10	7
L5	M	21.1	17	5
	F	18.4	18	8

Intra-operatively, the entry point is located in the lateral half of the oval area of the pedicle in the AP fluoroscopy.) This also includes measuring the transverse diameter of the pedicles (illustrated in Table 46.1). The *orientation of the pedicle* can be gauged in lateral radiographs or, even more precise, using CT-Scans (sagittal reconstructions for the cranial-caudal angle and coronary scans for the lateral deviation as illustrated in Table 46.1). The *pedicle length* also shows great variations. The correct screw length cannot be gauged intraoperatively in lateral fluoroscopy, as the anterior cortex has a convex shape. When deciding for a screw length, one must keep in mind that 60% of the pullout force is achieved in the pedicle and 15–20% additionally in the cancellous bone of the vertebra body. So the screw is rather chosen too short than too long!

46.5.1 Anatomical Specifications of the Thoracolumbar and Lumbar Spine

- Large pedicle diameter (average 8 mm in L1 to 18 mm in L5). Avoid using too small screws. The screw diameter should be 75–80% of the transverse pedicle diameter.
- Often, degenerative changes of the facet joints make it difficult to identify the proper entry point.
- Plain radiographs in two planes are enough to plan the instrumentation, if there are not any severe degenerative changes.

The patient is placed in a prone position with cushioning of the body parts in contact with the table. The definitive positioning depends on the case to be treated. In the case of decompression, the lumbar spine should be slightly kyphotic for an easier approach to the canal. On the other hand – in case of fractures – depending on the habits of the surgical team, extension/traction can be added. The patient should always be positioned in a lordotic position to ease the reduction. In scoliosis surgery, as there is no spinal canal decompression, the

patient is placed directly in the lumbar lordotic position. In cases of decompression and reduction surgery (e.g., spondylolisthesis), decompression can be realized in a kyphotic position with flexion of the hips of up to 60°. To avoid the risk of arthrodesis in a kyphotic position, the extension of the legs may be performed during the surgery. Whatever the position chosen there are always certain rules to respect:

- Avoid abdominal compression to decrease the pressure in the epidural veins.
- Positioning of the shoulders and elbows flexed with cubital nerve protection.
- Flexion of the knees to relax the sciatic nerves.
- Rest position of the head with eye protection and straight cervical spine.
- Follow the basic rules of prone position surgery.
- Cushioning of body parts in contact with the table.

46.6 Surgical Technique

46.6.1 Approach

- *Open access via a midline incision*: The incision should be one or two segments longer than the intended length of fusion. The subcutis is dissected to the fascia, and wound retractors are applied. The fascia is detached on both sides of the spinal processes using a diathermy knife close to the bone. The paraspinal structures are retracted with a raspatory. The muscles are retracted to expose the ends of the costal processes.
- *Alternative, paraspinal approach*: Two paramedian skin incisions are made two fingerbreadths laterally to the spinous processes. The fascia of the iliocostal muscles is split longitudinally. Blunt dissection through the muscles until the vertebral joint is palpated. Implementation of the retractor.

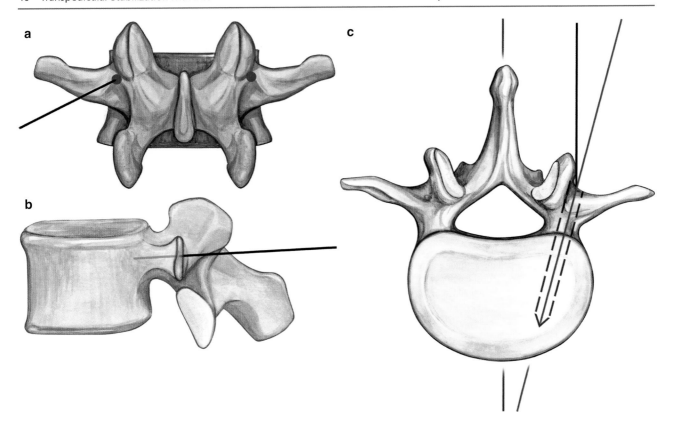

Fig. 46.1 *Converging screw placement* (**a**, **b**). The anatomical land-mark for converging screw placement is the transverse process (processus costarius). These *lines* are close to the midline of the transverse process (slightly above in the upper lumbar spine). The orientation of the trocar must be strictly in the longitudinal axis of the pedicle. Usually, an angle of about 15–25° to the sagittal plane is chosen for the lumbar spine (With permission from Aesculap AG, Tuttlingen, Germany [4]). *Standard screw placement* (**c**). In the so-called straightforward technique described by Roy Camille, the entry point is the downward projection of the posterior articular process 1 mm below the joint [3]

- *Percutaneous technique*: Marking of the entry points on the skin using fluoroscopy. Minimally invasive percutaneous approach to each pedicle. Marking of the intended screw position using K-Wires.

46.6.2 Instrumentation

46.6.2.1 Lumbar Spine

Entry point/trajectory: The entry point can be found at the intersection of the vertical line along the lateral edge of the superior articular process and the horizontal line through the middle of the transverse process. The bony crest on the entry point for the pedicle screw can be removed with a rongeur or, alternatively, with a high-speed drill; the subcortical cancellous bone of the pedicle entrance is exposed. The opening of the pedicle is then enlarged with a sharp center punch under lateral control to verify the correct entry point, and the sagittal angle or drilling of the pedicle is then performed with gentle pressure using a universal trocar or the adjustable trocar step by step under fluoroscopic control.

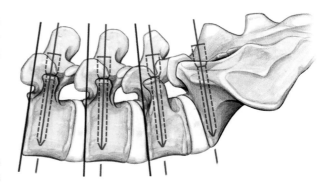

Fig. 46.2 For easier rod placement, the screws should be placed in one line and parallel to the upper endplates

- To detect the correct entry point, the "processus costarius" is a good landmark (see Fig. 46.1a–c) [1].
- Within the lumbar spine, the screws will have an increasing convergence toward the midline (10° in L1 to 20° in L5). The screws should be placed parallel to the superior endplate (see Fig. 46.2) [4].
- The pedicle is opened with a pedicle awl, followed by consecutive deepening with a pedicle trocar. The length of the

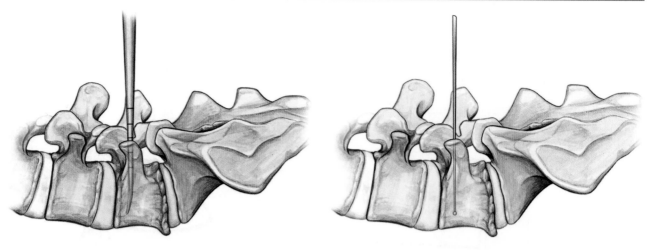

Fig. 46.3 The opening of the pedicle is then enlarged with a sharp center punch first under AP control for the entry point and then under lateral control to verify the correct sagittal angle

Fig. 46.4 Following the preparation of the screw hole, the channel can be checked using a dissector or pedicle sonde to disclose possible perforations of the pedicle wall

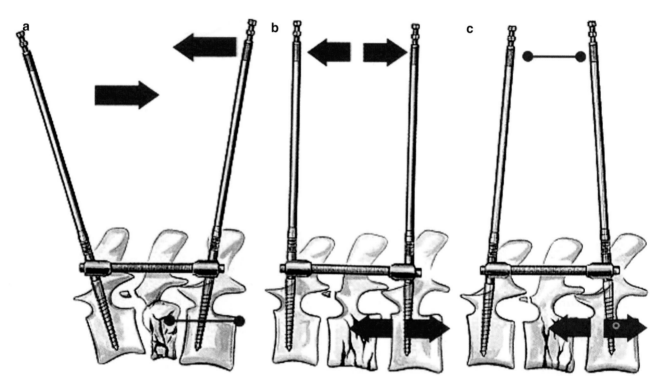

Fig. 46.5 (**a–c**) Repositioning examples ((**a**) repositioning, (**b**) parallel distraction (**c**) lordosation) with a pedicle screw system (With permission from Aesculap AG, Tuttlingen, Germany)

screw can be seen on the side of the trocar. To verify the intact pedicle walls, the walls of the canal can be tested with a ball-tipped pedicle probe (see Figs. 46.3 and 46.4).

• The pedicle screw systems allows movements/corrections in three directions, individually or combined, during the repositioning procedure: compression, angulation (see Fig. 46.5a, c), distraction (see Fig. 46.5b).

46.7 Sacrum

46.7.1 Entry Point/Trajectory

The entry point of the segment S1 is located on a vertical line along the lateral wall of the superior facet and right on the inferior border of the facet joint. Due to degenerative changes,

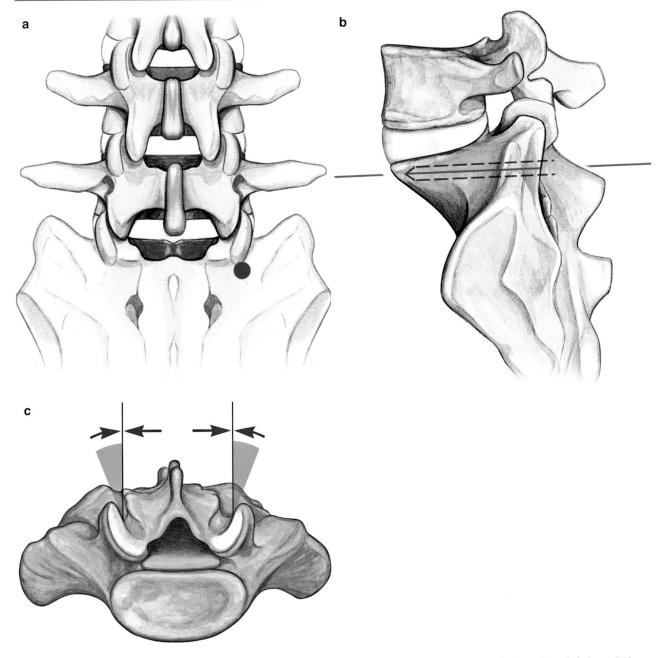

Fig. 46.6 (**a–c**) Preparation of the sacrum. The entry point for the converging screw channels in the sacrum is about 5 mm inferior and 10 mm lateral to the inferior border of the facet of S1

the identification of the exact entry point is sometimes quite difficult. A partial resection of the inferior facet of L5 is helpful in these cases.

There are two different trajectories in the sacrum:

- The most common is the trajectory aiming at the anterior corner of the promontorium with a 15–20° convergence of the screws. Superior strength of fixation is achieved by bicortical fixation of the screws along the pedicle axis in this "safe zone" (see Fig. 46.6b).

- The alternative safe zone is found in an angle of 45° deviation, aiming the screws toward the sacroiliacal joint. In this case, the screws should be no longer than 45 mm to avoid interference with the SI joint.

The sacrum has particular anatomical properties. Here, the values for the pullout strength are reversed, with anterior cortical fixation being responsible for 60%. Therefore, careful purchase of the anterior cortex is sometimes necessary for optimal fixation.

46.8 Tips and Tricks

- Start out by marking the entry points with K-wires or short pins using the fluoroscopy in the AP direction!
- For easy rod placement, the screws should be placed in one line and parallel to the upper endplates; the insertion depth should be the same for all pedicle screws to achieve aligned screw heads (see Fig. 46.2).
- Using pedicle markers, the screw channels can be checked under lateral X-ray control.

References

1. Ebraheim NA, Rollins JR, Xu R et al (1996) Projection of the lumbar pedicle and its morphometric analysis. Spine 21:1296–1300
2. Olsewski JM, Simmons EH, Kallen FC et al (1990) Morphometry of the lumbar spine: anatomical perspectives related to the transpedicular fixation. J Bone Joint Surg Am 71:541–549
3. Roy-Camille R, Saillant G, Mazel C (1986) Plating of thoracic, thoracolumbar, and lumbar injuries with pedicle screw plates. Orthop Clin North Am 17:147–159
4. Weinstein JN, Spratt KF, Spengler D et al (1988) Spinal pedicle fixation: reliability and validity of roentgenogram-based assessment and surgical factors on successful screw placement. Spine 13:1012–1018

Correction of Degenerative Scoliosis

47

Uwe Vieweg and Robert Morrison

47.1 Introduction and Core Messages

The degenerative scoliosis is the so-called de novo scoliosis. It is a form of secondary scoliosis in elderly patients (patients >65 years), as a result of gradual disc degeneration with a lateral deviation and rotated vertebral bodies. Surgical correction using a polyaxial internal fixation represents a possible treatment of a degenerative scoliosis. The correction is performed step by step using polyaxial pedicle screws, intercorporal fusion (generally using TLIF at the caudal level), a correction of the scoliosis using PLIF cages (box-like) following the resection of the facet joints and an intercorporal fusion using a TLIF cage (banana-like or kidney-shaped cage), again at the cranial end. The remaining malposition is corrected by restoration of the lumbar lordosis and the derotation of the vertebras using the prebent rods [1–7].

47.2 Indications

- Degenerative scoliosis >20°, with a significant progression of the scoliosis
- Persistent back pain and or leg pain that interferes with activities of daily living
- Failed conservative therapy and neurological deficits

47.3 Contraindications

- Severe osteoporosis, osteopenia, or osteomyelitis
- Poor psychological or medical situation of the patient

47.4 Technical Prerequisites

Fluoroscopy, special cushions (e.g., Wilson Frame), polyaxial screw system with cross connectors, PLIF and TLIF cages, distraction forceps, cell saver, radiolucent operating table, and bone grinder.

47.5 Planning, Preparation, and Positioning

Extensive radiological diagnostics such as conventional radiographs, functional radiographs (flexion, extension, lateral bending), MRI, and determination of the bone density are elemental. The lumbar myelography is a centerpiece of the

U. Vieweg, M.D., Ph.D. (✉)
Clinic for Spinal Surgery, Sana Hospital Rummelsberg,
90593 Schwarzenbruck, Germany
e-mail: uwe.vieweg@yahoo.de

R. Morrison, M.D.
Department of Spine Surgery, Sana Hospital Rummelsberg,
Rummelsberg 71, 90592 Schwarzenbruck, Germany
e-mail: dr.r.morrison@googlemail.com

U. Vieweg, F. Grochulla (eds.), *Manual of Spine Surgery*,
DOI 10.1007/978-3-642-22682-3_47, © Springer-Verlag Berlin Heidelberg 2012

diagnostics, as it shows the extent of the stenosis. These findings combined help to specify the extent of the instrumentation and the type as well as the location of the decompression. They are also elemental in planning the intercorporal fusion and reconstruction of the intervertebral height. During the operation, the patient is in a prone position on a radiolucent operating table. Different positioning systems can be used (Wilson frame, chest rolls, Relton hall frame, Hasting frame, Heffington frame). The patient should be positioned to minimize intra-abdominal pressure and thereby avoid venous congestion and excess intraoperative bleeding. The incision is planned using the fluoroscopy.

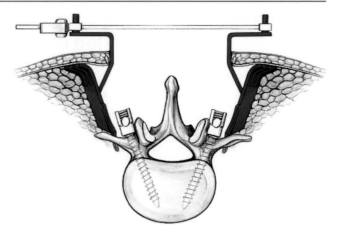

Fig. 47.1 Placement of the subcutaneous lumbar retractor system (SLR, Aesculap AG, Tuttlingen) in an axial view to reduce hematomas and postoperative pain (With permission from Aesculap AG, Tuttlingen, Germany)

47.6 Surgical Technique

47.6.1 Approach

- A midline posterior approach to the spine is performed with subperiosteal exposure of the posterior elements down to the transverse processes. For improved tissue protection and in order to use a smaller skin incision, a subcutaneous lumbar retractor system is advisable (see Figs. 47.1 and 47.2).
- The exposure of the spinous process should extend to at least one additional level above and below the levels to be instrumented. Care must be taken not to disrupt the facet joint capsules of the joints above and below the intended fusion segments.

47.6.2 Instrumentation

- Using the awl or Steinmann nail, the cortex is penetrated under fluoroscopy. The trajectory angle is determined preoperatively. Use the ball-tipped probe to make sure the pedicle is intact under fluoroscopy. The pedicle entry point is intersected by the vertical line that connects the lateral edges of bony crest extension of the pars interarticularis and the horizontal line that bisects the middle of the transverse process. Subsequently, transpedicular implantation of the polyaxial screws (see Fig. 47.3).
- After pedicle screw insertion, the superior and inferior articular processes of the caudal facet joint (in the most cases on the convex site) are resected with a high-speed drill and a Kerrison punch, and the intervertebral disc space is exposed. The disc is then resected subtotally using angled rongeurs, shavers, and curettes. After preparation of the end plates, the anterior part of the disc space

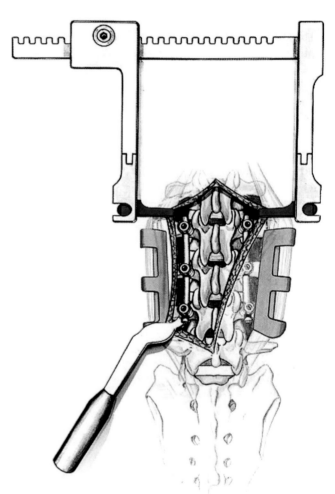

Fig. 47.2 Smaller skin incision with the SLR to reduce the operative trauma (With permission from Aesculap AG, Tuttlingen, Germany)

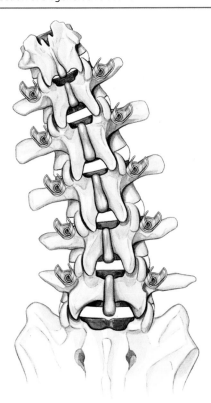

Fig. 47.3 Extensive instrumentation from L1 through L5 using a polyaxial internal fixateur (With permission from Aesculap AG, Tuttlingen, Germany)

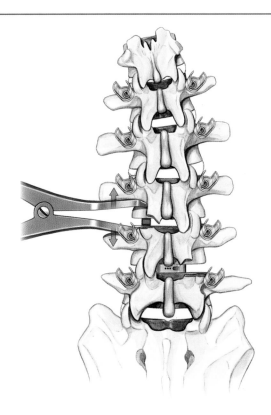

Fig. 47.5 Straightening of the scoliosis in the segment L3/4 by distracting the intervertebral space using a distraction forceps placed underneath the screw heads. Then, a PLIF cage is placed into the space (With permission from Aesculap AG, Tuttlingen, Germany)

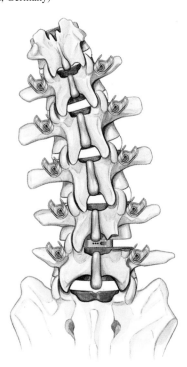

Fig. 47.4 First step of the correction by performing a intercorporal fusion using TLIF technique on the left side in the caudal segment (L4/5) (With permission from Aesculap AG, Tuttlingen, Germany)

is packed with autologous bone. A curved PEEK cage specially designed for the TLIF technique is also filled with autologous bone and inserted into the disc space (see Fig. 47.4).

- Now, the next facet joint on the concave site is resected using a high-speed drill and a Kerrison punch. The disc space is distracted with angulated distraction forceps. This distraction and the implantation of an additional interbody cage (PLIF) reconstruct the disc space (see Figs. 47.5 and 47.6).
- The cranial disc space is resected coming from the contralateral side. Here, we also recommend a reconstruction using the TLIF technique described above (see Fig. 47.7).
- The appropriate-sized rod is bent to match the sagittal contour of the spine using the rod bender. Place the rod into the screws, and then lock it in place with the set screws. By using this specific screw design with the removable tabs, an additional correction can be achieved (lordosis, reposition of a spondylolisthesis as well as a derotation) (see Figs. 47.8a, b).

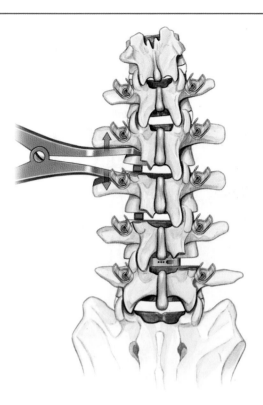

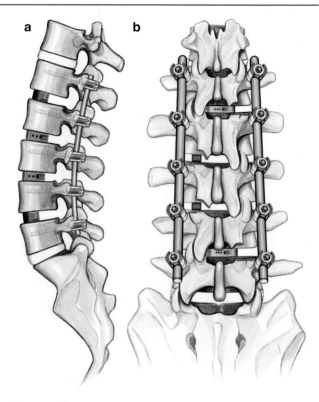

Fig. 47.6 Next step is the same procedure in the segment L2/3 (With permission from Aesculap AG, Tuttlingen, Germany)

Figs. 47.8 a, b Additional correction of the lumbar lordosis and derotation using an accordingly bent rod. (**a**) lateral (**b**) AP view (With permission from Aesculap AG, Tuttlingen, Germany)

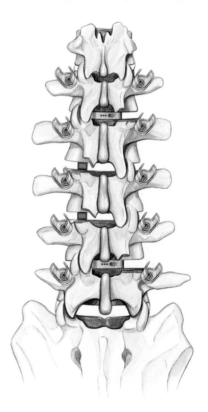

47.7 Tips and Tricks

- Pedicle screw augmentation for the upper and lower end of the instrumentation.
- Note the sagittal balance not only the anterior Cobb angle.
- Note the junction regions with instrumentation of lower thoracic spine (T10, T11, T12) or with S1 with or without a ilium screw.
- Position the fluoroscopy to where it is parallel to the instrumented segment; the end plates of the vertebra will be depicted as parallel lines.
- Guide pins are available and can be used to mark the pedicle before the pedicle screws are implanted. This allows a perfect pedicle screw placement.

Fig. 47.7 To complete the correction, a TLIF cage is placed into the segment L1/2, coming from the left side (With permission from Aesculap AG, Tuttlingen, Germany)

Fig. 47.9 (**a**) Lateral and (**b**) AP x-ray of a patient with a degenerative scoliosis (mild idiopathic component), visual analog scale seven back pain, and six leg pain

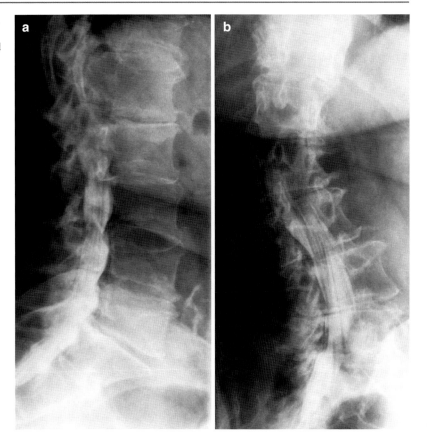

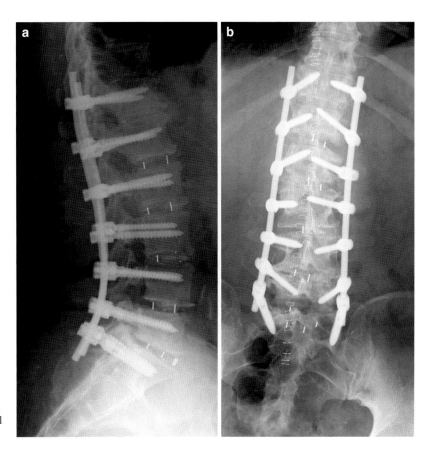

Fig. 47.10 Postoperative lateral (**a**) and (**b**) AP x-ray after correction of the degenerative scoliosis with an internal fixator (T12 to S1) with additional interbody fusion

References

1. Aebi M (2005) The adult scoliosis. Eur Spine J 14:925–948
2. Akbarnia BA, Ogilvie JW, Hammerberg KW (2006) Debate: degenerative scoliosis: to operate or not to operate. Spine 9(Suppl):S195–S201
3. Bradford DS, Tay BK, Hu SS (1999) Adult scoliosis: surgical indications, operative management, complications and outcome. Spine 24:2617–2629
4. Glassman SD, Bridwell K, Dimar JK (2005) The impact of positive sagittal balance in adult spinal deformity. Spine 30:2024–2029
5. Daffner SD, Vaccaro AR (2003) Adult degenerative lumbar scoliosis. Am J Orthop 32:77–82
6. Dick W, Widmer H (1993) Degenerative Lumbalskoliose und Spinalkanalstenose. Orthopade 22:232–242
7. Tribus CB (2003) Degenerative lumbar scoliosis: evaluation and management. J Am Acad Orthop Surg 11:174–183

Correction of Spondylolisthesis

Uwe Vieweg

48.1 Introduction and Core Messages

The goals of surgical treatment of spondylolisthesis are: decompression of neuronal structures, stabilization of spondylolytic instability, reduction of slippage, restoration of the disc height, and restoration of the sagittal alignment [1, 2]. With the appropriate instruments, it is possible to instrument a single compartment and in most cases, to completely reduce the spondylolisthesis. This technique allows an instrumented monosegmental slippage reduction of low- and middle-grade isthmic spondylolisthesis via fusion with a polyaxial internal fixator, titanium spacer, and cross-link connector.

48.2 Indications

- Spondylolytic spondylolisthesis Meyerding grade I–III (IV) L5/S1 and L4/L5
- Significant progression of the slip spondylolisthesis
- Persistent back pain and/or leg pain that interferes with activities of daily living
- Failed conservative therapy
- Neurological deficits [1–5]

48.3 Contraindications

- Reduction should not be attempted in patients with spondyloptosis
- Osteoporosis, osteopenia, or osteomyelitis
- Poor psychological and/or poor general medical state of the patient [1–5]

48.4 Technical Prerequisites

Fluoroscopy, positioning device (e.g., Wiltse frame), adequate implants, and instruments with the following technical requirements:
- Simultaneous correction of translation and slip angle.
- Reduction with single-level fusion and sparing adjacent healthy vertebrae.
- Reduction of the listhetic vertebral body along the same curved displacement route. This minimizes interference with anatomical structures and eliminates the neurological deficits that typically result from initial overdistraction of an already stretched nerve root.

U. Vieweg, M.D., Ph.D.
Clinic for Spinal Surgery, Sana Hospital Rummelsberg,
90593 Schwarzenbruck, Germany
e-mail: uwe.vieweg@yahoo.de

U. Vieweg, F. Grochulla (eds.), *Manual of Spine Surgery*,
DOI 10.1007/978-3-642-22682-3_48, © Springer-Verlag Berlin Heidelberg 2012

Fig. 48.1 The S⁴ SRI spondylolisthesis reduction instrument (SRI) has a *right* and a *left* component. Each has two pedicle screw attachments. One attaches to the cephalad vertebral screw that will be repositioned and the other to the caudal vertebral screw (With permission from Aesculap AG, Tuttlingen, Germany)

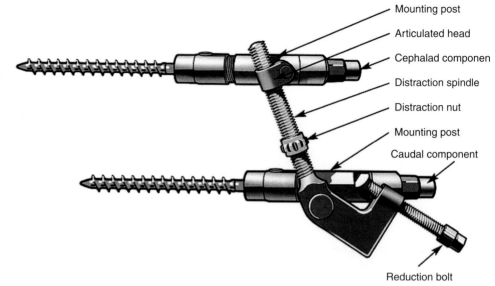

- Mounting post
- Articulated head
- Cephalad componen
- Distraction spindle
- Distraction nut
- Mounting post
- Caudal component
- Reduction bolt

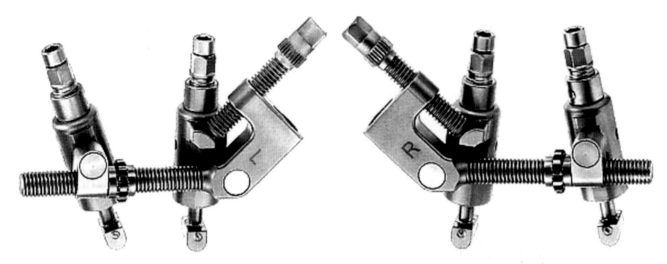

Fig. 48.2 The *right* and the *left* component of the S⁴ SRI (With permission from Aesculap AG, Tuttlingen, Germany)

The S⁴ SRI = spondylolisthesis reduction instrument is one possible method of reducing a spondylolisthesis (see Figs. 48.1 and 48.2). Other possibilities are Krypton (Ulrich, Ulm, Germany), TSRH 3D Plus MPA (Medtronic, USA), Xia (Stryker, USA), Pathfinder (Abbott Spine, USA), SOCON (Aesculap, Tuttlingen, Germany), and USS Click'X (Synthes, Umkirch, Germany).

48.5   Planning, Preparation, and Positioning

Prior to surgery, the patient's X-rays are reviewed to access pedicle diameter, length, and orientation. Knowledge of normal pedicle anatomy is essential to proper placement of pedicle screws, especially in L5. The patient is positioned prone on a radiolucent operating table. The abdomen is permitted to hang freely. The hips are extended to enhance lumbar lordosis.

48.6   Surgical Technique

48.6.1 Approach

A midline posterior approach to the spine is performed with subperiosteal exposure of the posterior bony elements to the level of the transverse processes. On the lateral side, the posterior segments are exposed including the facet joints. (Access to L5/S1 should generally be made large enough to ensure reliable instrumentation.)

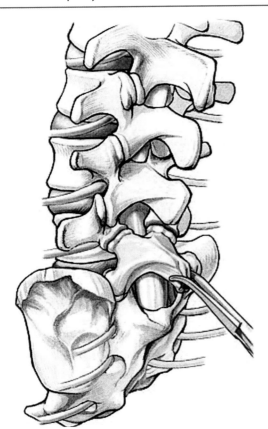

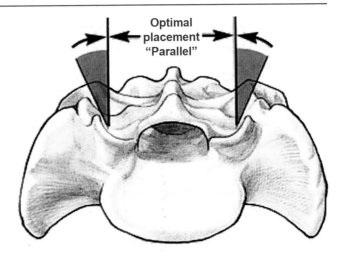

Fig. 48.4 Optimal parallel placement of the pedicle screws in the sacrum (With permission from Aesculap AG, Tuttlingen, Germany)

Fig. 48.3 Standard Gill procedure (With permission from Aesculap AG, Tuttlingen, Germany)

48.6.2 Instrumentation

- Perform a standard Gill procedure (see Fig. 48.3).
- Using the awl, the cortex is penetrated under C-arm control. The drilling angle is determined. Use the ball-tipped probe to make sure the pedicle is intact.
- Screws in the sacrum are best placed parallel to its superior end plate and as parallel to each other as possible (see Fig. 48.4, see pedicle access, pedicle preparation, and screw placement, Chap. 46).
- Place the caudal screws so that they are parallel to the cephalad vertebra screws in both planes. This differs from the standard convergent manner (see Fig. 48.5).
- *An alternative technique – instrumentation with polyaxial screws, allows a standard convergent positioning and easier attaching of the S⁴ SRI.*
- In the case of an L5/S1 reduction, the chosen length at S1 should achieve bicortical purchase. In most cases, this is 45 mm in length and 7 mm diameter.
- During the decompression, perform a complete resection of the pars interarticularis defects to fully decompress the exiting nerve roots. This may include removal of the Gill fragment.

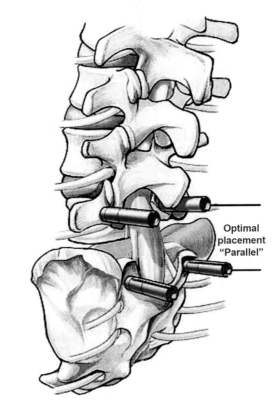

Fig. 48.5 Parallel placement of the caudal vertebral screws to the cephalad vertebra screws in both planes and complete decompression of the exiting nerve roots (with permission from Aesculap AG, Tuttlingen, Germany)

- Perform a complete resection of the residual superior articular processes in preparation for the PLIF. A wide decompression allows access to the intervening disc space, lateral to the thecal sac.

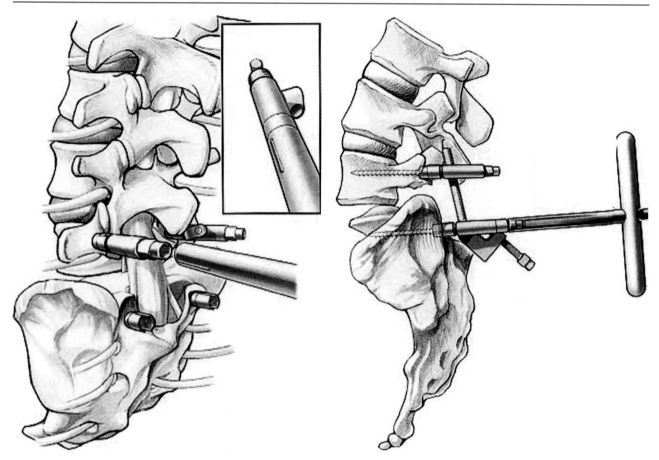

Fig. 48.6 Insert the mounting post into the tulip of the screw and finger tighten. Attach the cephalad component first (With permission from Aesculap AG, Tuttlingen, Germany)

Fig. 48.7 The instrument is attached and positioned properly. Tighten the caudal and cephalad components using the T-handles (With permission from Aesculap AG, Tuttlingen, Germany)

- On the caudal components, make sure the distraction nuts are of a point of minimal distraction (toward the most caudal position of the S^4 SRI).
- On the caudal components, make sure the reduction bolts are backed out to the point of minimal reduction.
- Attach the cephalad component first (see Fig. 48.6).
- Insert the mounting post into the tulip of the screw and finger tighten (Fig. 48.7).
- The caudal components are labeled "R" for right and "L" for left. For alternative placement of SRI medially to the pedicle screws, (see Figs. 48.8 and 48.9).
- Ensure that the articulated head is positioned inferiorly and insert the distraction spindle (caudal component) into the articulated head of the cephalad component. At the same time, insert the mounting post into the tulip of the pedicle screw of the caudal vertebra and finger tighten.
- Once the instrument is attached and positioned properly, tighten the caudal and cephalad components using the T-handles.

- Hold the smaller inner T-handle and use it to apply counter-torque while tightening with the larger outer T-handle.
- The mounting post on polyaxial screws should be tightened enough to lock slightly the polyaxial head.
- The mounting post on monoaxial screws need to be tightened enough to cover the break-off tabs and part of the screw head.
- Using the distraction forceps, slowly spread the SRI device to achieve the desired distraction. Then, lock the distraction nut on the threaded distraction spindle (see Fig. 48.10).
- Using the larger outer T-handle on the reduction bolt, turn clockwise to carefully reduce the spondylolisthesis under fluoroscopy control (see Fig. 48.11).
- Monitor the nerve root tension during reduction. Typically, a decrease in the nerve root tension will be observed.
- Remove the SRI from one side if required to provide room to work and perform a routine PLIF (TLIF). If the decompression is great enough, the SRI can be left in place.

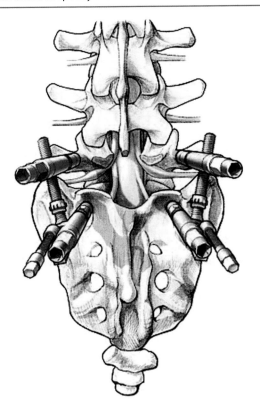

Fig. 48.8 Lateral placement of the reduction instrument (With permission from Aesculap AG, Tuttlingen, Germany)

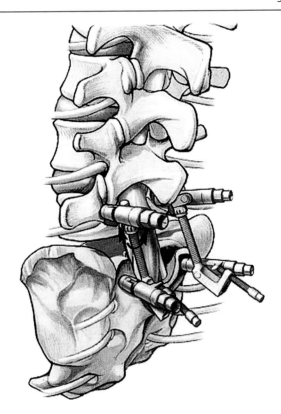

Fig. 48.10 First perform distraction with spreading of the SRI device with distraction forceps or with the distraction nut. Then, lock the distraction in place with the distraction nut on the threaded distraction spindle (With permission from Aesculap AG, Tuttlingen, Germany)

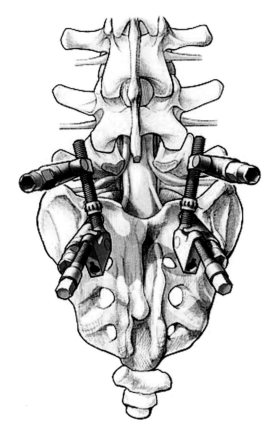

Fig. 48.9 Medial placement of the reduction instrument (alternative) (With permission from Aesculap AG, Tuttlingen, Germany)

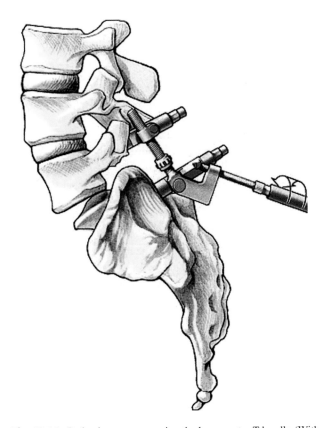

Fig. 48.11 Reduction progress using the larger outer T-handle (With permission from Aesculap AG, Tuttlingen, Germany)

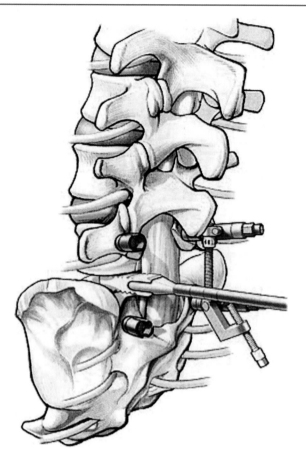

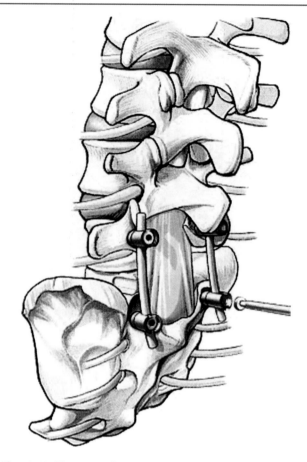

Fig. 48.12 Interbody fusion with PLIF cage (With permission from Aesculap AG, Tuttlingen, Germany)

Fig. 48.13 Placement of the rod and locking into place with set screws (With permission from Aesculap AG, Tuttlingen, Germany)

- Retract the dura and upper nerve root carefully in the desired direction using the nerve root retractors.
- Besides retracting, the nerve root retractor provides protection for the surrounding tissues during the following operative steps.
- In order to make room for the insertion of the distractor of the PLIF instruments, resection of disc material is now carried out using rongeurs and forceps on both sides of the disc.
- The PLIF implant (see Prospace Titan Spacer) should be inserted in the disc space 2–3 mm beyond or anterior to the rear edge of the vertebral body (Fig. 48.12).
- During insertion of the spacer or cage, the provided retractor can be used to ensure that the dura and nerve roots are carefully protected.
- Position the rod, and then lock in place with the set screws (Figs. 48.13 and 48.14).

48.7   Tips and Tricks

- In the event that the space lateral to the pedicle screws is not sufficient for introduction of the distraction spindle, both SRI components (right/left) can also be transposed laterally.
- Medial placement of the reduction instruments is the preferred method. This usually allows for easier reduction and less soft tissue impingement from the device itself. Lateral placement sometimes allows an easier interbody placement, but can make the reduction maneuver more difficult.
- In order to avoid breaking of the tab during reduction, make sure to fully tighten the SRI device to the pedicle screw prior to performing the reduction.
- Prepare the small pedicle L5 with cannulated instruments and use cannulated screws in L5.

Fig. 48.14 (**a**) Lateral radiological X-ray of a spondylolytic spondylolisthesis at L5/S1, (**b**) lateral postoperative radiograph after repositioning with the S^4 SRI and interbody fusion with the PLIF cage

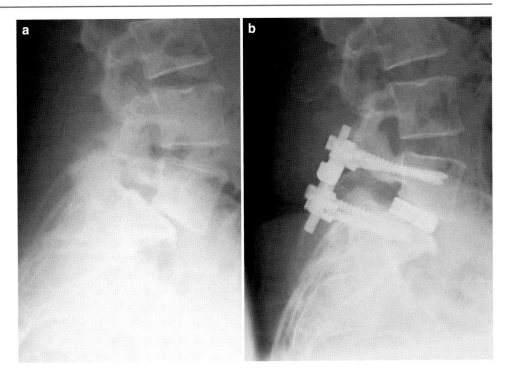

References

1. Harrington PR, Dickson JH (1976) Spinal instrumentation in the treatment of severe progressive spondylolisthesis. Clin Orthop 117:157–163
2. La Rosa G, Germano A, Conti A et al (1999) Posterior fusion and implantation of the SOCON-SRI system in the treatment of adult spondylolisthesis. Neurosurg Focus 7(6):E2
3. La Rosa G, Cacciola F, Conti A et al (2001) Posterior fusion compared with posterior interbody fusion in segmental spinal fixation for adult spondylolisthesis. Neurosurg Focus 10(4):E9
4. Majcher P, Fatyga M, Skwarcz A (2000) Internal fixation systems in the surgical treatment of spondylolisthesis. Ortop Traumatol Rehabil 30:65–68
5. Periasamy K, Shah K, Wheelwright EF (2008) Posterior lumbar interbody fusion using cages, combined with instrumented posterolateral fusion: a study of 75 cases. Acta Orthop Belg 74: 240–248

Microsurgical Monosegmental Fusion with Internal Fixator and Interbody Fusion

49

Uwe Vieweg and Stefan Kroppenstedt

49.1 Introduction and Core Messages

The methods described here (Method I: ipsilateral transpedicular instrumentation and interbody fusion about a lateral paraspinal approach and contralateral percutaneous transpedicular instrumentation, Method II: instrumentation and interbody fusion about both paraspinal lateral approaches) allow the surgeon to perform less-invasive spinal instrumentation with short operating time, less blood loss, and small skin incisions. The technique of transforaminal lumbar interbody fusion involves facetectomy, discectomy, and interbody fusion, carried out with the aid of a high-speed reamer, microsurgical instruments, and an operating microscope or endoscope. Patients benefit from reduced trauma, less pain, and shorter hospitalization and recovery times.

49.2 Indications

- Spondylolisthesis that has not responded, or has responded inadequately, to non-operative treatment of symptoms
- Discogenic low-back pain with or without paresis [1, 2, 4]

U. Vieweg, M.D., Ph.D. (✉)
Clinic for Spinal Surgery, Sana Hospital Rummelsberg,
90593 Schwarzenbruck, Germany
e-mail: uwe.vieweg@yahoo.de

S. Kroppenstedt, M.D., Ph.D.
Department of Spinal Surgery, Center of Orthopedic Surgery,
Sana Hospital Sommerfeld, Waldhausstraße 44,
16766 Kremmen, Germany
e-mail: s.kroppenstedt@sana-hu.de

49.3 Contraindications

- Severe spinal canal stenosis
- Higher grade spondylolisthesis (Meyerding grade III–IV) and deformities
- Absent, fractured, or atrophic pedicles and severe osteopenia that limits secure screw purchase
- Signs of current active infection

49.4 Technical Requirements

C-arm fluoroscope, microscope or endoscope, supporting pads and cushions to aid positioning, radiolucent surgical table, high-speed burr, and retractor systems (METRx X-TUBE MicroDiscectomy Retraction System (Medtronic), MLD retractor system (Aesculap), ProView Minimal Access Portal System (Blackstone), Luxor (Stryker), MIRA (Synthes)). Internal fixator systems (top loading system) with cannulated screws (CD Horizon Sextant I/II and CD Horizon Longitude, Medtronic; S^4 internal fixator, Aesculap). Other systems for minimally invasive screw and rod insertion for posterior stabilization are spirit with cannulated Click'X (Synthes), REVOLVE Stabilization System (Globus Medical), SpheRx-DBR system (NuVasive), EXPEDIUM and VIPER (DePuy), Silverbolt (Via 4 Spine). abd Mispas (Synthes) Spinal navigation is an additional option.

49.5 Planning, Preparation, and Positioning

The patient is placed in a prone position on a radiolucent table under general anesthesia (see Fig. 49.1) and prepared and draped in the conventional manner. The abdomen is permitted to hang freely. The hips are extended to enhance lumbar lordosis. The skin incision is planned under X-ray control with a C-arm fluoroscope using anteroposterior and lateral beam directions. Four needles are placed at the level of the pedicles to ascertain the level (see Fig. 49.2). The Ferguson arrangement

Fig. 49.1 Positioning of the patient (With permission from Aesculap AG, Tuttlingen, Germany)

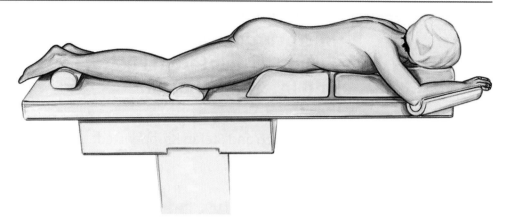

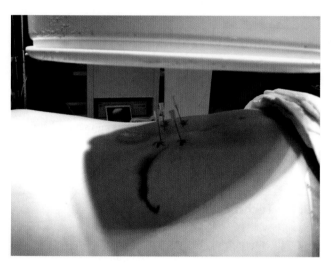

Fig. 49.2 Planning of the skin incision with C-arm fluoroscope

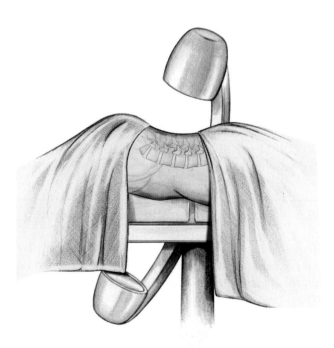

Fig. 49.3 Ferguson arrangement/positioning of the C-arm for the L5/S1 level

provides the best image, focusing correctly on the S1 pedicle (see Fig. 49.3). Biplanar fluoroscopy with two C-arms facilitates safer and easier radiographic assessment (see Fig. 49.4). *Note*: When planning the approach, the spinous processes should appear exactly in the middle between the two pedicles, and the superior end plates should appear exactly parallel when viewed in AP X-rays. Care should be taken to ensure that the superior end plates are also parallel in lateral X-rays.

49.6 Surgical Technique

49.6.1 Method I: Ipsilateral Mini-Open and Contralateral Percutaneous Instrumentation [1–3]

Mini-Open Access

- After radiological planning incisions are made in the skin (4–5 cm long) and the lateral fascia of the pedicle.
- The retractor system (METRx, Medtronic) is delivered via the dilatation tubes at approximately the angle at which the pedicle screws are to be inserted.
- The expansion and position of the retractor system are confirmed by imaging.
- A Jamshidi needle is inserted. After locating the entry point on the pedicle, the Jamshidi needle needs to be aligned with the pedicle trajectory. The needle is driven in as far as the anterior edge of the vertebral body. It should not extend beyond the medial edge of the pedicle (see Figs. 49.5 and 49.6a, b). If necessary, the needle must be reinserted and realigned. The position is fixed by slightly pushing the Jamshidi needle into the cortex.
- The pedicle is prepared with the appropriate tap. The tap must correspond to the screw type and diameter.
- The Kirschner wire is replaced with a marker pin or about 3 cm of wire (see Fig. 49.8b).
- The second pedicle is prepared as described above.
- The microscope is swung into place.
- Transforaminal access to the disc is typically performed on the most symptomatic side. The facet is resected with

Fig. 49.4 Using two C-arm fluoroscopes for percutaneous instrumentation

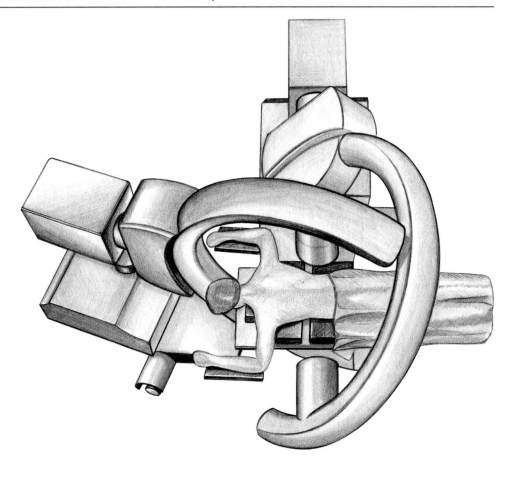

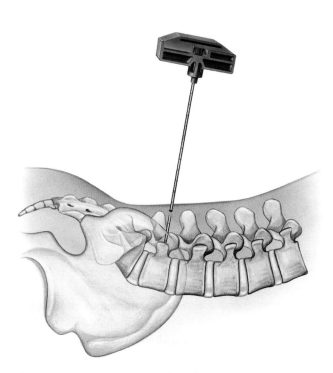

Fig. 49.5 Positioning the Jamshidi needle

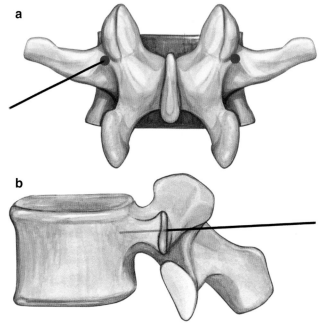

Fig. 49.6 AP (**a**) and lateral (**b**) X-ray views of the ideal positioning of the cannula in the pedicle

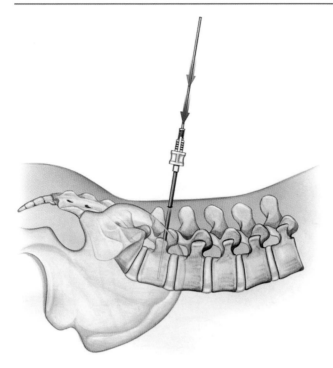

Fig. 49.7 Insertion of the K-wire

a high-speed reamer. *Note*: Bone removal should begin caudally between the two pedicles, directly over the disc space.

- A diamond reamer is then used. This is subsequently replaced with a punch. The nerve roots leaving the vertebra are viewed microscopically.
- The end plate is prepared for interbody fusion.
- Once the disc space has been meticulously prepared, cancellous bone is inserted into the disc space using angled and straight forceps (or a funnel). A cage or spacer is then inserted with autologous bone or bone substitute.
- The marker pin is removed, and the pedicle screws are screwed in. The rod is inserted either using the conventional technique or with a rod inserter (below).

Percutaneous Instrumentation of the Contralateral Side

- Skin incisions 1–2 cm long are made, as planned, slightly lateral to the pedicle. Incisions are also made in the fascia to make tissue dilatation easier.
- Using C-arm fluoroscopy, the pedicle is accessed with a Jamshidi needle. The correct entry point should be identified in both AP and lateral X-ray views (see Fig. 49.5).
- After placing the Jamshidi needle at the intersection of the facet and the transverse process, the needle may be driven partially through the pedicle using a hammer. When the Jamshidi needle reaches the medial wall on the

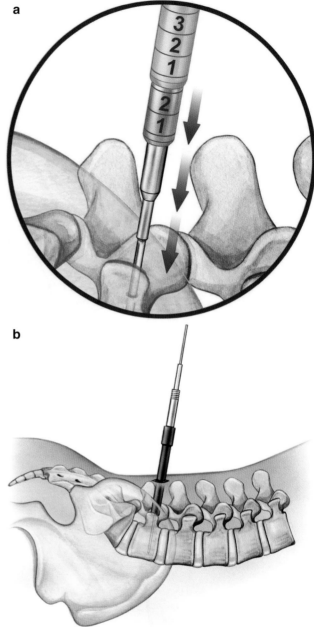

Fig. 49.8 (**a, b**) Insertion of the dilatation sheath

AP view, its position needs to be verified in the lateral view to ensure that the needle is in the bony canal of the pedicle (see Fig. 49.6a, b).

- The handle and inner trocar are removed from the Jamshidi needle, and a K-wire is inserted. The position of the K-wire is verified with fluoroscopy to ensure that it extends through 2/3 of the vertebral body (see Fig. 49.7). *Note*: During advancement of the K-wire, its progress must be checked using continuous radiological monitoring.

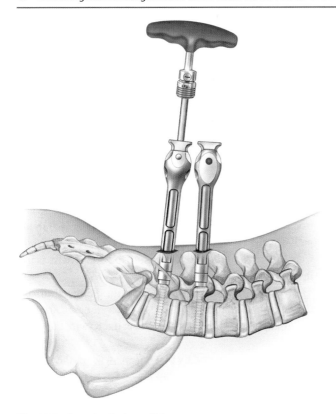

Fig. 49.9 Screwing in the pedicle screws

- An incision is made in the skin and fascia around the K-wire. The incision is dilated with dilatation tubes (see Fig. 49.8a, b).
- The pedicle is prepared by placing an awl over the K-wire or, if the bone is too hard, a tap may be used to prepare the pedicle screw canal. The K-wire must be held in position when removing the awl or tap. *Note*: The axis of the tap must be kept constant to avoid bending the wire. The K-wire must not advance during tapping and must not become displaced when instruments are removed.
- Using the additional extender, the pedicle screws are driven over the K-wire into the prepared pedicle. Fluoroscopy must be used to monitor screw insertion and placement (Fig. 49.9). Once the screw reaches the posterior aspect of the vertebral body, the wire can be removed.
- *Note*: The screw assembly must not be inserted too far. The K-wire must not be allowed to advance.
- The second screw is inserted in the same way. *Note*: After inserting additional bone screws, the heads of the bone screws should be at the same height.
- The extenders are connected.
- The rod inserter is attached.
- A trocar is used to prepare the way through the fascia and muscle (see Fig. 49.10a). The trocar is inserted through a small skin incision and pushed through the muscle, checking its position on the image converter, until it reaches the first screw.

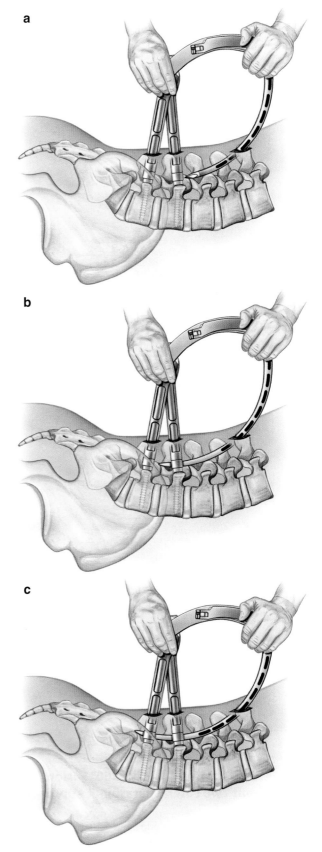

Fig. 49.10 Swinging items into place: trocar (**a**), rod (**b**), and final position (**c**)

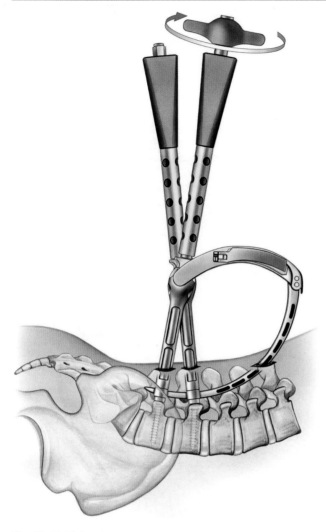

Fig. 49.11 Fixing the setscrews

- A rod-measuring instrument is used to determine the correct rod length.
- Using the rod inserter, the rod is then pushed into the heads of the polyaxial screws (see Fig. 49.10b, c). *Note*: The AP view must also be used to check whether the rod has been inserted into both the screw heads.
- The rod is then fixed with setscrews (see Fig. 49.11). *Note*: Fixation must start with the deepest screw. The firmness of the connection must be checked by pulling on the inserter.

49.6.2 Method II: Less-Invasive 360° Fusion About Two Lateral Paraspinal Approaches

- A 4–5-cm skin incision is made approximately 3 cm from the midline, and the fascia is incised and divided (see Fig. 49.12a and 49.21).
- Using the fingers, the muscles are bluntly dissected, and an MLD retractor (Aesculap) is introduced (see

Fig. 49.12b, c). Upon insertion, the retractor exposes portions of the lamina, facet joints, and transverse process.

- *Conventional screw technique with uncannulated screws.* Under X-ray control and using a Steinmann nail, the pedicles are drilled open and polyaxial screws (S4 internal system, Aesculap) are then placed transpedicularly (see Fig. 49.13).
- *Cannulated screw technique.*
  After the screw entry point has been determined, the pedicle is accessed. The guiding instrument is inserted at the junction between the facet and the transverse process. The trocar is then removed, leaving the targeting device in the pedicle. The K-wire is inserted to guide the screws. *Note*: Care must always be taken to ensure that the K-wire is not inserted too far.
- The working area must be dilated with the metal dilatation sheath so that the implant screws can be positioned. The dilatation sheath is guided in via the K-wire targeting device.
- The pedicle is prepared by placing an awl over the K-wire or, if the bone is too hard, a tap may be used to prepare the pedicle screw canal.
- Using the additional extender, the pedicle screws are driven over the K-wire into the prepared pedicle.
- The disc space is distracted with angulated distraction forceps.
- After pedicle screw insertion, the superior and inferior articular processes are resected with a high-speed drill and Kerrison punch. In cases of unilateral nerve root compression, the facet joint is resected on that side only.
- The intervertebral disc is exposed and is subtotally resected using angled rongeurs, shavers, and curettes (see Fig. 49.14a, b and 49.15).
- After scraping off the end plates, bone or bone substitute is packed into the anterior part of the disc space. Insertion of a trial to measure the hight of the implant (see Fig. 49.16).
- A curved PEEK cage specially designed for the TLIF technique is packed with bone or bone substitute and inserted into the disc space (see Fig. 49.17a–d).
- The tulips heads of the bone screws are aligned using a screw head adjuster to facilitate rod insertion.
- The appropriate rod is loaded into a fixed rod holder.
- A rod is inserted into the heads of the polyaxial screws and fixed with setscrews. The precontoured bullet-nosed rod is inserted.
- The polyaxial head is given 42° angulation to provide optimal and easy rod placement. To reposition the vertebra in cases with spondylolisthesis, the setscrew of the higher pedicle is fixed first. Only then is the setscrew of the lower pedicle fixed. *Note*: Rod position and advancement must be verified using fluoroscopy until fully seated (see Fig. 49.18a).

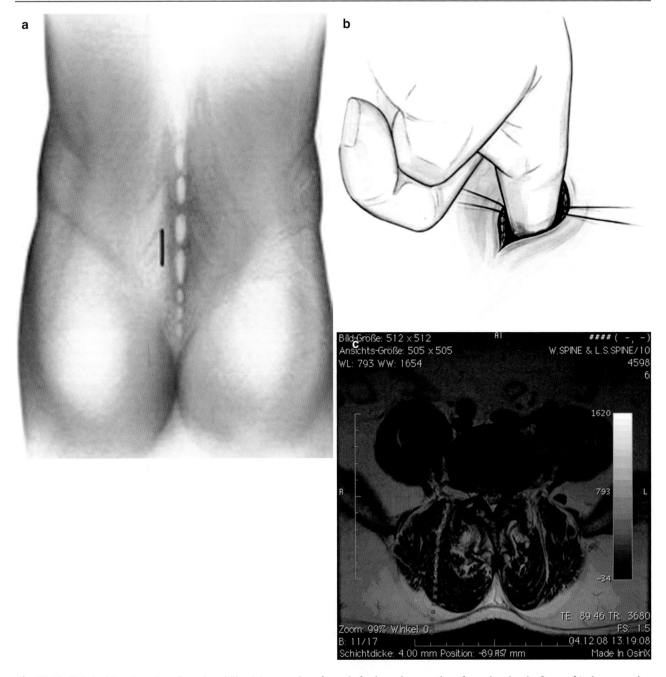

Fig. 49.12 Skin incision about 3 cm from the midline (**a**), separation of muscle fascia, and preparation of muscle using the fingers (**b**), demonstration of the lateral paraspinal approach on an MRI scan (**c**)

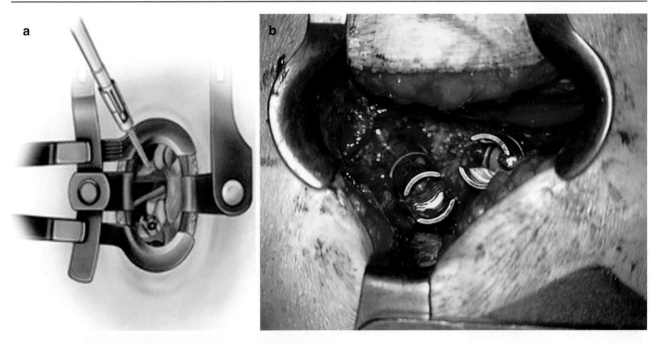

Fig. 49.13 Insertion of MLD retractor and transpedicular positioning of pedicle screws (**a**), intraoperative situation (**b**)

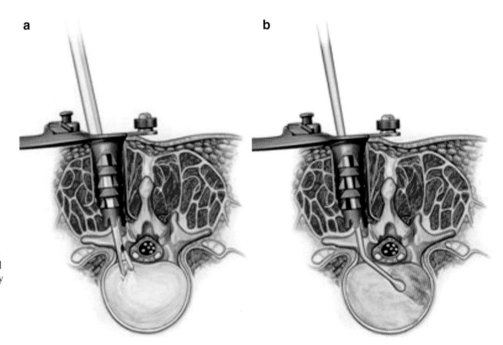

Fig. 49.14 (**a**) Discectomy and debridement of the intervertebral surfaces of the (**b**) vertebral body as far as the contralateral side using angled instruments (With permission from Aesculap AG, Tuttlingen, Germany)

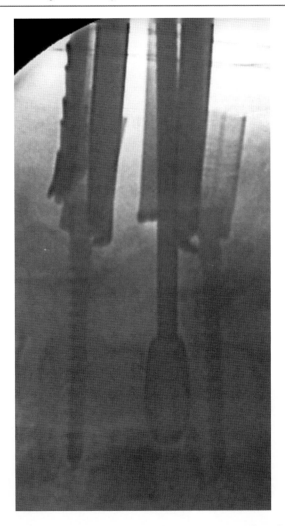

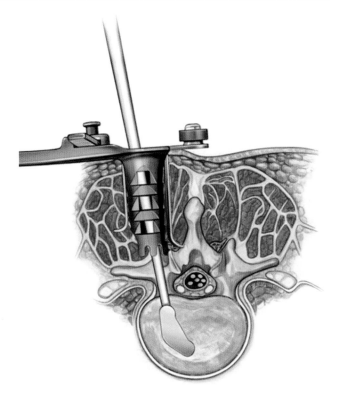

Fig. 49.16 Insertion of a trial to measure the height of the implant (With permission of Aesculap AG, Tuttlingen, Germany)

Fig. 49.15 Intraoperative X-ray demonstrats the preparation of the endplates with plate shavers

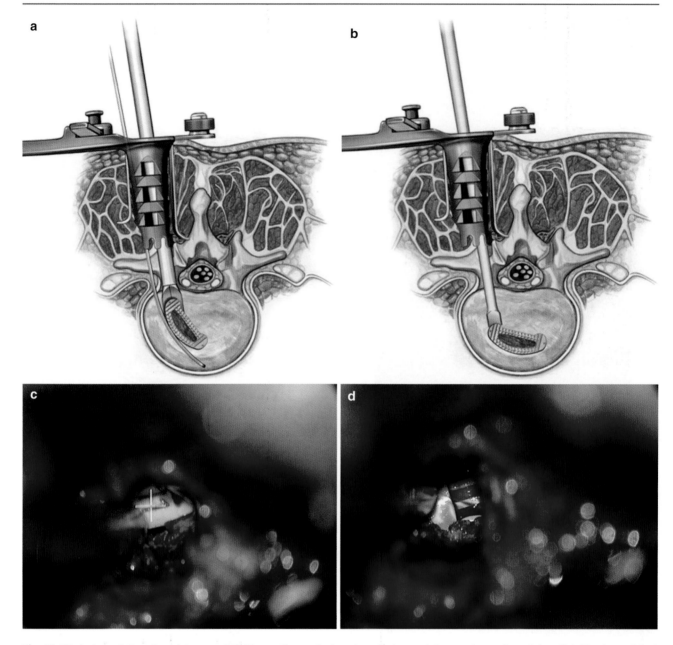

Fig. 49.17 (**a**, **b**, **c**, **d**) Insertion of the curved TLIF cage. Bone substitute is packed around the cage (ventrally and dorsally). Turning and final positioning of the cage (intraoperative situation)

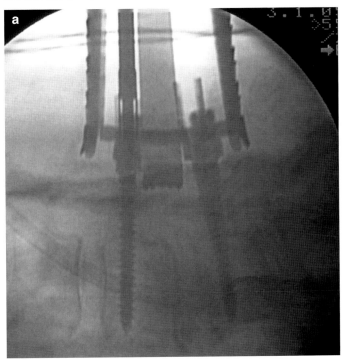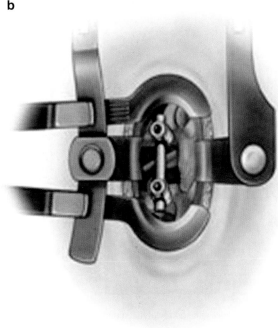

Fig. 49.18 Fixing of the rod (**a**) intraoperative X-ray (**b**) illustration

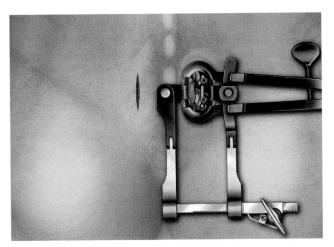

Fig. 49.19 Contralateral pedicle screw instrumentation (With permission of Aescupap AG, Tuttlingen, Germany)

• After closure of the fascia and skin, an identical procedure is carried out on the contralateral side (see Figs. 49.19, 49.20 and 49.21).

49.7 Tips and Tricks

• The K-wires should remain securely in position throughout the entire procedure and must not slip out before the screws are inserted. The wires are long enough to be held in place by hand during the different surgical steps.
• The tip of the K-wire should be monitored fluoroscopically to ensure that it does not penetrate the anterior wall of the vertebral body.
• The K-wires should be kept parallel to one another during insertion.

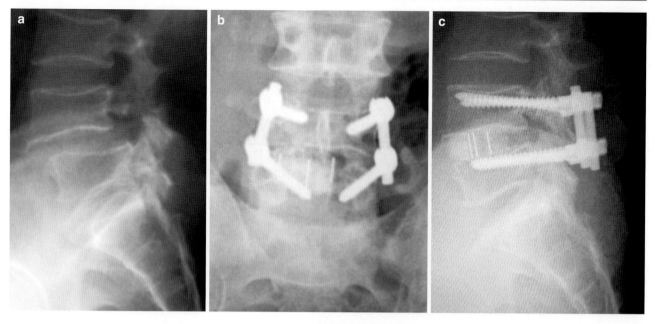

Fig. 49.20 Patient with spondylolytic spondylolisthesis: preoperative X-ray at L4/L5 (**a**) and postoperative AP (**b**) and lateral (**c**) X-rays

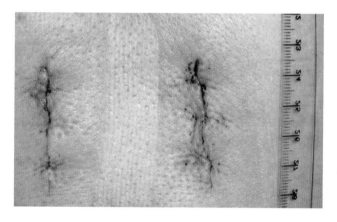

Fig. 49.21 Length of the two scin incision (3–4 cm) postoperativly

References

1. Foley KT, Holly LT, Schwender JD (2003) Minimally invasive lumbar fusion. Spine 28(suppl):26–35
2. Jong JS, Lee SH (2005) Minimally invasive transforaminal lumbar interbody fusion with ipsilateral pedicle screw and contralateral facet screw fixation. J Neurosurg Spine 3:218–223
3. Khoo LT, Palmer S, Loich OT (2005) Minimally invasive percutaneous posterior lumbar interbody fusion. Neurosurgery 51(Suppl 2): 166–181
4. Wimmer C, Pfandlsteiner T, Walochnik N (2006) Less invasive spine fusion. A comparison study. Eur Spine J 10:179–182

Cement Augmentation of Pedicle Screw Fixation

50

Jürgen Nothwang

50.1 Introduction and Core Messages

Reduced bone quality is a particular problem of spine surgery in elderly people. Anchorage of pedicle screws can be improved with cement augmentation to achieve increased pull-out strength and greater stability of the pedicle screws. In principle, augmentation of the screw can be achieved using two different techniques: (1) cement insertion through cannulated pedicle screws with slots (either open or minimally invasive) or (2) vertebroplasty followed by insertion of the pedicle screw into the cement (either open or minimally invasive).

50.2 Indications

- Osteoporosis or history of osteoporosis treatment
- Past osteoporotic fracture
- Decrease of bone mineral density to ≤ 90–100 mg/cm^3
- Rarification of trabecular pattern in CT scan
- Need for multisegmental stabilisation in older patient
- Multilevel osteolytic destruction of the vertebral bodies (i.e., multiple myeloma, plasmocytoma, NHL)

50.3 Contraindications

- Reduced general condition of the patient: pulmonary and cardiac risk factors (ASA $\geq$ IV, NYHA IV)
- Allergy to radiopaque cement
- Severe pre-existing deformity with high degree of osteoporosis of the whole vertebral column

50.4 Technical Prerequisites

- Fluoroscopy, radiolucent operating table, (in multilevel stabilisation – i.e., de novo scoliotic deformity – a slidable operating table is helpful).
- Cannulated pedicle screws with slots or holes (see Figs. 50.1 and 50.3a–c).

J. Nothwang, M.D.
Department of Traumatology and Orthopedics,
Rems-Murr-Kliniken gGmbH, Schlichener Strasse 105,
73614 Schondorf, Germany
e-mail: jnothwang@khrmk.de

U. Vieweg, F. Grochulla (eds.), *Manual of Spine Surgery*,
DOI 10.1007/978-3-642-22682-3_50, © Springer-Verlag Berlin Heidelberg 2012

Fig. 50.1 Augmentable cannulated monoaxial pedicle screw (SOCON, Aesculap) (With permission from Aesculap AG, Tuttlingen, Germany)

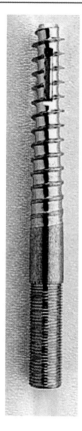

the functional spine unit can bear about 8,000 N (1,800 lbf) of compressive load. Between 40 and 60 years, the strength decreases to 55% of this value, and above 60 years it decreases to 45% [6].

- Compression forces generated by various loading conditions affect the end plates of the vertebral bodies more than the vertebral walls. Fatigue of the end plate is an important cause of cut out of pedicle screws and adjacent level disease.
- By using 2–3 cm^3 cement to augment a screw, we can increase the strength to greater than that of larger diameter screws in normal density bone (~1,600 N) [3, 4, 8].
- Recent clinical studies confirm the biomechanical results of cement augmentation and indicate high levels of reliability and safety [2].

50.6 Planning, Preparation, and Positioning

- Preoperative X-rays and CT scans are analysed to evaluate the diameter and direction of the pedicles and the integrity of the vertebral wall.
- Patient lies in a prone position (see Fig. 50.4).
- The position of the pedicles should be verified preoperatively by fluoroscopy.
- The pedicle is exposed symmetrically with the spinous processes in the midline.

50.7 Operating Technique

50.7.1 Approach

The skin incision depends on the surgical technique chosen. To avoid the risk of higher blood loss especially in older patients, percutaneous minimally invasive instrumentation techniques are becoming more and more important. In our experience, they have also influenced the assessment of the risks to the patient arising from the anaesthetic and the operation.

I *Minimally Invasive Technique*
- We use the same technique as for vertebro- or kyphoplasty: the skin incision is at the lateral border of the pedicle.
- The incision should have a length of 10 mm to provide enough space for later insertion of the rod.
- Blunt dissection of the soft tissue leads to the cross-section of transverse process and facet joint.
- For subsequent steps, the soft tissue should be protected by a sleeve.

- For the minimally invasive technique, cannulated instruments are essential.
- Connecting device for cement delivery to the pedicle screw (Luer lock connector).
- Radiopaque low viscosity slow setting cement.
- Trocars for cannulation and vertebroplasty augmentation.

50.5 Basic Biomechanical Messages

- The strength of the vertebrae decreases with age [1], with a definite relationship between failure stress and vertebral bone quality.
- A 25% decrease in bone quality results in a decrease of more than 50% in the strength of a vertebra.
- There is a high correlation between the risk of screw loosening and the density of the bone [7]. The quality of the bone is more important than the design of the pedicle screws. Below a critical bone density (≤90–100 mg/cm^3), early loosening of the screws is to be expected. Clinical trials confirmed these biomechanical results [5].
- Reduced bone mineral density must be addressed in early end plate failure under axial load. Below 40 years of age,

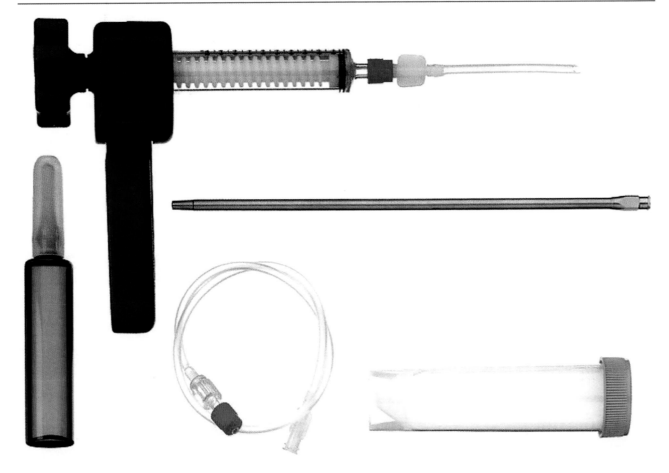

Fig. 50.2 Application set for pedicle screw augmentation (Aesculap) (With permission from Aesculap AG, Tuttlingen, Germany)

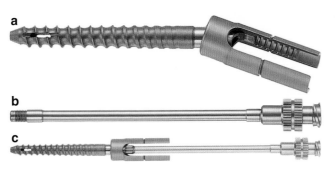

Fig. 50.3 Cannulated polyaxial pedicle screw for cement augmentation (**a**) (S4, Aesculap), with delivery cannula (**b**) and connected to the pedicle screw (**c**) (With permission from Aesculap AG, Tuttlingen, Germany)

II *Open Procedure*
- Under fluoroscopic control, we mark the beginning and end point of the planned extent of instrumentation.
- The midline incision has to respect these end points and should allow the instrumentation of the pedicles without stressing the skin.

- The preparation then follows the typical steps as already described in previous chapters.
- A blunt retractor exposes the field of operation.

50.7.2 Instrumentation

I *Minimally Invasive Technique*
Trocar Technique
- When the trocar has reached the lateral border of the pedicle, the lateral cortex is opened.
- The trocar is inserted towards the medial border of the pedicle using AP imaging.
- In the lateral plane, the trocar should penetrate a little way past the posterior margin of the vertebral body.
- Having ensured the correct position, the trocar can be replaced with a long threaded wire.
- With a soft tissue dilator, the access to the pedicle should be expanded.
- The pedicle is opened towards its entrance into the vertebral body with a tap.

Fig. 50.4 Positioning of the patient

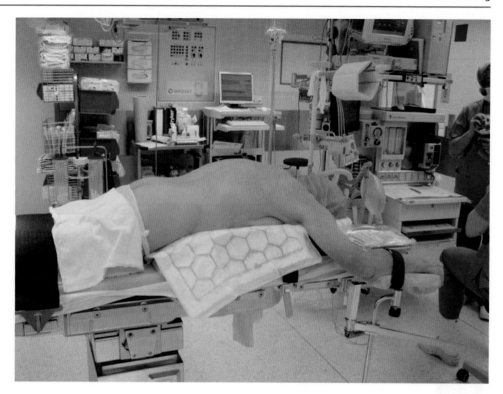

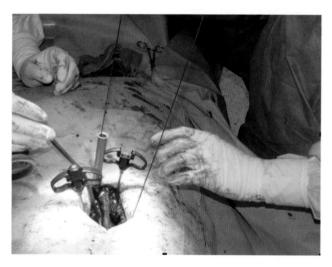

Fig. 50.5 Instrumentation in a cannulated technique

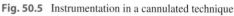

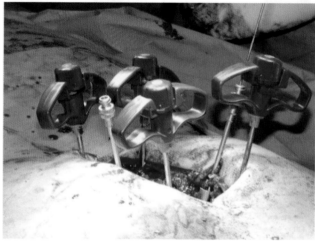

Fig. 50.6 Adaption of the connector guided by the K-wire

- The tap is removed and the trocar is again inserted at least into the first third of the vertebral body.
- The length of the screws (i.e., 45–50 mm) should be measured and prepared by the operating nurse.
- The low-viscosity cement is prepared. The right moment for application of the cement is comparable to the viscosity characteristics for vertebro- or kyphoplastic cement application (with or without application set) (see Fig 50.2).
- The trocar is filled with cement. The cement is then injected into the vertebral body under controlled conditions using the inserter. Usually, 2–3 cm³ is required for each side (Fig. 50.8).

- *Attention*: Avoid cement extrusion into the disc and spinal canal. Stop cement insertion if cement flow into a vessel is observed.
- The threaded wire is inserted through the trocar, and the trocar can be removed.
- Then, the prepared screws can be inserted along the threaded wires.

Direct Screw Augmentation

- New pedicle screw designs allow cement to be delivered after the cannulated and perforated pedicle screws have been positioned (Fig. 50.3a).

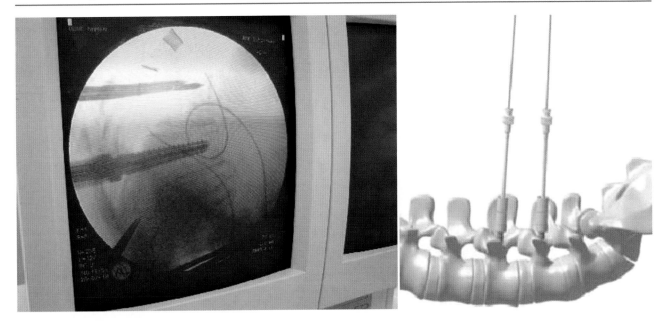

Fig. 50.7 Jamshidi needles and slot screw with K-wire: schema and X-ray imaging

Fig. 50.8 Jamshidi augmentation technique and X-ray imaging

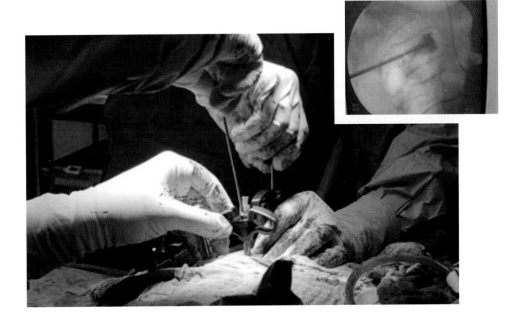

- (Advantage: more stable connection between the cement and the pedicle screws through the side-opening holes or slots of the screw.)
- After insertion of the screws, a connector is fixed to the pedicle screw, and the cement is injected into the screw (Figs. 50.3a, b and 50.7).
- The cement flow and anchorage must be observed using fluoroscopy (Fig. 50.9).
- *Attention*: Do not perforate the anterior cortex of the vertebral body. Do not allow cement to enter the central vertebral vein which leads directly into the spinal canal.

Because of reduced bending stability, polyaxial screws are not suitable for bisegmental four-point fixation.

II *Open Procedure*
- The entrance point on the pedicle is identified, and the pedicle is then opened and penetrated using an awl or trocar. Correct positioning must be checked with fluoroscopy.
- The integrity of the pedicle must be confirmed using the ball-tipped probe.
- The subsequent steps are as for the trocar or direct-screw application technique described above.

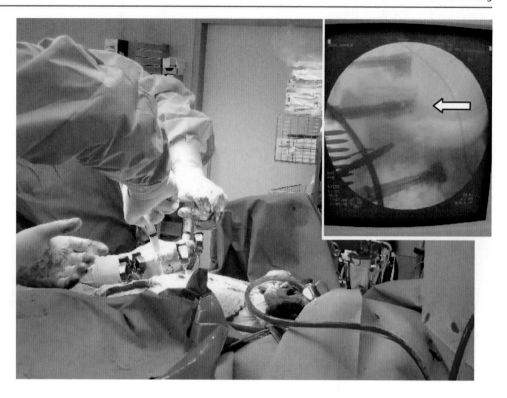

Fig. 50.9 Slot-screw augmentation technique and X-ray imaging

- Non-cannulated screws can be inserted into the tapped pedicle canal.
- In open approaches, cannulated pedicle screws allowing direct cement injection are preferred. The screws must not perforate the anterior cortex.
- The low-viscosity cement can be inserted with an adapter device and a Luer lock connection. A cement gun is helpful.
- *Attention*: Following the line of least resistance, the cement leaves the screw first through the most proximal lateral holes (beware: central vein and posterior venous sinusoids). If there is a slot in the screw, the valve effect is lower. The distribution of the cement seems to be better, but the risk of central cement leakage still remains. In our experience, the safest position of the screws is close to the anterior wall. Notice that even under high caution cement augmentation technique includes a respectable rate of complications. In an own one year investigation of 39 cases with 100 augmented pedicle instrumentations, the rate of complications due to cement application reached 15% and included paravertebral cement extrusion, lung embolism and in 2 cases temporary radicular deficiency.

50.8   Tips and Tricks

- For cement application, the pedicle screws must be perfectly seated. For instrumentation and cement insertion, fluoroscopic control is essential. If possible, simultaneous fluoroscopy in both planes provides maximum safety.

- Tapping should only extend as far as the pedicle root and should not be continued into the vertebral body. The trocar for cement delivery should then be anchored in the cancellous bone of the anterior vertebral body. This prevents the cement from flowing along the tapped canal towards the pedicle.
- The time of cement application often depends on individual experience and special knowledge of the cement being used. It is likely that this problem can be solved in future with the help of a viscometer which is provided by several companies. It must, of course, be remembered that these viscometers are normally calibrated to the cement of the particular company.
- In our experience, the trocar insertion technique is the safest method of controlling the flow of cement. After pushing the inserter into the trocar, the distribution of the cement can be followed under fluoroscopy.
- If there are any doubts concerning the precise position of the trocar, it can be checked in relation to the 45-degree "Scottie dog projection". Especially in L5 with a very lateral pedicle entrance, this fluoroscopic control is helpful to confirm correct pedicle penetration.
- In cases of generalised decrease of bone mineral density due to osteoporosis or tumour diseases (plasmocytoma, multiple myeloma, NHL), the spine surgeon should consider prophylactic adjacent level vertebroplasty.
- In accordance with the traditional rules governing the treatment of spinal deformities, instrumentation should not terminate within the apex of the kyphotic or scoliotic deformity to avoid progression of the deformity and adjacent level collapse.

References

1. Bell GH, Dunbar O, Beck JS et al (1967) Variation in strength of vertebrae with age and their relationship to osteoporosis. Calcif Tissue Res 1:75–86

2. Chang MC, Liu CL, Chen Th (2008) Polymethylmethacrylate augmentation of pedicle screws for osteoporotic spinal surgery: a novel technique. Spine 33(10):317–324

3. Cohen DB, Cullinane D et al: Biomechanics of pedicle screw augmentation using polymethylmethacrylate. New Orleans, LA: North American Spine Society 15th Annual Meeting 2000 p 167

4. Frankel B (2007) Segmental polymethylmethacrylate-augmented pedicle screw fixation in patients with bone softening due to osteoporosis and metastatic tumor involvement. A clinical evaluation. Neurosurgery 61:531–538

5. Okuyama K, Abe E, Suzuki T et al (2001) Influence of bone mineral density on pedicle screw fixation, a study of pedicle screw fixation augmenting posterior lumbar interbody fusion in elderly patients. Spine J 1:402–407

6. Perey O (1957) Fracture of the vertebral end plate in the lumbar spine: an experimental biomechanical investigation. Acta Orthop Scand Suppl 25:1–101

7. Wittenberg RH, Shea M, Swartz DE et al (1991) Importance of bone mineral density in instrumented spine fusions. Spine 16:647–652

8. Zindrick MR, Wiltse LL, Widell EH et al (1986) A biomechanical study of intrapeduncular screw fixation in the lumbosacral spine. Clin Orthop 203:99–112

Less-Invasive Pedicle Screw Instrumentation of Lumbar Spine Fractures

51

Ulrich Hahn

51.1 Introduction and Core Messages

The distinctive feature of the minimally invasive posterior dorsal instrumentation is not so much the less-invasive placement of mono- or polyaxial pedicle screws, but rather the fact that it allows a genuine distraction and lordosis reduction, the real benefit of the procedure described here. However, this minimally invasive reduction requires a special instrumentation and the mandatory use of monoaxial pedicle screws since only such screws can sustain the preload resulting from the reduction. The goals of the minimally invasive posterior instrumentation with S4 fracture reduction instruments are almost no soft tissue damage because muscle attachments are not detached, same reduction results as in open procedures, same implants as for open procedures, reduced postoperative pain, shorter operation time, and negligible blood loss.

51.2 Indications

- Anterior compression fractures with kyphosis angle and unstable fractures of the lumbar spine [1]
- Only restricted indication in AO C-type fractures (see contraindications [3])
- Only relative indications in multilevel injuries [6]

51.3 Contraindications

- Severe osteoporosis, osteopenia, or osteomyelitis
- Transverse connector required in cases of rotational instability
- Same contraindications as for open procedures [2, 7]

51.4 Technical Prerequisites

Fluoroscopy, radiolucent operating table, cannulated pedicle screws (S4 Spinal System, Aesculap AG), special fracture reduction instruments (e.g., S4 spinal system with fracture reduction instrument – FRI, Aesculap, see Fig. 51.1). If kyphosis correction is intended, the use of monoaxial fracture screws is required because only these screws can sustain the preload of the reduction maneuver. There are other devices available for percutaneous dorsal instrumentation (e.g., Sextant, Medtronic), but at the moment, only the FRI device allows genuine fracture reduction.

U. Hahn, M.D.
Department for Trauma and Orthopedic Surgery,
Medical Center Geldern,
Clemensstr. 4, 47608 Geldern, Germany
e-mail: u.hahn@aoz-geldern.de

U. Vieweg, F. Grochulla (eds.), *Manual of Spine Surgery*,
DOI 10.1007/978-3-642-22682-3_51, © Springer-Verlag Berlin Heidelberg 2012

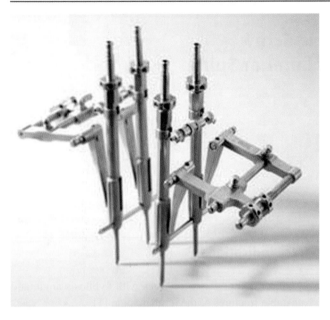

Fig. 51.1 S4 fracture reduction instrument (Aesculap AG) (With permission from Aesculap AG, Tuttlingen, Germany)

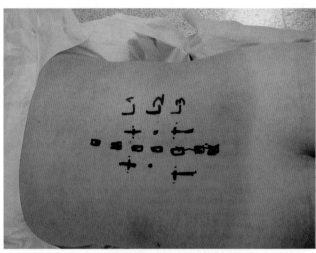

Fig. 51.2 Preoperative fluoroscopy-based planning of the skin incision

51.5 Planning, Preparation, and Positioning

During the operation, the patient is in a prone position on a radiolucent operating table. Different positioning systems can be used (Wilson frame, chest rolls, Relton-Hall frame, etc.).

Exact C-arm-controlled planning of the approach is mandatory (see Fig. 51.2).

51.6 Surgical Technique

51.6.1 Approach

- Access is obtained by an incision of the thoracolumbar fascia between the multifidus and the longissimus muscles. The muscles are dissected bluntly only in the fiber direction. As a rule, this procedure can be carried out without bleeding or with minimal blood loss. With the help of an appropriate cannulated guiding device (see Fig. 51.3), the entry point is selected at the junction of the facet and the transverse process.
- Remove the trocar; the K-wire aiming device remains in the pedicle (see Fig. 51.4).
- To guide the cannulated pedicle screw, insert the K-wire into the aiming device. As alternative, you can use a K-wire protection sleeve (see Fig. 51.5).

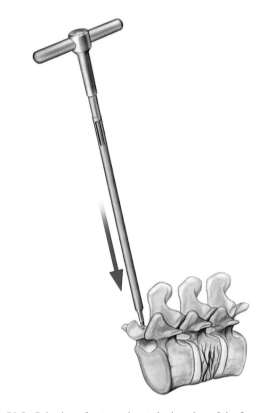

Fig. 51.3 Selection of entry point at the junction of the facet and the transverse process and decortication with cannulated guiding device (With permission from Aesculap AG, Tuttlingen, Germany)

- *Note*: The Kirschner wire should be inserted so far that its tip represents the end position of the pedicle screw tip.
- You must be absolutely certain that the Kirschner wire is not inserted too far to avoid damaging soft tissue and vessels. Use intraoperative fluoroscopy!

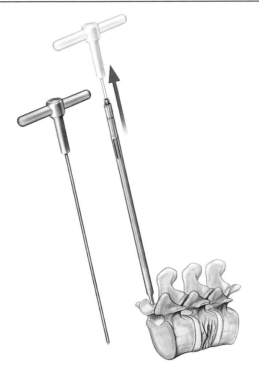

Fig. 51.4 Removal of trocar, the K-wire aiming device remains in the pedicle (With permission from Aesculap AG, Tuttlingen, Germany)

- Insert dilatation sleeves via the K-wire aiming device to create sufficient space for the pedicle screw (see Fig. 51.6).
- Slide the blue tissue protection sleeve over the dilatation sleeve (see Fig. 51.7).

51.6.2 Instrumentation [1–7]

- If necessary, use a pedicle reamer to further prepare the pedicle (see Fig. 51.8) or, in the case of sclerotic bone, a thread cutter with the appropriate diameter (see Fig. 51.9).
- To determine the length of the screw, insert the screw length-measuring instrument, with the calibration markings turned upward, via the K-wire and place it on the vertebral body with the distal end (see Fig. 51.10). The length of the screw can be read from the markings on the K-wire (see Fig. 51.10).
- Insert the screws with the cannulated screwdriver under fluoroscopy guidance in lateral and anteroposterior projections.
- *Note*: If necessary, after 3–4 turns of the screw, the K-wire should be removed to avoid its rotation and ventral perforation.

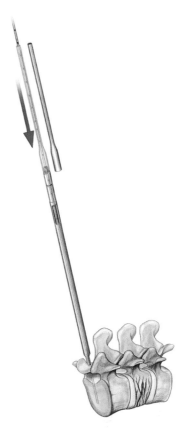

Fig. 51.5 Insertion of K-wire, if necessary, a K-wire protection sleeve is used (With permission from Aesculap AG, Tuttlingen, Germany)

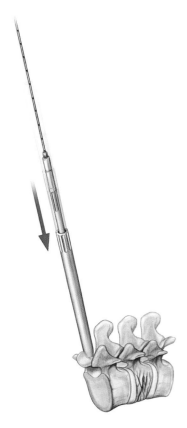

Fig. 51.6 Insertion of dilatation sleeves via the K-wire aiming device (With permission from Aesculap AG, Tuttlingen, Germany)

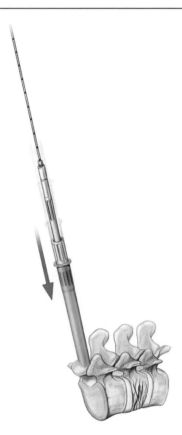

Fig. 51.7 Sliding of the blue tissue protection sleeve over the dilatation sleeve (With permission from Aesculap AG, Tuttlingen, Germany)

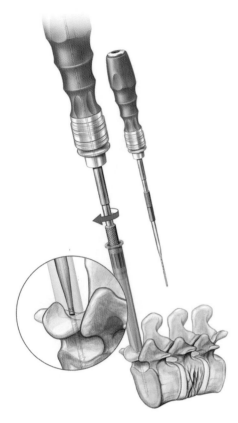

Fig. 51.9 Preparation of pedicle using a thread cutter in the case of sclerotic bone (With permission from Aesculap AG, Tuttlingen, Germany)

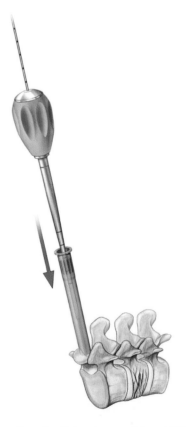

Fig. 51.8 Preparation of pedicle using a pedicle awl (With permission from Aesculap AG, Tuttlingen, Germany)

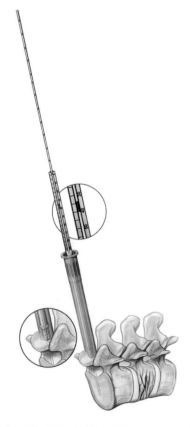

Fig. 51.10 Length determination using the cannulated measuring instrument (With permission from Aesculap AG, Tuttlingen, Germany)

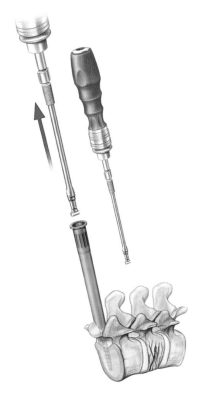

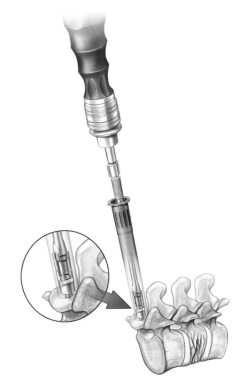

Fig. 51.11 Correct alignment of the screw slot, using the wings of the alignment device (With permission from Aesculap AG, Tuttlingen, Germany)

Fig. 51.12 As alternative, a special alignment device can be used (With permission from Aesculap AG, Tuttlingen, Germany)

- Align the screw to the cranio-caudal axis. Both sides of the screwdriver must show in the cranio-caudal direction (see Fig. 51.11). If necessary, a special top piece can be used (Fig. 51.12).
- Measure the length of the rod with the rod length–measuring instrument (see Fig. 51.13). If a distraction is necessary, a longer rod should be used accordingly. If you use prebent rods, add ca. 10 mm.
- Then, insert the FRI outer sleeves through the tissue protection sleeves. Align the longitudinal slit of the outer sleeve caudally. Then, remove the protection sleeves and insert the transverse rod with the rod inserter (see Fig. 51.14).
- *Note*: Before placing the FRI outer sleeves, the surgical field can be kept free using a Langenbeck hook; the rod can then be inserted through this aperture (see Fig. 51.15).
- Put the reduction lever in place, the setscrew is received; then insert the construct through the FRI sleeve in the pedicle screw (see Fig. 51.16). Screw the construct as far as it will go into the flanks of the pedicle screw (see Fig. 51.17).
- *Note*: Make sure the setscrew does not block the rod to avoid blocking the distraction (s. b.). If necessary, loosen the setscrews a quarter of a turn.

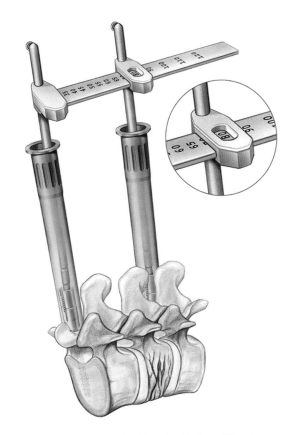

Fig. 51.13 Measurement of rod length with the rod length–measuring instrument (With permission from Aesculap AG, Tuttlingen, Germany)

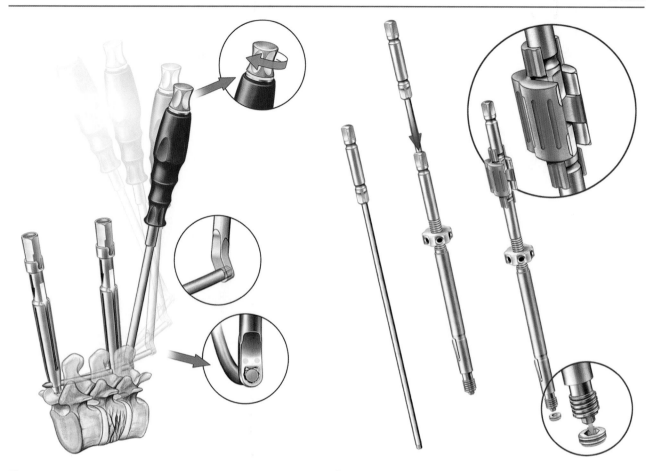

Fig. 51.14 Representation of screw with two Langenbeck hooks (With permission from Aesculap AG, Tuttlingen, Germany)

Fig. 51.16 Assembly of reduction lever (With permission from Aesculap AG, Tuttlingen, Germany)

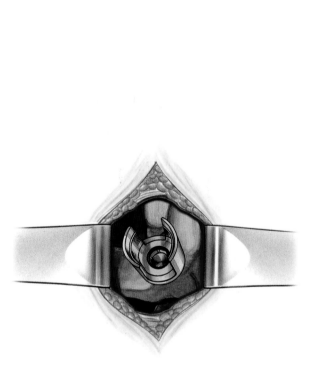

Fig. 51.15 Insertion of rod with rod inserter (With permission from Aesculap AG, Tuttlingen, Germany)

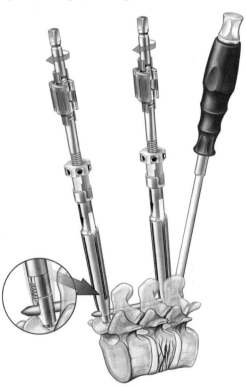

Fig. 51.17 Turning of setscrew down to contact. If necessary, loosen a quarter of a turn (With permission from Aesculap AG, Tuttlingen, Germany)

Fig. 51.18 (**a**)
Installation of
distractor and
(**b**) reduction of
vertebral height
(With permission
from Aesculap AG,
Tuttlingen, Germany)

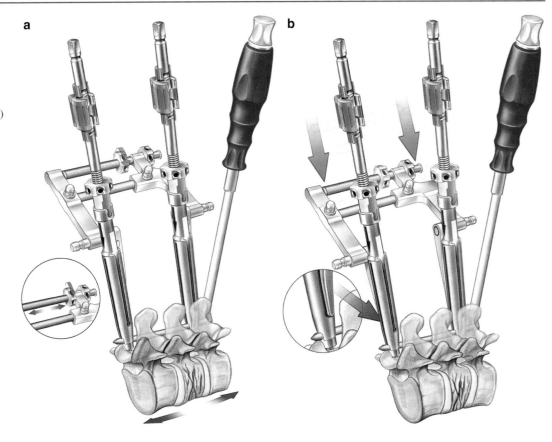

51.6.3 Reduction

- Now, the installation of the distraction tool follows. The
  distractor is inserted via the bolt in the guiding groove of
  the cranial and caudal outer sleeve. The distraction blades
  must be aligned parallel to the outer sleeves (see
  Fig. 51.18a, b). The distraction is carried out consecu-
  tively (1 surgeon) or simultaneously (surgeon and assistant) under C-arm guidance.
- To reconstruct the natural lordosis, insert the spindle distractor into the corresponding nut and, by activating the
  control knob, adjust the lordosis under fluoroscopy guidance (see Fig. 51.19a, b).
- Using the regulating screw on the threaded tube, press
  the rod firmly. You must loosen the regulating crew a
  quarter of a turn to avoid blocking of the setscrew. Then,
  tighten up the setscrew with the screwdriver (see
  Fig. 51.20).
- Remove the screwdriver and unscrew the threaded tube
  with the ratchet handle (see Fig. 51.21).
- Final tightening of the construct is carried out with a
  countering instrument and a 10-Nm (90-in/lb) torque
  wrench (see Fig. 51.22). Finally, the flanks are broken
  off using the flank breaking forceps (Fig. 51.23).

51.7   Tips and Tricks

- Accurate positioning of patient, carefully aligned anterio-
  posteriorly to the perpendicular line of the room axis, is
  enormously helpful for the surgeon's spatial orientation
  and facilitates the initial pedicle screw alignment.
- If the instrumentation "is stuck," then loosen the setscrew
  or regulating screw little bit.
- If the insertion of prebent rods is planned, then it is helpful to position the cranial pedicle screws at an angle of ca.
  10° cranially and the caudal pedicle screws at an angle of
  ca. 10° caudally.

51.8   Results

The example of a LWK 1 AO-A3.1 fracture shows that,
through a minimally invasive procedure, the FRI instrumentation allows to achieve an anatomical reduction in
spite of restricted access. It permits a clearly more expedi-
tious postoperative mobilization of the patients while causing them less pain in comparison to the open procedure
(Figs. 51.23).

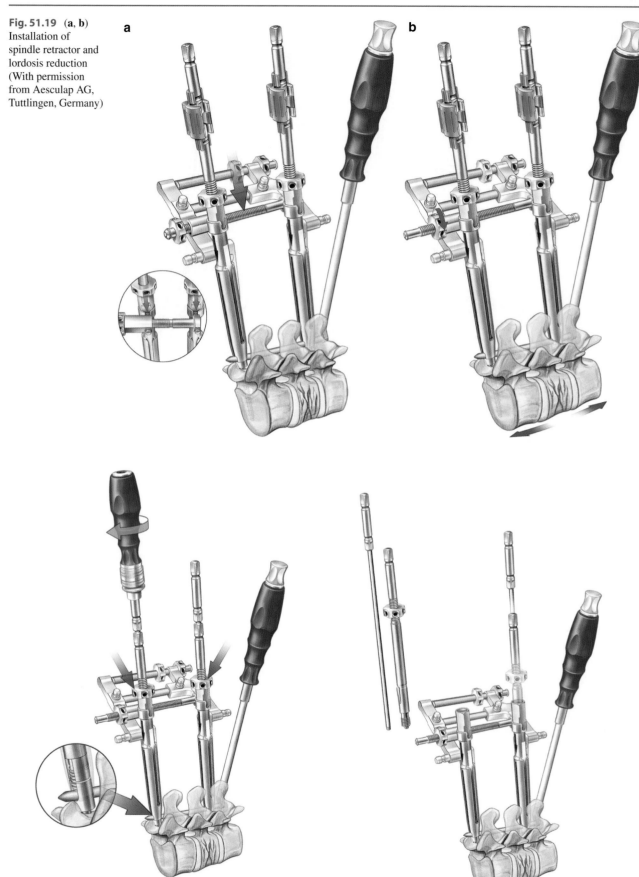

Fig. 51.19 (**a**, **b**) Installation of spindle retractor and lordosis reduction (With permission from Aesculap AG, Tuttlingen, Germany)

a

b

Fig. 51.20 Tightening the regulating screw and loosening a quarter of a turn. Tightening up the setscrew (With permission from Aesculap AG, Tuttlingen, Germany)

Fig. 51.21 Removal of screwdriver and threaded tubes (With permission from Aesculap AG, Tuttlingen, Germany)

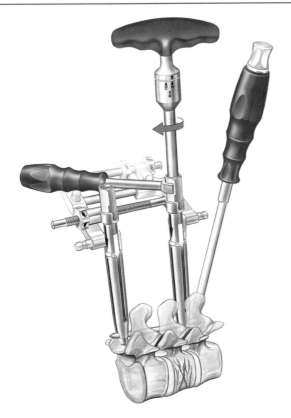

Fig. 51.22 Final tightening with prescribed torque (With permission from Aesculap AG, Tuttlingen, Germany)

References

1. Foley KT, Gupta SK (2002) Percutaneous pedicle screw fixation of the lumbar spine: preliminary clinical results. J Neurosurg 97(1 suppl):7–12
2. Grass R, Biewener A, Dickopf A et al (2006) Percutaneous dorsal versus open instrumentation for fractures of the thoracolumbar border. a comparative, prospective study. Unfallchirurg 109:297–305
3. Hahn U, Andermahr J, Prokop A, Rehm KE (2006) Minimal-invasive Operationstechniken an der Wirbelsäule. Mediathek der Deutschen Gesellschaft für Chirurgie: Aesculap Akademie
4. Korovessis P, Hadjipavlou A, Repantis T (2008) Minimal invasive short posterior instrumentation plus balloon kyphoplasty with calcium phosphate for burst and severe compression lumbar fractures. Spine 33:658–667
5. Merom L, Raz N, Hamud C et al (2009) Minimally invasive burst fracture fixation in the thoracolumbar region. Orthopedics 32(4):pii
6. Palmisani M, Gasbarrini A, Brodano GB et al (2009) Minimally invasive percutaneous fixation in the treatment of thoracic and lumbar spine fractures. Eur Spine J 18(suppl 1):71–74
7. Prokop A, Lohlein F, Chmielnicki M, Volbracht J (2009) Minimally invasive percutaneous instrumentation for spine fractures. Unfallchirurg 112:621–626

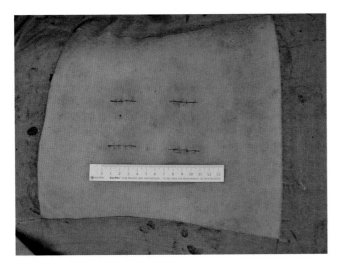

Fig. 51.23 Scars after less-invasive transpedicular stabilization

Transforaminal Lumbar Interbody Fusion

52

Stefan Kroppenstedt and Uwe Vieweg

52.1   Introduction and Core Messages

Interbody fusion performed by placing spacers or graft materials via a transfacetar route is named transarticular lumbar interbody fusion (TLIF). TLIF is typically performed via a unilateral approach and can be performed via a standard open approach with a midline lumbar incision or in a less-invasive mini-open fashion (see Chap. 49). Because the TLIF approach uses a unilateral facetectomy, it is typically combined with screw fixation (see Fig. 52.1). Advantages compared to bilateral PLIF are contralateral facet joint and posterior laminar arch are preserved and iatrogenic contralateral scar formation is eliminated. Further, exposure of the disc space requires less or no medial dural retraction.

This can be particularly advantageous in the face of scarring after prior surgery and in the thoracolumbar area, where the myelon restricts the retraction of the thecal sac. Other potential advantages are less bleeding and a shorter operation time. Compared to bilateral PLIF, TLIF has potentially the following disadvantages. In case of high-grade spondylolisthesis, extended segmental mobilization may be necessary to achieve a proper reduction. This can be done worse. Although contralateral decompression via undercutting is possible, it is technically more challenging. Since for TLIF generally one cage is used theoretically, the risk for cage migration and loss of correction is higher compared to bilateral PLIF using two cages, and thereby having a larger cage contact area to only approach an additional posterior decompression is possible in the bone face.

52.2   Indications

The indications and contraindications for TLIF are similar to those for posterior lumbar interbody fusion (PLIF).

- Degenerative diseases from the thoracolumbar area down to S1
- Degenerative pathologies that require complete facetectomies
- Isthmic spondylolisthesis
- Pseudoarthrosis after posterolateral fusion

S. Kroppenstedt, M.D., Ph.D. (✉)
Department of Spinal Surgery, Center of Orthopedic Surgery,
Sana Hospital Sommerfeld, Waldhausstraße 44,
16766 Kremmen, Germany
e-mail: s.kroppenstedt@sana-hu.de

U. Vieweg, M.D., Ph.D.
Clinic for Spinal Surgery, Sana Hospital Rummelsberg,
90593 Schwarzenbruck, Germany
e-mail: uwe.vieweg@yahoo.de

U. Vieweg, F. Grochulla (eds.), *Manual of Spine Surgery*,
DOI 10.1007/978-3-642-22682-3_52, © Springer-Verlag Berlin Heidelberg 2012

Fig. 52.1 Illustration of the transarticular or transforaminal interbody fusion (TLIF). (**a**) preserved facet joint (**b**) resected facet joint

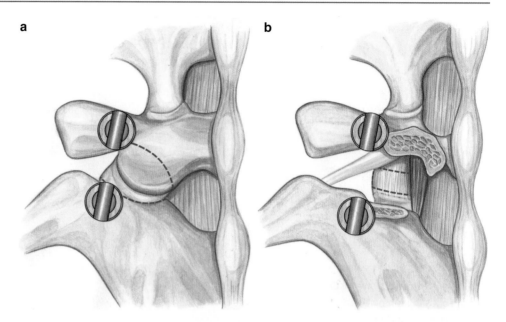

52.3   Contraindications

- High angulation of the level L5/S1
- Destruction of the end plates

52.4   Technical Prerequisites

Fluoroscopy, positioning device (e.g., Wiltse frame), adequate implants (e.g., kidney-shaped or banana-designed PEEK or titanium cages or spacer; see Fig. 52.2), and different instruments (Fig. 52.3a–c).

52.5   Planning, Preparation, and Positioning

The patient is positioned prone on a radiolucent operating room table with chest and hip rolls/pillows in order to enhance lumbar lordosis and to permit the abdomen to hang freely. For L5–S1 fusions, the operating table is moved in 20–30° of reverse Trendelenburg to allow the surgeon to have a more convenient view into the L5–S1 disc space. The level of the incision is verified fluoroscopically.

52.6   Surgical Technique [1–4]

52.6.1 Approach

A midline posterior approach to the spine is performed with subperiosteal exposure of the posterior bony elements to the level of the transverse processes.

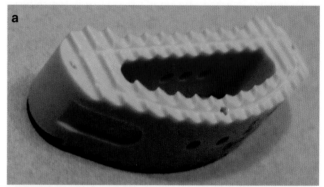
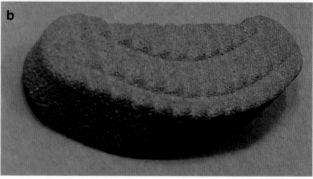

Fig. 52.2 Different TLIF cages T-Space PEEK (**a**) and titanium allow (**b**) (Aesculap AG, Germany)

52.6.2 Instrumentation

Pedicle Preparation
- The pedicle is instrumented using clinical and radiological landmarks.
- The pedicle screw entry points (junction of the midpoint of the transverse process with the lateral facet) are identified and marked under fluoroscopy.

Fig. 52.3 (**a–e**) Different TLIF instruments: angled bone curette (**a**), angled curette (**b**), and trial implant (**c**)

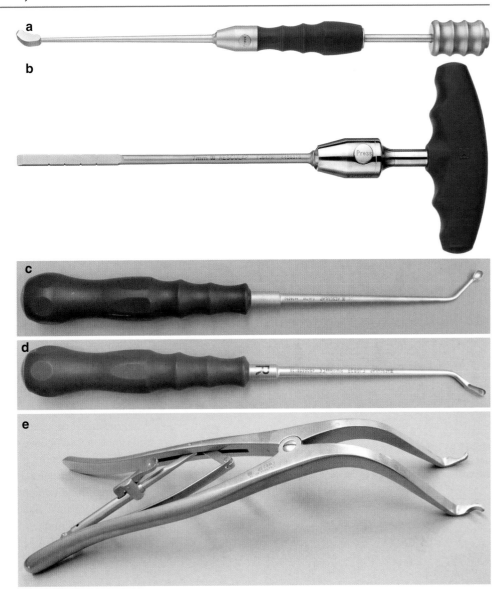

- The pedicles are probed and tapped, and screws are inserted on the side ipsilateral to the decompression.

Decompression and End Plate Preparation
- On the symptomatic side, a total facetectomy is performed using a combination of osteotomes, Kerrison rongeurs, and a high-speed burr.
- Using a big bone rongeur, the top of the facet joint is removed until the gap of the facet joint is clearly seen. This is of importance for the later use of the osteotome.
- With an osteotome, the inferior articular facet is removed (Fig. 52.4). The direction of the osteotome is from medial to lateral and from cranial to caudal orienting on the gap of the facet joint. Care must be taken not to break the pedicle or to injure the intraspinal structures.

- Using bone rongeurs, Kerrison punches, and/or a drill, the superior articular facet is removed (Fig. 52.1a, b). Care must be taken not to injure the exiting nerve root.
- The working corridor is the space defined by the thecal sac medially, exiting nerve root superiorly, and pedicle wall inferiorly. Care should be taken to protect the exiting and traversing nerve root during the remainder of the surgery.
- The annulotomy and discectomy is performed in the standard technique with standard pituitary rongeurs.
- Distraction and if necessary removal of the posterior lip of both end plates open a wider window to the posterolateral disc space and thereby facilitates extensive disc excision.

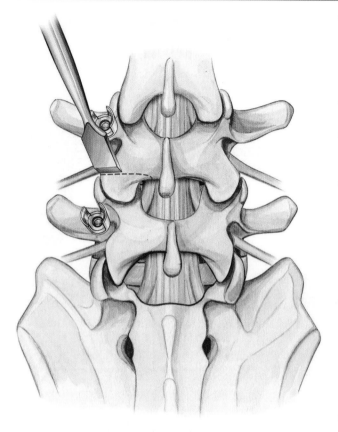

Fig. 52.4 Using a big bone rongeur, the top of the facet joint is removed until the gap of the facet joint is clearly. With an osteotome, the inferior articular facet is removed. The direction of the osteotome is from medial to lateral and from cranial to caudal orienting on the gap of the facet joint

- Special-angled rongeurs, bone curettes, shavers, and rasps aid in cleaning of the disc space and end plates from the cartilaginous surface (Fig. 52.5a–d).
- Special care should be taken not to penetrate the anterior part of the annulus with the curettes in order to avoid vascular injury.

Interbody Fusion
- The desired restoration of the natural disc height can be set using distractors. They are available in heights from 7 to 17 mm in 2-mm increments (see Fig. 52.6).
- In addition to the osteoinductive graft material, a structural interbody spacer should be placed in the interbody space to maintain intervertebral body and neuroforaminal height and sagittal balance.

- Depending on the shape of the end plates and the spinal profile, it has been our practice to use either boomerang or rectangular spacers in case of TLIF. For example, in case of segmental kyphosis, we prefer to position a rectangular cage laterally at the affected side.
- The appropriate size of the spacer is selected using specifically designed trials.
- Before placement of a cage, milled local autograft from the facet joint (and lamina) is inserted into the disc space using a special funnel or a syringe (see Fig. 52.7).
- After autograft insertion, the cage is inserted under distraction into the intended position. Distraction can be achieved by placing a spreader under the screw heads of the ispi- or contralateral pedicel screws. Placement of a lamina spreader at the base of the spinous process is a further option in case of a midline approach.
- Using a boomerang cage, it is impacted until it is completely inside the disc space and then it is gradually rotated into position using an impactor (Fig. 52.8). If the cage is already in midline position and further anterior placement is needed, a hockey-stick-shaped impactor is placed onto the concave surface of the cage in order to push the cage straight anterior.
- After the cage is placed, the distraction is released and the rods are attached and fixed.
- A further option is the placement of a translaminar facet screw from the ipsilateral side. If lumbar lordosis needs to be restored, mild compression of the screws can be performed before final fixation of the rods. Overdo of the pedicle screw compression may create a contralateral foraminal stenosis. A standard closure in layers is performed (Fig. 52.9).

52.7 Tips and Tricks

- Cage position is an important factor to avoid cage migration. Mapping the structural properties of the lumbosacral vertebral end plates has shown that the rigidity of the end plates varies significantly. In general, the strongest region is located posterolaterally, just in front of the pedicles, with more than twice the strength of the central end plate. Due to difficulties in preparation of the anterior end plates and especially in case with anterior lips, it is often very difficult to position a boomerang cage on the anterior cortical ring. Thus, contrary to a rectangular cage, a frequent position of a boomerang cage is in the "weaker" anterior-central end plate region. If this fact is associated with a

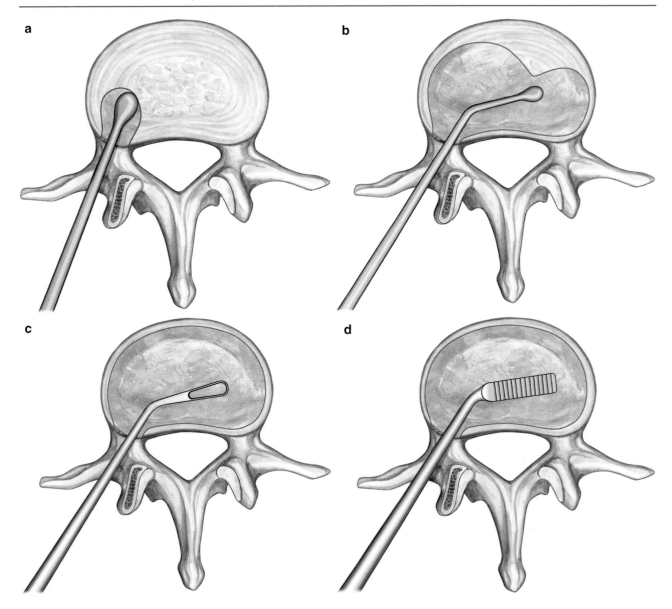

Fig. 52.5 Disc space and end plate preparation (**a–d**)

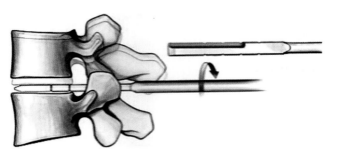

Fig. 52.6 Restoration of the disc height using a distractor

higher rate of cage migration, associated loss of correction has so far not been investigated in the clinical setting. Using a long rectangular cage might overcome this potential problem.

- If too much autograft is packed ventrally into the disc space, adequate anterior positioning of a boomerang cage might not be possible. If it is intended to place an rh-BMP-2 sponge into the disc space, the sponge should be placed into the anterior disc space before cage placement to avoid inducing of heterotopic bone formation near the dura mater.

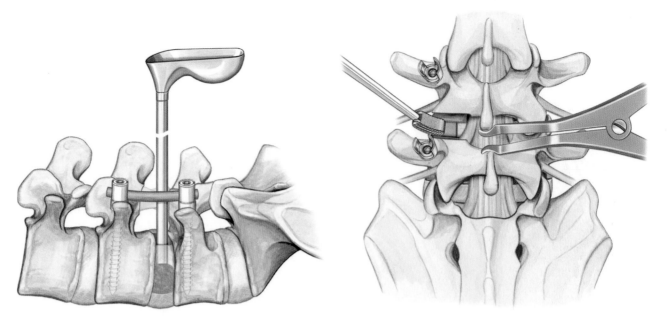

Fig. 52.7 Insertion of cancellous bone graft or bone substitute into the disc space using a funnel

Fig. 52.8 Introduction under interspinous distraction of a boomerang cage (TLIF Cage) with an implant holder into the disc space. Alternatively, distraction with an angled distraction forceps over the ipsilateral side fixed on the pedicle screws

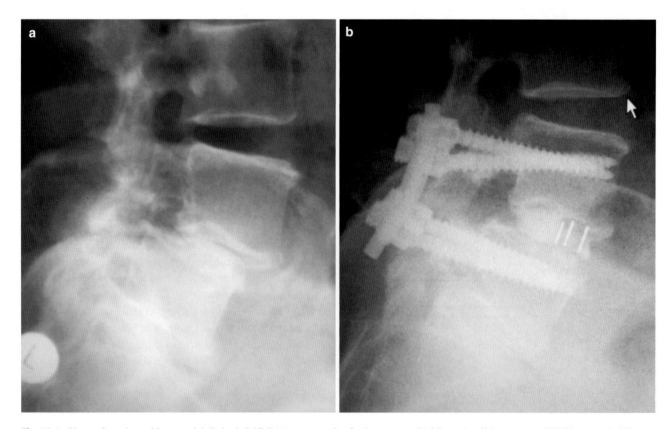

Fig. 52.9 X-ray of a patient with a spondylolisthesis L4/L5 (**a**), postoperative final construct with bilateral pedicle screws and TLIF cage and additional bone substitute (anterior, posterior, and inside the cage) (**b**, **c**); CT scans: level L4 (**d**), disc space level L4 (**e**) and level L5 (f) (**f**)

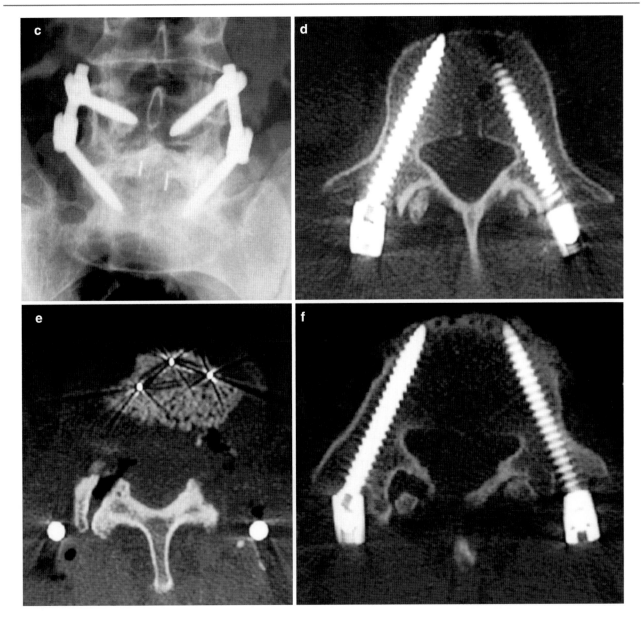

Fig. 52.9 (continued)

References

1. Rosenberg WS, Mummaneni PV (2001) Transforaminal lumbar interbody fusion: technique, complications, and early results. Neurosurgery 48:569–574
2. Mummaneni PV, Rodts GE (2005) The mini-open transforaminal lumbar interbody fusion. Neurosurgery 57:256–261
3. Dhall SS, Wang MY, Mummaneni PV (2008) Clinical and radiographic comparison of mini–open transforaminal lumbar interbody fusion with open transforaminal lumbar interbody fusion in 42 patients with long-term follow-up. J Neurosurg Spine 9:560–565
4. Hackenberg L, Halm H, Bullmann V (2005) Transforaminal lumbar interbody fusion: a safe technique with satisfactory three to five year results. Eur Spine J 14:551–558

Posterior Lumbar Interbody Fusion with an Interbody Fusion Spacer or Cage

53

Uwe Vieweg and Steffen Sola

53.1 Introduction and Core Messages

Posterior lumbar interbody fusion (PLIF) is a treatment option currently used for degenerative disc diseases [1] and was introduced by Cloward in the 1940s [2]. Interbody fusion probably results in the most stable construction for intersegmental spinal fusion. Anterior column support is provided via a posterior approach, and the disc height is restored in order to open the neural foramen. A PLIF procedure is especially attractive in cases where a posterior approach is needed anyway, for example, for nerve root or spinal canal decompression. Different devices are available including allograft spacers, titanium spacers with or without a Plasmapore coating, tantalum spacers, and titanium or PEEK cages. This chapter describes the posterior technique for implanting an interbody spacer or cage. These implants are used to obtain 360° fusion.

53.2 Indications

- Degeneration of lumbar segments (L2 to sacrum)
- Discogenic low-back pain
- Degenerative spondylolisthesis
- Pseudarthrosis of a posterolateral fusion
- Isthmic spondylolisthesis grade I–II (III)

53.3 Contraindications

- Severe osteoporosis
- Infection
- Severe epidural scarring
- Unstable burst fractures and compression fractures
- Destructive tumors

53.4 Technical Prerequisites

Fluoroscopy, positioning device (e.g., Wilson frame), adequate instruments, and implants to meet the following requirements: primary stability, restoration of natural lordosis, and long-term maintenance of spinal balance. Intersomatic devices: allograft spacers (Vertigraft VG2 PLIF, DePuy Spine; ProSpace spacer, Aesculap; PLIF allograft spacer, Synthes), titanium cages (CONTACT Fusion Cage, Synthes; Ray cage, Surgical Dynamics, LT cage, Medtronic; OIC PL, Stryker), titanium Plasmapore-coated spacers (ProSpace, Aesculap) (see Fig. 53.1a), tantalum spacers (Zimmer Spine), and PEEK cages (ProSpace, Aesculap, see Fig. 53.1b; Plivios, Synthes; Coda, Mercy Health System; Tetris, Signus; Oria Natura/Adonys, Alphatec Spine/Scient'X; Pezo-P, Ulrich; Luna Cage, Bricon; OIC PL, Stryker; Lumbo-Space PLIF, Intromed).

U. Vieweg, M.D., Ph.D. (✉)
Clinic for Spinal Surgery, Sana Hospital Rummelsberg,
90593 Schwarzenbruck, Germany
e-mail: uwe.vieweg@sana.de,
uwe.vieweg@spine-therapy-surgery.com

S. Sola, M.D.
Department of Neurosurgery, University of Rostock,
Schillingallee 35, 18057 Rostock, Germany
e-mail: solastef@med.uni-rostock.de

U. Vieweg, F. Grochulla (eds.), *Manual of Spine Surgery*,
DOI 10.1007/978-3-642-22682-3_53, © Springer-Verlag Berlin Heidelberg 2012

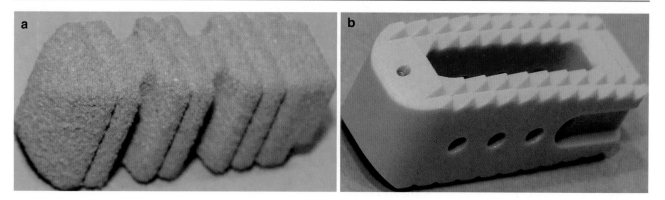

Fig. 53.1 ProSpace titanium spacer with Plasmapore coating (**a**) and ProSpace PEEK cage (**b**) (Aesculap AG, Tuttlingen, Germany)

Plasmapore-Coated Spacer

The heart of the disc implant is a solid core. The core is coated with Plasmapore to increase the area of contact between the implant and the end plates. The implant is made of ISOTAN F, a titanium alloy which also has a Plasmapore coating. Plasmapore is a well-established pure titanium coating material which offers an optimal foundation for the ingrowth of bone due to its balanced relationship between pore depth, porosity, and roughness. Plasmapore promotes osteointegration and osteoconduction without requiring additional bone graft material [1].

The aim of the Plasmapore coating is to achieve both primary and secondary stability. The increased surface roughness of the Plasmapore coating, in combination with a posterior fixation device, ensures immediate primary stability of the motion segment. Bone growth into the coating is rapid, owing to the optimal properties of Plasmapore. This results in bone fusion between vertebrae and implant (secondary stability).

PEEK Cages

PEEK stands for polyetheretherketone. The use of PEEK as an orthopedic device material has become increasingly popular in recent years owing to the material's unique combination of characteristics. Its properties include radiolucency, high mechanical strength, bio-compatibility, and compatibility with standard sterilization methods. The intrinsic radioscopic transparency of the material gives it permeability on X-rays and CT scans, making it possible to view bone growth adjacent to the implant. Of particular interest is the modulus of elasticity of PEEK which is 3.6 GPa and thus similar to that of cortical bone. This specific stiffness encourages load sharing between implant

material and natural bone, thereby stimulating bone healing activity (see Fig. 53.2).

53.5 Planning, Preparation, and Positioning

The patient is placed in a prone position. A radiolucent operating table is recommended to ensure unobstructed intraoperative fluoroscopic visualization in the anteroposterior (AP) and lateral planes. The elbows and knees are appropriately padded. The abdomen must be free. The lumbar spine should be in natural lordosis.

53.6 Surgical Technique

53.6.1 Approach

A midline incision is performed over the levels to be instrumented. The muscle should not be stripped more laterally than the lateral aspects of the facet joints unless posterolateral fusion between transverse processes is planned.

53.6.2 Instrumentation [1–7]

With a Plasmapore-Coated Titanium Spacer

- Bone resection
  The bone is resected using an osteotome and Kerrison bone punch to gain access to the intervertebral space. Alternatively, bone can be removed at the joints using a chisel or high-speed burr. The bone that has been removed is stored in a container under gauze to serve as graft material.

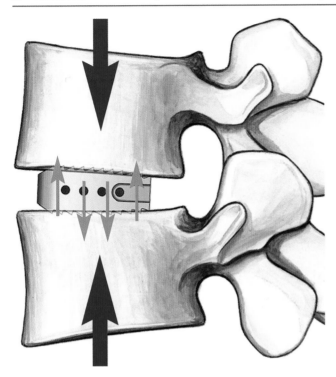

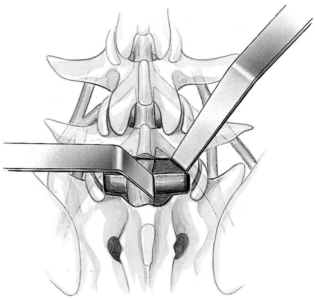

Fig. 53.3 After appropriate laminectomy, the nerve root and dura mater should be protected and the disc sufficiently exposed. Retraction of the dura and upper nerve root with nerve root retractors

Fig. 53.2 Load sharing between PEEK implant material and natural bone stimulates bone healing activity (With permission from Aesculap AG, Tuttlingen, Germany)

- Revealing the disc space

  The dura and upper nerve root are carefully retracted in the desired direction using the nerve root retractors (see Fig. 53.3). Often, large epidural veins need to be cauterized to permit visualization of the posterolateral disc annulus. This must be done carefully, using bipolar cautery to prevent damage to the nerve roots.

- Restoration of disc height

  In order to make room for the insertion of the distractor, the disc material is now resected using rongeurs and forceps. Distraction can be set to the required height using the distractors (see Fig. 53.4). The distractors are inserted one after the other on alternate sides of the disc until the desired distraction is obtained (see Fig. 53.5).

- Clearance of the intervertebral space

- Besides rongeurs and curettes, reamers and rasps can also be used to prepare the intervertebral space. Turning the instrument will remove disc material (see Fig. 53.6). Using the rasps, the cartilaginous end plates are refreshed (see Fig. 53.7). The anulus has to be cleaned out as completely as possible, and the end plates need to be freed from cartilage, taking care not to perforate the bone.

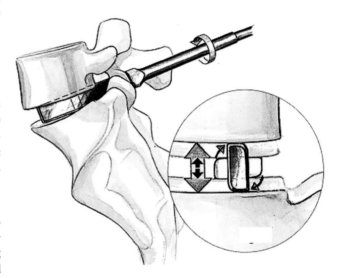

Fig. 53.4 Restoration of the disc height using different distractors (With permission from Aesculap AG, Tuttlingen, Germany)

- Preparation of the implant bed
- Any unevenness of the borders of the implant bed can be smoothed using the broach. The sharp leading edge of the instrument permits simple bone resection to the dimensions required (see Figs. 53.7 and 53.8). The implant bed is now prepared, and the implant can be inserted.
- Insertion of the cage

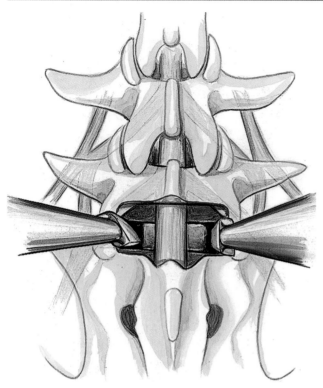

Fig. 53.5 The distractors are inserted one after the other on alternate sides (With permission from Aesculap AG, Tuttlingen, Germany)

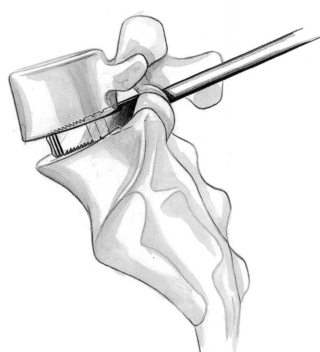

Fig. 53.7 Preparation of the implant bed using a broach (With permission from Aesculap AG, Tuttlingen, Germany)

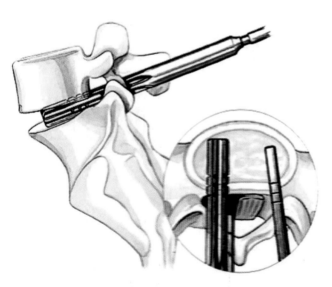

Fig. 53.6 Clearance of the intervertebal space with curettes, reamers, and rasps (With permission from Aesculap AG, Tuttlingen, Germany)

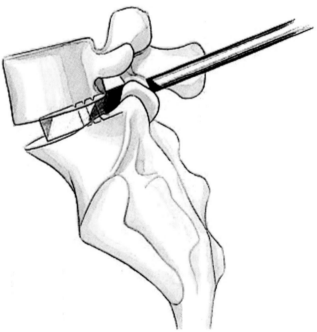

Fig. 53.8 Preparation of the implant bed using a broach (With permission from Aesculap AG, Tuttlingen, Germany)

- Either a straight implant (0°) or a lordotic implant (5° or 8°) can be used, depending on the particular level and anatomy. The implant is connected to the inserter by engaging the thread using the Allen key connected to the instrument (see Fig. 53.9). The spacer is introduced on the flat side and turned clockwise in order to spread the disc space. The implant is then brought into its final vertical position. The position of the implant can be corrected with the impactor (see Fig. 53.10).

- Insertion on the contralateral side
- The operative steps described above are now repeated for the contralateral side. Bone material can be packed between both implants. Additional posterior stabilization of the segment should be performed (see Figs. 53.10 and 53.11).

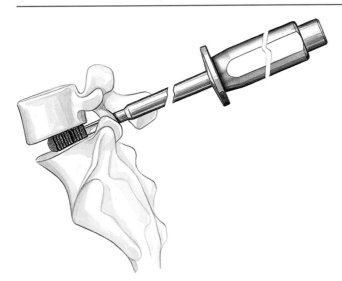

Fig. 53.9 Insertion of the spacer with the insertion instrument and impactor (With permission from Aesculap AG, Tuttlingen, Germany)

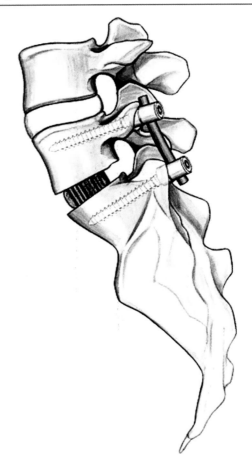

Fig. 53.10 Additional posterior stabilization of the motion segment is necessary

With a PEEK Spacer

(Operating steps are comparable to those for the titanium cages.)
- Bone resection
- The bone is resected using an osteotome and a Kerrison bone punch to gain access to the intervertebral space. Alternatively, bone can be removed at the joints using a chisel or high-speed burr.
- Revealing the disc space
- The dura and upper nerve root are carefully retracted in the desired direction using the nerve root retractors (see Fig. 53.3).
- The sharp leading edge of the instrument permits simple bone resection to the dimensions required.
- Restoration of disc height

- Distraction can be set to the required height using the distractors (see Figs. 53.11 and 53.12). The distractors are inserted one after the other on alternate sides of the disc until the desired distraction is obtained.
- Clearance of the intervertebral disc

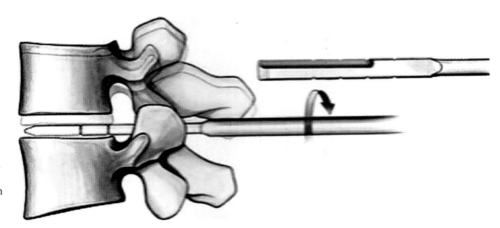

Fig. 53.11 Restoration of disc height using different distractors. Positioning of contralateral distractor (With permission from Aesculap Ag, Tuttlingen, Germany)

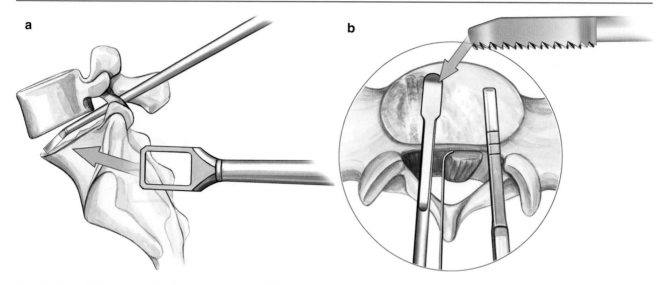

Fig. 53.12 (**a**, **b**) Clearance of the intervertebral space (With permission from Aesculap AG, Tuttlingen, Germany)

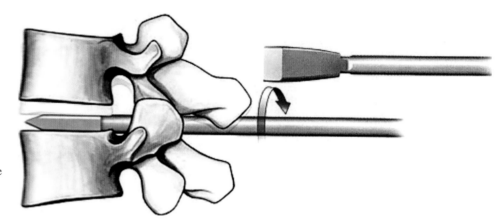

Fig. 53.13 Determination of the implant size using trial implants (With permission from Aesculap AG, Tuttlingen, Germany)

- The disc space is cleared using rongeurs, bone curettes, and rectangular curettes. Bone rasps are used to refresh the cartilaginous end plates (see Figs. 53.12 and 53.13).
- Determination of implant size using trial implants
- Trial implants are available in different sizes and with different angulations. Trial implants are inserted in turn, starting with the smallest size. Each is inserted horizontally and rotated clockwise (see Figs. 53.13 and 53.14). Progressively, taller trial implants are inserted until the required distraction has been achieved. The trial implant now in place indicates the height, angle, and length of the implant to be inserted.
- Insertion of the PEEK cage

- After filling the PEEK implant with bone graft or artificial bone substitute, the implant is clamped to the PEEK insertion instrument (see Figs. 53.14 and 53.15) and inserted in the intervertebral space (see Figs. 53.15 and 53.16). The cage is filled with finely milled autologous bone (the resected bone from the spinous processes and the facet joints will generally be sufficient).
- Insertion on the contralateral side.
- The operative steps described are now repeated for the contralateral side. Bone material can be packed between both implants.
- Posterior stabilization
- Additional posterior stabilization of the segment should be performed.

Fig. 53.14 The implant is clamped to the insertion instrument (With permission from Aesculap AG, Tuttlingen, Germany)

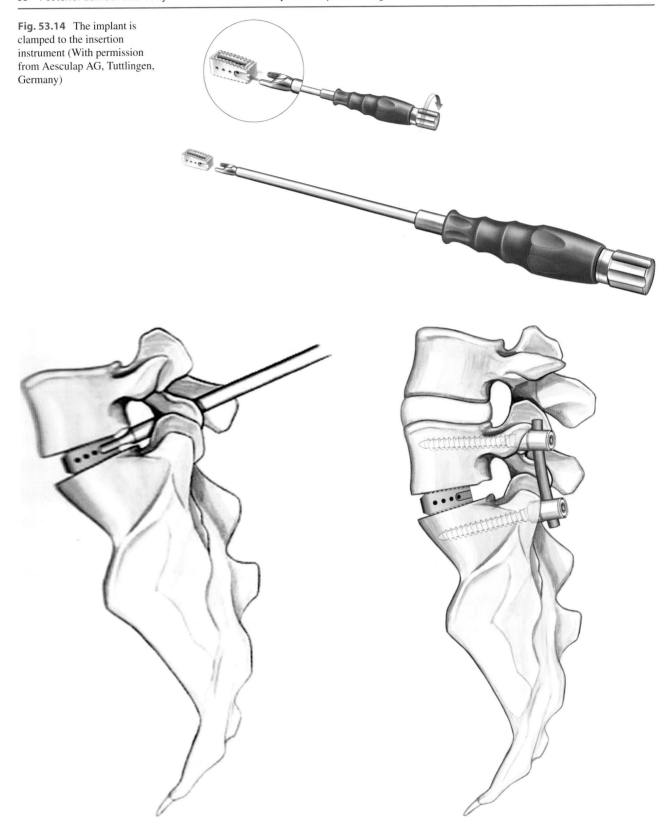

Fig. 53.15 Insertion of the PEEK cage with the insertion instrument (With permission from Aesculap AG, Tuttlingen, Germany)

Fig. 53.16 Three-column stabilization with anterior column fusion with PEEK cage and posterior column fixation with internal fixator (With permission from Aesculap AG, Tuttlingen, Germany)

References

1. Bronsard JJ, Tropiano P, Louis C et al (2002) Three–column spinal fusion using ProSpace intervertebral blocks. In: Kaech DL, Jinkins JR (eds) Spinal restabilisation procedures. Elsevier Science, Amsterdam, pp 153–170
2. Cloward RB (1981) Spondylolisthesis: treatment by laminectomy and posterior lumbar interbody fusion. Clin Orthop 154:74–82
3. Freemann BJ, Licina P, Mehdina SH (2000) Posterior lumbar interbody fusion combined with instrumented posterolateral fusion: 5 year results in 60 patients. Eur Spine J 9:42–46
4. La Rosa G, Germano A, Conti A et al (1999) Posterior fusion and implantation of the SOCON-SRI system in the treatment of adult spondylolisthesis. Neurosurg Focus 7(6):E2
5. La Rosa G, Cacciola F, Conti A et al (2001) Posterior fusion compared with posterior interbody fusion in segmental spinal fixation for adult spondylolisthesis. Neurosurg Focus 10(4):E9
6. Periasamy K, Shah K, Wheelwright EF (2008) Posterior lumbar interbody fusion using cages, combined with instrumented posterolateral fusion: a study of 75 cases. Acta Orthop Belg 74:240–8
7. Potel A, Welch WC (2000) Posterior lumbar interbody fusion with metal cages: current techniques. Oper Tech Orthop 10:311–319

Transsacral Screw Fixation for High-Grade L5/S1 Spondylolisthesis Including Spondyloptosis

54

Palaniappan Lakshmanan and Sashin Ahuja

54.1 Introduction and Core Messages

The goals of treatment of high-grade spondylolisthesis including spondyloptosis are to relieve back pain by stabilizing the segmental instability, to achieve 360° fusion to prevent instability and pseudarthrosis to relieve leg pain by decompressing the neuronal structures, and to minimize risks to neuronal structures by avoiding reduction. Using different methods, a circumferential 360° fusion can be achieved in high-grade spondylolisthesis including spondyloptosis through an all-posterior approach [1–5]. The technique outlined in this chapter employs two transsacral HMA (hollow modular anchorage) screws (Inventors Jean Hupp, Thierry Marnay, Marc Ameil 1995) filled with bone graft and supplemented with posterolateral fusion with pedicle screw instrumentation.

P. Lakshmanan (✉)
Sunderland Royal Hospital,
Sunderland, SR4 7TP, UK
e-mail: lakunns@gmail.com

S. Ahuja
University Hospital of Wales,
Heath Park, Heath CF14 4XW, Cardiff, UK
e-mail: sashinahuja@doctors.org.uk

54.2 Indications

- High-grade spondylolisthesis Meyerding grade III–V L5/S1 including spondyloptosis
- Persistent back pain and/or leg pain affecting quality of life
- Failed nonoperative treatment

54.3 Contraindications

- Infection
- Medically unfit for operation and general anesthesia
- Poor bone quality – osteoporosis (poor screw purchase)

54.4 Technical Prerequisites

- Fluoroscopy with live screening
- Radiolucent table
- Patient positioning device like Wilson's frame, Jackson's table, etc.
- Hollow modular anchorage (HMA) screw (Aesculap Ltd, Tuttlingen) and instrumentation
- Polyaxial pedicle screw system with implants and instrumentation (Figs. 54.1 and 54.2)
- Drill sleeve from any bone drill set

54.5 Planning, Preparation, and Positioning

The patient's X-rays are reviewed to assess the length of the transsacral screw from the posterior body of S1 to the superior corner of the anterior margin of L5 vertebral body

U. Vieweg, F. Grochulla (eds.), *Manual of Spine Surgery*,
DOI 10.1007/978-3-642-22682-3_54, © Springer-Verlag Berlin Heidelberg 2012

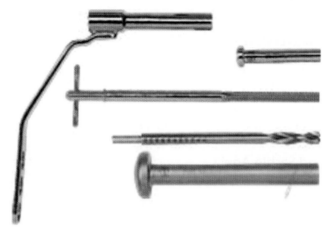

Fig. 54.1 Instruments for transsacral screw fixation (With permission from Aesculap AG, Tuttlingen, Germany)

Fig. 54.2 HMA (hollow modular anchorage) screw. (**a**) Fixation nut, (**b**) sleeve, (**c**) locking nut (With permission from Aesculap AG, Tuttlingen, Germany)

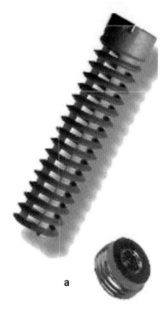

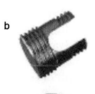

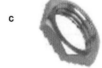

on the lateral view and taking away 1 cm from the measurement. The length and thickness of the pedicle screws at L4 and S1 can be preoperatively determined by reviewing the axial sections of the MRI scans. Further, by analyzing the

pedicular anatomy, it will aid the surgeon in proper placement of the pedicle screws in the L4 and S1 vertebral bodies.

The patient is positioned prone under general anesthesia on a radiolucent operating table, and the image intensifier is used to check whether adequate anteroposterior (AP) and lateral imaging of the lumbosacral spine can be obtained. Also, the abdomen should be free to avoid venous impediment.

54.6 Surgical Technique

54.6.1 Approach

The approach is via a posterior midline longitudinal incision approximately from L3 to S2 spinous processes. The posterior elements up to the transverse processes are exposed by subperiosteal elevation of the paraspinal muscles on either side. Care is taken not to disrupt the facet joint of L3/4.

54.6.2 Instrumentation

- Perform adequate decompression by removing the posterior element of L5 with removal of the fibrous tissue around the pars defect. Also, the bony and soft tissue elements compressing the L5 nerve root are removed until the L5 nerve root is completely free under the L5 pedicle (Gill's procedure).
- The posterior part of the sacrum is deroofed, and an extensive posterior spinal decompression is performed to expose the S1 and S2 nerve roots.
- The S1 nerve root and the theca are carefully freed up from any underlying adhesions.
- The S1 nerve root is retracted laterally with a nerve root retractor, while the theca with the rest of the nerve roots is retracted medially. Care is taken not to retract forcefully to avoid postoperative neurological complications.
- During periods of inactivity, the retraction must be released to avoid constant traction on the nerve roots for long periods.
- The entry point on the posterior wall of the body of S1 between the S1 and S2 nerve roots is identified lateral to midline using C-arm and confirmed on the lateral view depending on the angle it penetrates the L5 vertebral body to reach the anterosuperior corner of L5 vertebral body (Fig. 54.3).
- The guide wire is passed using a drill sleeve under image guidance from the posterior wall of S1 vertebral body through the L5–S1 disc space and then into the L5 vertebral body to end 5 mm short of penetrating the anterosuperior corner of L5 vertebral body (Fig. 54.7).

Fig. 54.3 Decision for a posterior transsacral approach. *Note*: Laminectomy S1/S2 is required to visualize the nerves

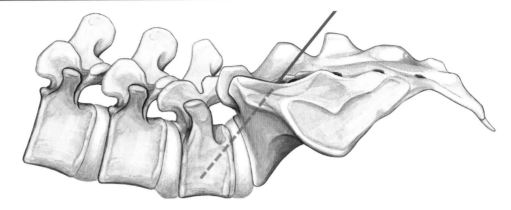

Fig. 54.4 Preparation of the sacrum and the disc L5/S1

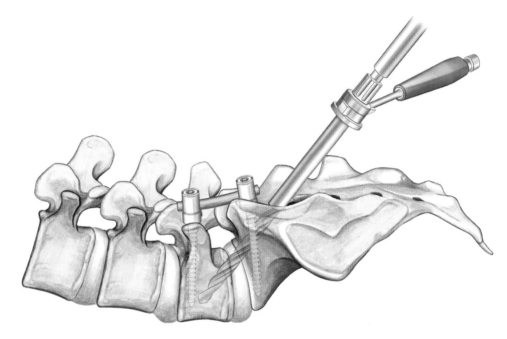

- A cannulated drill is then passed over the guide wire with a drill sleeve in position. To prevent the drill sleeve from slipping, the tip can be buried in the posterior cortex of S1 vertebral body by nibbling away the cortex to avoid catching the dura or the S1 nerve root (Fig. 54.4).
- The drill hole must be tapped adequately depending on the size of the screw chosen. The size of the HMA screw is determined by the size of the sacral vertebra and should be in such a way that two screws on either side can be used with no difficulty.
- A depth gauge is used to find the length of the HMA screw, and the closest available length is used.
- The hollowness in the HMA screw is then filled with cancellous bone graft procured from the posterior elements of the spine during decompression with or without posterior iliac crest bone grafting. It can also be supplemented with bone graft substitutes.
- The screw with the bone graft is then inserted to anchor the L5 on S1 to produce an in situ fixation for high-grade spondylolisthesis including spondyloptosis.

- The same procedure is repeated on the other side to insert another HMA screw parallel to the previous one.
- To supplement the transsacral HMA screw construct, a pedicle screw fixation from L4 to S1 is performed as detailed below (see Figs. 54.5 and 54.6).
- The entry point for the pedicle screw of L4 is identified, and the cortex is nibbled away to show the bleeding cancellous bone.
- The awl is then used to make entry for the pedicular probe. However, in some cases where the anatomy is distorted, C-arm can be used to guide the awl and subsequently the pedicular probe in the appropriate angle both in the AP and lateral planes. A ball-tip probe is then used to confirm the intactness of the walls on all four sides and also the anterior wall. The graduations on the ball-tip probe can give the length of the screw.
- A separate depth gauge can be used to measure the length of the screw up to the anterior cortex of the vertebral body.
- The polyaxial pedicle screw is then inserted in a converging direction.

Fig. 54.5 Implant in place

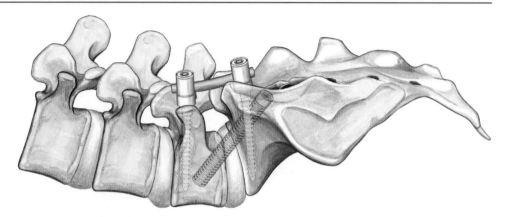

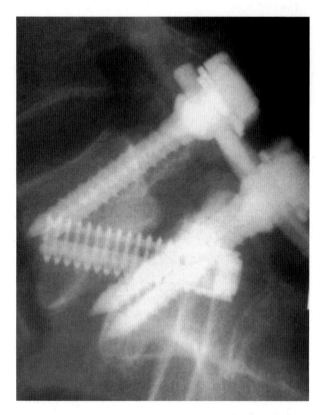

Fig. 54.6 Fusion of the level L5–S1 with internal fixator and HMA screw

- The same technique is repeated on the other side of L4.
- At S1, the pedicle screws are inserted as above, but the screws are aimed toward the promontory of the sacrum, and they are medialized as much as possible. Further, a bicortical purchase is achieved with each sacral screw.
- The transverse processes of the vertebral bodies and the ala of the sacrum are decorticated to act as a bed for the posterolateral bone graft.
- The titanium rods usually >5.5 mm in diameter are contoured and fixed to the pedicle screws using setscrews or grub screws without attempting any reduction.

- The bone graft obtained from the removed posterior elements and/or the posterior iliac crest is packed on either side to give a posterolateral fusion. This can be supplemented with bone graft substitutes if needed.

## 54.7	Tips and Tricks

- If the posterior body of the sacrum is indenting the dura significantly, then the posterosuperior corner of the sacral dome can be carefully osteotomized or nibbled away to prevent any compression on the dura.
- Care must be taken while drilling over the guide wire, and repeated C-arm pictures are needed, or even live screening is required as there is a potential for the guide wire to be pushed anteriorly inadvertently which can result in serious injury to the neurovascular structures in the front.
- Also, as the guide wire passes through three cortices (Fig. 54.7) and if the bone is strong, then the guide wire may gently curve. This results in the drill rotating against the guide wire, thereby heating it up and ultimately breaking the guide wire. Hence, we advice to frequently take X-rays while drilling, for smooth passage of the drill over the guide wire (Fig. 54.8).
- If, however, the guide wire breaks inadvertently, then instruments like narrow pituitary rongeur or grasper must be readily available to retrieve the broken part.
- Adequate and appropriate tapping of the HMA screw is needed as otherwise the screw may break while inserting if not adequately tapped.
- If the posterior body of the sacrum is small and looks like it may not take up two HMA screws, then a midline large single HMA screw can be used instead of two HMA screws on either side.
- The HMA screws are not strong enough to use them as stand-alone devices and needs posterior supplementation with pedicle screws and posterolateral fusion (Fig. 54.9) as otherwise the HMA screws may break.

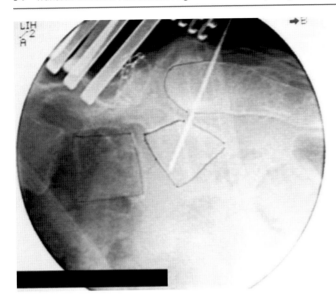

Fig. 54.7 Interoperative X-ray demonstrating the guide wire. The guide wire is passed using a drill sleeve under image guidance from the posterior wall of S1 through L5–S1 disc space

Fig. 54.8 Drill on the guide wire with the drill sleeve

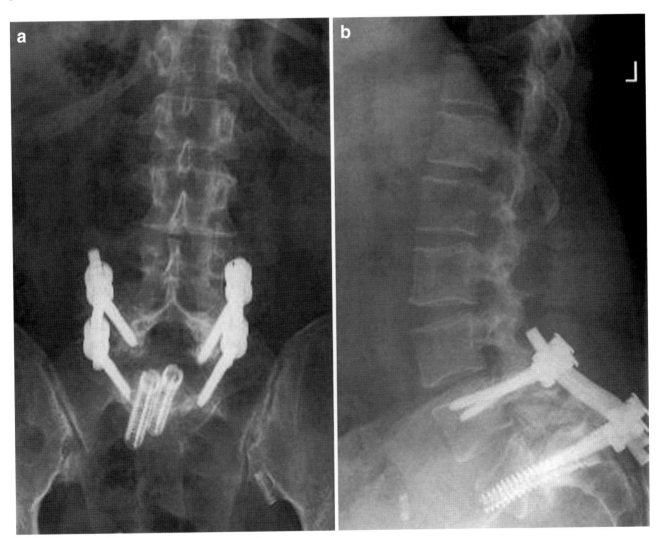

Fig. 54.9 Final postoperative AP X-ray (**a**) and (**b**) lateral view with the 2 HMA screws and pedicle screws

References

1. Bohlman HH, Cook SS (1982) One-stage decompression and posterolateral and interbody fusion for lumbosacral spondyloptosis through a posterior approach. Report of two cases. J Bone Joint Surg Am 64(3):415–418

2. Esses SI, Natout N, Kip P (1995) Posterior interbody arthrodesis with a fibular strut graft in spondylolisthesis. J Bone Joint Surg Am 77(2):172–176

3. Lakshmanan P, Ahuja S, Lewis M et al (2009) Achieving 360 degrees fusion in high-grade spondylolisthesis using HMA screws. Surg Technol Int 18:219–222

4. Roca J, Ubierna MT, Cáceres E et al (1999) One-stage decompression and posterolateral and interbody fusion for severe spondylolisthesis. An analysis of 14 patients. Spine (Phila Pa 1976) 24(7):709–714

5. Whitecloud TS 3rd, Butler JC (1988) Anterior lumbar fusion utilizing transvertebral fibular graft. Spine (Phila Pa 1976) 13(3): 370–374

Guided Oblique Lumbar Interbody Fusion (GO-LIF®)

55

Christof Birkenmaier

55.1 Introduction and Core Messages

While a pedicle screw needs to truly fill the pedicle and – in cases of reduced bone quality – to purchase the anterior vertebral cortex for optimum stability, a transpedicular, transdiscal screw finds strong purchase in three cortices (pedicle, superior end plate of inferior vertebra, inferior end plate of superior vertebra) without anterior cortical penetration. Grob et al. [1] was the first to present a series of 16 cases, in which direct transpedicular, transdiscal screw fixation of isthmic or degenerative spondylolisthesis without the use of an additional pedicle screw construct was successfully performed at the L4/5 and L5/S1 levels. Zagra et al. [4] published his series of 62 patients operated on with the Grob technique for isthmic spondylolisthesis at the L3 through S1 levels. Despite high clinical success rates, the screw-related complications in these 2 series included inadvertent anterior cortical penetration, nerve root compression in the foramen and iliac artery compression, all requiring screw removal and repositioning.

These complications already hint at the difficulty of safely drilling the transpedicular, transdiscal trajectories under fluoroscopy guidance with optimum screw purchase, but without compromising neural or vascular structures. The newly developed "Guided Oblique Lumbar Interbody Fusion" (GO-LIF) procedure overcomes these problems by means of robotic-assisted navigation [2, 3], and it expands on the original Grob procedure in three important ways, which greatly enhances the range of possible applications. First, it makes minimally invasive, percutaneous screw placement possible; second, it allows for the combination with intervertebral cage fusion techniques, and third, it does not require the presence of spondylolisthesis. The exact biomechanics of GO-LIF are not yet fully understood. Cadaveric and biomechanical studies, performed at the Cleveland Clinic, Ohio, USA, and in two independent biomechanical laboratories in Germany and in the USA, have shown the construct to be at least as stable as a pedicle screw construct. With its implants being loaded considerably closer to the instantaneous axis of rotation than with a pedicle construct, the GO-LIF construct might even offer superior stability (Fig. 55.1).

55.2 Indications

A multicenter study is currently underway to demonstrate the safety and efficacy of this instrumentation technique. During this evaluation period, the suggested indications and the contraindications are as follows.

C. Birkenmaier, M.D.
Department of Orthopedic Surgery,
Großhadern Medical Center, University of Munich,
Marchioninistr. 15, 81377 Munich, Germany
e-mail: christof.birkenmaier@med.uni-muenchen.de

U. Vieweg, F. Grochulla (eds.), *Manual of Spine Surgery*,
DOI 10.1007/978-3-642-22682-3_55, © Springer-Verlag Berlin Heidelberg 2012

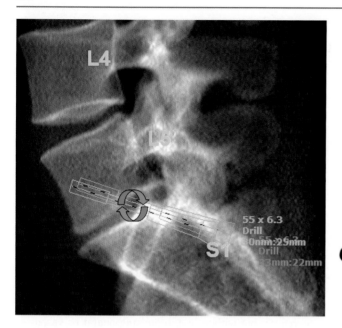

Fig. 55.1 GO-LIF planning at L5/S1. The instantaneous axis of rotation (IAR, *rotating arrows*) lies within the trajectory of the implants

Clinical indication for monosegmental lumbar or lumbosacral fusion (with or without decompression) based on a diagnosis of:
- Painful disc degeneration (black disc)
- Painful erosive osteochondrosis
- Segmental instability
- Recurrent disc herniation
- Spinal canal stenosis
- Foraminal stenosis

55.3 Contraindications

- Hyperlordosis (>70° between superior end plates of L1 and S1)
- Spinal deformities (not asymmetric disc space collapse)
- Spondylolisthesis >2nd degree (Meyerding)
- Poor bone quality

Surgeons are free to combine any fusion technique they prefer with the GO-LIF procedure in order to achieve a definitive fusion.

55.4 Technical Requirements

Preoperative CT scan for planning and navigation, fluoroscopy unit with a video-out port, operating table with (ideally) a central carbon plate for the region of interest, SpineAssist®

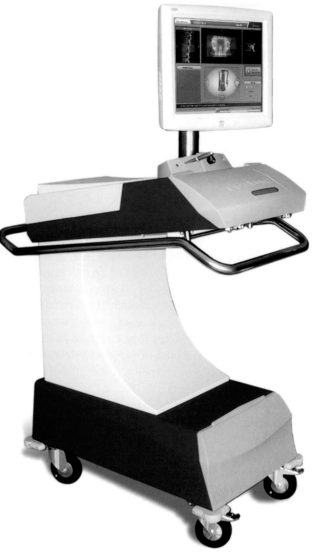

Fig. 55.2 SpineAssist® workstation

workstation, robotic unit (Mazor Surgical Technologies, Caesarea, Israel, Figs. 55.2 and 55.3), GO-LIF instruments set, bilateral bed mount, and GO-LIF implants (Mazor Surgical Technologies, Caesarea, Israel).

55.5 Planning, Preparation, and Positioning

A preoperative CT scan of the relevant spinal region is obtained and imported into the SpineAssist planning software, either on the SpineAssist workstation or on a PC. This allows for the examination of all relevant anatomical details and for the planning of screw trajectories with both

Fig. 55.3 SpineAssist®
miniature robotic device with
attached arm and guide sleeve

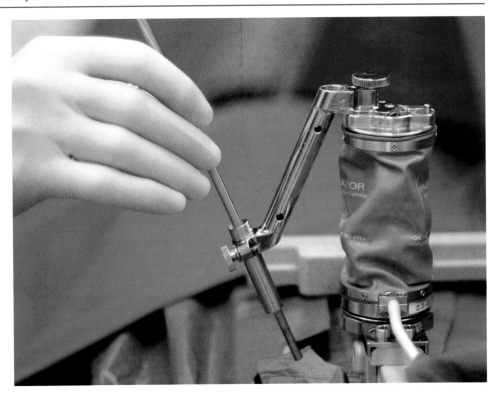

optimum screw purchase and maximum safety with regards to neural structures. Patient positioning follows the clinical requirements. Ideally, a carbon plate without metal sidebars should be used for the region of interest as to not interfere with fluoroscopy. For the same reason, gel-filled positioning pads are to be avoided in the area of surgery. It is recommended to check whether an anteroposterior (AP) and a 60° oblique fluoroscopy shot can be acquired with reasonable quality and without interference. In cases of advanced disc space collapse ("bone-on-bone") with the remaining micro-instability as the likely cause of back pain and without the need for neural decompression, fixation can be performed percutaneously.

55.6   Surgical Technique

- Position the patient prone.
- Check whether an AP and a 60° oblique fluoroscopy shot of the region of interest can be obtained without interference.
- Perform standard surgical skin prep and draping (must allow for the fluoroscopy unit to freely switch from AP to oblique and lateral). For a percutaneous procedure, the bilateral bed mount and the robotic device are set

up in the next step. For an open procedure, exposure and – if required – decompression are performed first.

55.6.1   Percutaneous In Situ Fixation

- Set up the bilateral bed mount far enough caudally so that it does not interfere with the fluoroscopy unit, yet can secure the pelvis.
- Use the attached pelvic paddles to firmly secure the patient's pelvis between the bed mount posts.
- Connect the two bed mount posts with the crossbar.
- Place a percutaneous K-wire into the spinous process of the vertebra that is two levels above the superior vertebra to be instrumented (e.g., L3 for L5/S1).
- Attach the bilateral Hover-T and the calibration target and then acquire the calibration fluoroscopy images (one anteroposterior and one oblique) according to the protocol.
- Follow through the software-guided steps so that the SpineAssist navigation unit matches your preoperative CT planning to the fluoroscopy images.
- Mount the robotic device onto the Hover-T.
- Choose which trajectory to start with and let the navigation software tell you which base position for the robotic device and which drill sleeve are the best choice.

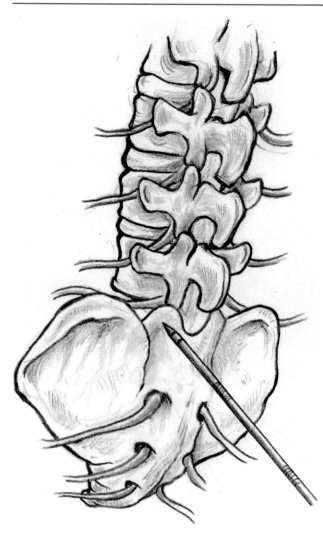

Fig. 55.4 Schematic of the sharp drill guide being tapped onto bone to precisely mark the entry point for the drill

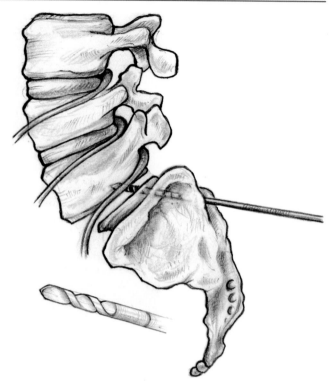

Fig. 55.5 Schematic of the implant trajectory being drilled

55.6.2 Open Fixation

For cases requiring open surgery, the exposure and decompression follows standard surgical procedure. The robot-guided placement of the GO-LIF implant is performed either between the exposure and the decompression or between the decompression and the preparation of the fusion mass. The setup of the bilateral bed mount and of the robotic device is then done just prior to the placement of the GO-LIF implants. By doing so, these items do not present an obstacle for the surgeon during the preceding steps and the chance of decalibrating the guidance by accidentally shifting a component is minimized. A posterolateral fusion may be performed after the placement of the GO-LIF implants. The individual steps to be followed are nearly identical to the ones for percutaneous fixation.

- Let the robotic device position itself.
- Mount the selected drill sleeve, lock it firmly using the support arm, and mark the skin entry point.
- Perform a stab incision and a small fascia split.
- Advance first the dilator and then the drill guide onto bone, remove the dilator, and tap the drill guide so it is securely attached to the posterior elements (Fig. 55.4).
- Drill the trajectory under lateral fluoroscopy control for depth. Steinmann pins can be used to hold the drilled holes until the next step (Figs. 55.5, 55.6, and 55.7).
- If the bone is very hard/sclerotic, a tap is used (Fig. 55.8).
- Then place the GO-LIF implant (Fig. 55.9).
- Perform the identical sequence for the contralateral side.
- If deemed necessary, facet fusions or posterolateral fusions can additionally be performed through separate mini-incisions.

55.6.3 Combination with an Interbody Device

Interbody fusion and the use of load-sharing devices (PLIF, TLIF, etc.) combined with pedicle screw fixation have become the preferred standard for spinal arthrodesis in many parts of the world. The SpineAssist software allows for the combination of these techniques with GO-LIF. It is important, however, to incorporate the desired interbody device in the preoperative planning in

Fig. 55.6 Drilling of the GO-LIF trajectory under lateral fluoroscopy control

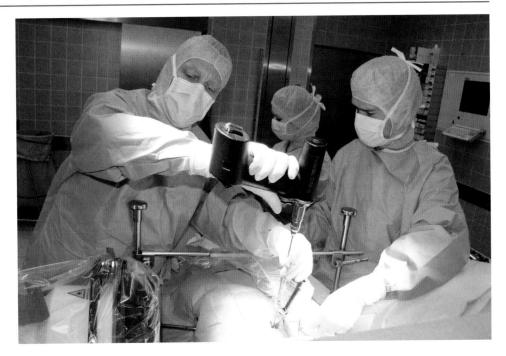

Fig. 55.7 Both trajectories have been drilled, and Steinmann pins are inserted to hold the drill holes for the next step

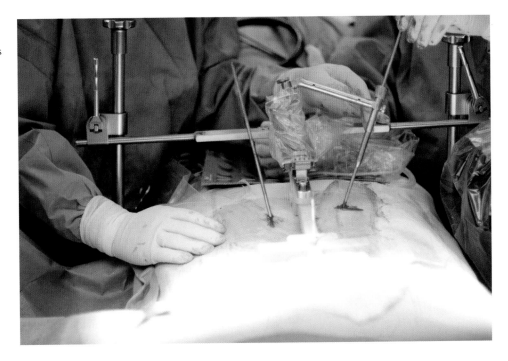

order to rule out a possible interference of the device with one or both GO-LIF trajectories. Depending on the GO-LIF trajectories and the specific anatomical situation, a single, oblique PLIF cage (Figs. 55.10, 55.11, and 55.12) or an anteriorly placed TLIF cage may represent the best solution (Figs. 55.13, 55.14, and 55.15). Minimally invasive PLIF or TLIF approaches can be combined with percutaneous GO-LIF. The sequence

of the individual steps for these procedures is however somewhat more complex:

- Set up the bilateral bed mount far enough caudally so that it does not interfere with the fluoroscopy unit, yet can secure the pelvis.
- Use the attached pelvic paddles to firmly lock the patient's pelvis between the bed mount posts.
- Connect the two bed mount posts with the crossbar.

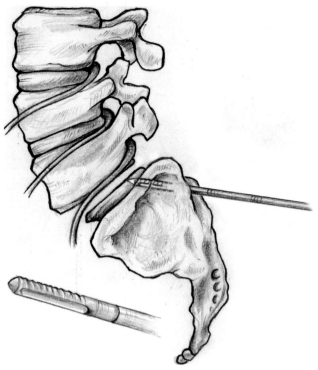

Fig. 55.8 Schematic of a tap being used to prepare the trajectory for the implant

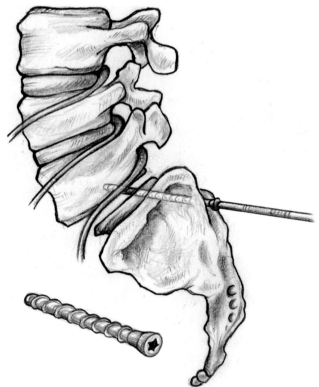

Fig. 55.9 Schematic of the GO-LIF screw implant being placed

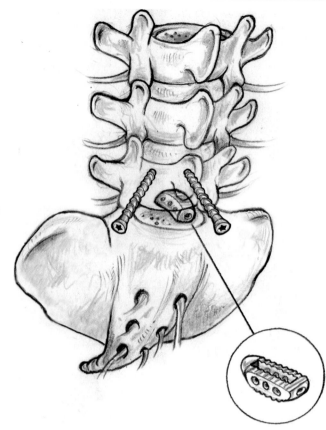

Fig. 55.10 Schematic of a single PLIF cage in an oblique position being used in conjunction with the GO-LIF procedure

- Place a percutaneous K-wire into the spinous process of the vertebra that is two levels above the superior vertebra to be instrumented (e.g., L3 for L5/S1).
- Attach the bilateral Hover-T and the calibration target and then acquire the calibration fluoroscopy images (one anteroposterior and one oblique) according to the protocol.
- Follow through the software-guided steps so that the SpineAssist navigation unit matches your preoperative CT planning to the fluoroscopy images.
- Mount the robotic device onto the Hover-T.
- Choose which trajectory to start with and let the navigation software tell you which base position for the robotic device and which drill sleeve are the best choice.
- Let the robotic device position itself.
- Mount the selected drill sleeve, lock it firmly using the support arm, and mark the skin entry point.
- Perform a stab incision and a small fascia split.
- Advance first the dilator and then the drill guide onto bone, remove the dilator, and tap the drill guide so it is securely attached to the posterior elements.

Fig. 55.11 Pre-op planning of a single oblique PLIF cage in combination with GO-LIF (**a** AP and **b** lateral view). There is no collision between the cage and the screw implants

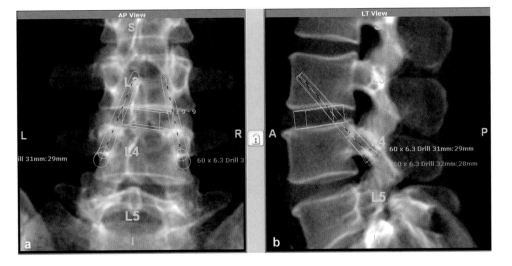

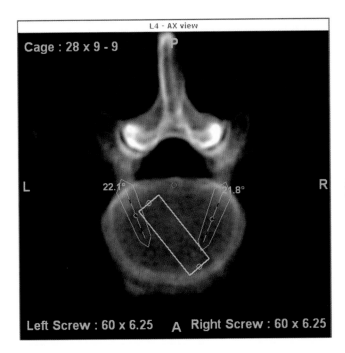

Fig. 55.12 Same pre-op planning as above, selected axial view incorporating the disc space and both adjacent end plates. There is no collision between cage and screws

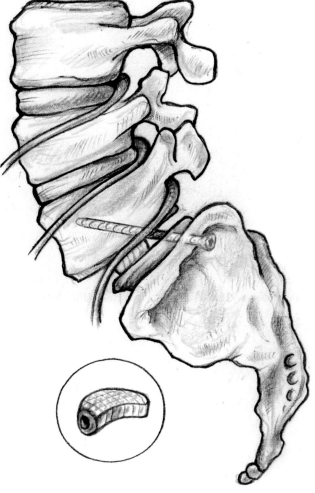

Fig. 55.13 Schematic of a TLIF cage being used in conjunction with the GO-LIF procedure

Fig. 55.14 Pre-op planning of TLIF cage in combination with GO-LIF (**a** AP and **b** lateral view). There is no collision between the cage and the screw implants

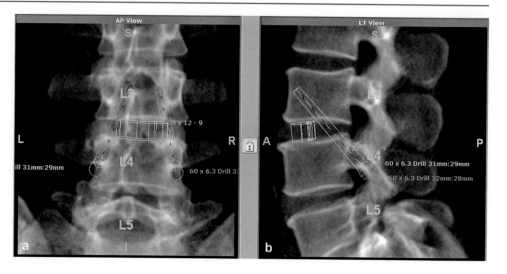

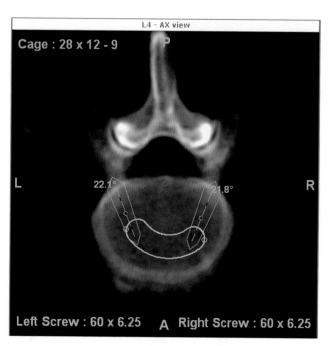

Fig. 55.15 Same pre-op planning as above, selected axial view incorporating the disc space and both adjacent end plates. There is no collision between cage and screws

- Drill the trajectory under lateral fluoroscopy control until you reach the disc space.
- Perform the identical sequence for the contralateral side.
- Now, perform your approach and the decompression required. Gaining access to the disc space from one side should be sufficient, but a facetectomy may be needed.
- Adequately prepare your disc space and clear it of disc material and cartilage.

- Place bone graft or bone substitute anteriorly.
- Position the cage (TLIF or single PLIF) according to the planning.
- Probe through the predrilled GO-LIF trajectories with a long Steinmann pin to check whether the interbody device interferes with a trajectory. If this is the case, the position of the cage must be corrected (Figs. 55.16 and 55.17).
- Extend the trajectories into the superior vertebra and place the GO-LIF implants.
- Additional bone graft can now be added.

Alternatively, the decompression steps and the preparation of the disc space can come first. By doing so, the surgeon is not bothered by the bilateral bed mount and the Hover-T during this part of the surgery. The robotic guidance setup is performed next, and the distal GO-LIF trajectories (inferior vertebra of the fusion segment) are then drilled prior to placing the bone graft and the interbody device. The other steps are then as laid out above (Figs. 55.18–55.21).

55.7 Tips and Pitfalls

- The GO-LIF trajectories are a very different concept from pedicle screw trajectories, and it takes some time to get a full understanding of this technique.
- It is recommended to adequately (re)familiarize oneself with the pertinent anatomy and to dedicate some time to the planning software prior to performing the first case.
- The miniature robot is a sensitive device that requires proper handling. Insensitive operation can force the drill sleeve away from the optimum trajectory and hence lead to reduced accuracy.

Fig. 55.16 Pre-op planning of TLIF cage in combination with GO-LIF (**a** AP and **b** lateral view). The cage is positioned in an oblique fashion, and the planning software warns of a collision between the cage and the left screw implant (*red star* symbol)

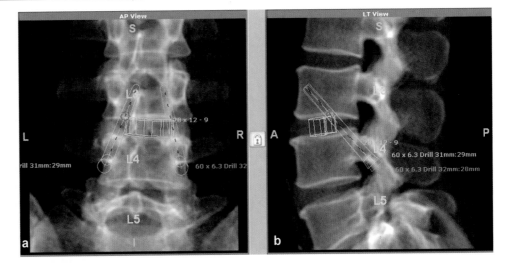

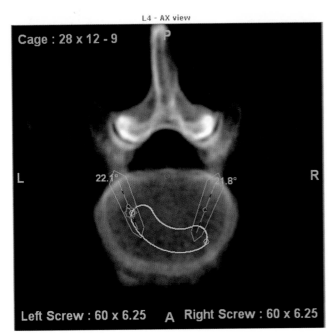

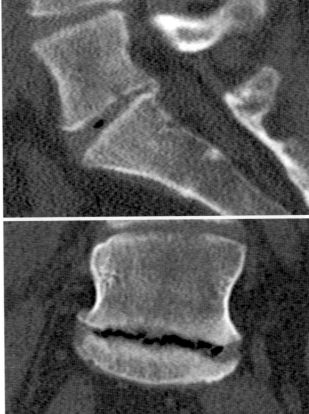

Fig. 55.17 Same pre-op planning as above, selected axial view incorporating the disc space and both adjacent end plates. The *red star* symbol indicates where the collision between the TLIF cage and the left screw would occur. The position of the cage needs to be corrected

Fig. 55.18 Case example of painful L5/S1 erosive osteochondrosis, corroborated by staged infiltration testing. The CT scan shows initial posterior and lateral bony bridging as well as gas in the disc space, an indicator of residual instability

**Figs. 55.19 and
55.20** Pre-op planning (AP, lateral, and axial) of the two GO-LIF trajectories and of two additional trajectories for facet fusion. The procedure was performed through four small incisions without any major soft tissue dissection

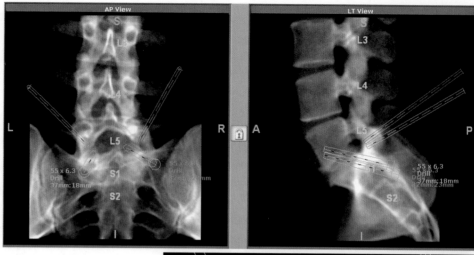

Fig. 55.19

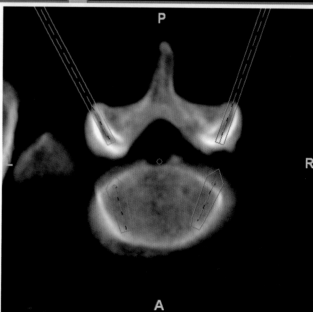

Fig. 55.20

Fig. 55.21 Postop standing radiographs of the above case (**a** AP and **b** lateral view)

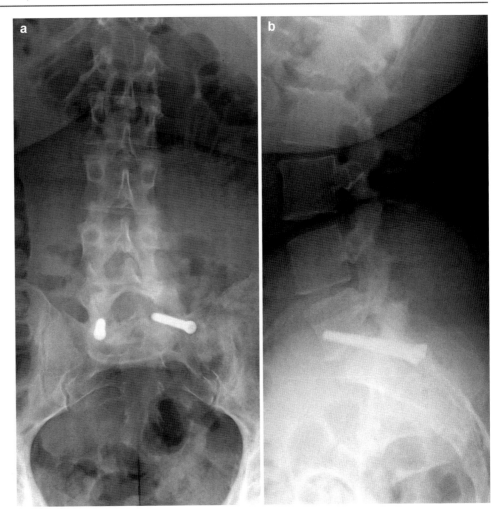

References

1. Grob D, Humke T, Dvorak J (1996) Direct pediculo-body fixation in cases of spondylolisthesis with advanced intervertebral disc degeneration. Eur Spine J 5:281–285
2. Lieberman IH, Togawa D, Kayanja MM et al (2006) Bone-mounted miniature robotic guidance for pedicle screw and translaminar facet screw placement: part I-technical development and a test case result. Neurosurgery 59:641–650; discussion 641–650
3. Sukovich W, Brink-Danan S, Hardenbrook M (2006) Miniature robotic guidance for pedicle screw placement in posterior spinal fusion: early clinical experience with the SpineAssist. Int J Med Robot 2:114–122
4. Zagra A, Giudici F, Minoia L et al (2009) Long-term results of pediculo-body fixation and posterolateral fusion for lumbar spondylolisthesis. Eur Spine J 18(suppl 1):151–155

Index

U. Vieweg, F. Grochulla (eds.), *Manual of Spine Surgery*,
DOI 10.1007/978-3-642-22682-3, © Springer-Verlag Berlin Heidelberg 2012